Ultimate Back Fitness and Performance

Fourth Edition

Stuart McGill, PhD

Professor of Spine Biomechanics
University of Waterloo
Canada

Backfitpro Inc. (formerly Wabuno Publishers)
Waterloo, Ontario, Canada
2009

ISBN: 0 – 9735018 – 1 – 2

Printing   1   2   3   4   5   6   7   8   9   10

Printed in Canada

Wabuno Publishers, Backfitpro Inc.
292 Beechlawn Dr.,
Waterloo. Ontario, Canada
N2L 5W7

www.backfitpro.com

Copies of this book can be purchased in bulk quantities at reduced rates. Contact:

email: kathryn@backfitpro.com

Cover Photos:

Front Cover - Spine image courtesy of Primal Pictures.

Back Cover - Top image courtesy of Steve Brooks (University of Waterloo), middle image with permission of my friend and dancer/choreographer Indy Tyler, bottom image with permission of my friend and world champ Jerzy Gregorek.

Disclaimer: No exercise can be deemed "safe" or "dangerous". However inappropriate exercise has an increased risk for harm. The information in this book is to assist in wise exercise choice. The author and publisher are not responsible for poor choices or any harm that may result.

Ultimate Back Fitness and Performance

Table of Contents

Part I Scientific Foundation

The Ultimate approach
    The concept of tolerance and capacity
Current low back disorder myths
    The myths associated with stretching
    The myths associated with strengthening – rehabilitation vs training for performance
    Motion and motor changes from back injury – pain inhibits optimal motor patterns
    What distinguishes the best athletes?
    Focusing on multifidus, or transverse abdominis or any other single muscle - Misdirected clinical effort
    The confusion between rehabilitation and performance training
    The pollution of body building approaches in low back training
    Athletic bad backs: Dealing with the cause and the role of prevention
    The mind and performance
    The doctor says the pain is in your head – don't believe it!
    Each person is an individual – there are no approaches that work with all
    Are back troubles a life sentence?
How we obtain the evidence to improve back training – Our unique approach
    In-vitro lab
    The in vivo lab
References for the modeling process
References

Introduction
Training affects all systems
Preliminary issues for designing a program
    Strength
    Factors that limit training outcome
    Biomechanics and training
        The concept of the moment
    Muscle mechanics
    The Russian philosophy of training
    A note on Plyometrics

Strength and posture
Proprioception training
The science of flexibility
Progression of a program with younger athletes
Training balance
The popularity of the Olympic lifts: Justifiable or misdirected
Training with machines – a discussion
The principle of dynamic correspondence
Safety Issues – a generic discussion
Principles for designing a good warm-up
Specific Considerations for Rehabilitative Back Exercise
Back Flexibility
Strength and Endurance
Spine Power – integration of flexibility and strength discussions
Motor patterns
Eliciting volitional movement
Aerobic exercise
Studies on the connection between fitness and injury disability
Order of exercises within a session
Establishing grooved patterns
Breathing
Time of day for exercise
Clinical Relevance for the Rehabilitative Exercise
The process of injury: Tissue response to mechanical load
References

Some anatomically based facts
Basic neural structure – activating back muscles
Are you a master of your motor control domain?
The full spine
The vertebrae
Vertebral endplate fractures
Posterior elements of the vertebrae and neural arch fracture
Optimizing health of the intervertebral disc
Avoiding disc herniation
Muscles
The proprioceptive function of the small rotators and the intertransversarii
The back extensors have several important roles: Longissimus, iliocostalis and multifidus
Latissimus dorsi is a critical performance muscle
Abdominal muscles
Abdominal fascia
Rectus abdominis
Abdominal wall – Obliques and transverse abdominis
Psoas

A classic- viewing instability and injury
Illustrating the important conditions for stability
Stability myths, facts, and clinical implications
Ensuring sufficient stability usually only needs modest levels of muscle activation
The special case of transverse abdominis
Abdominal bracing vs. hollowing
Breathing and stability
Summary: The lesson for athletes
References

Part II Individualizing Programs

Section 1. Identifying the fundamental movement patterns
Section 2. Identifying movement errors and correcting their cause
Finding optimal movement and performance techniques
Principles for optimizing performance
Summation and continuity of joint forces and moments
Production of linear impulse
Direction of force application
Principle of stability
Summation of segment velocities
Production of angular impulse (rotational motion)
Conservation of momentum
Manipulation of moment of inertia
Eliminate energy leaks
Principles for safety
Minimization of tissue stress
Optimal joint positioning
Minimization of fatigue
Qualitative biomechanics to analyze the movement – putting the principles
together
Final thoughts: Control feedback and proprioception
Section 3. Understanding the stages of motor skill development to better teach motor
skills

Preparing the athlete
Reducing the risk in athletes – guidelines
What coaches need to know
References

The first consultant-athlete (with back symptoms) meeting
So what have we learned?

The first meeting for those without back troubles
Some additional performance-specific tests
    Assess posture
    Basic Movement – The squat
    Basic Movement – The squat – Choosing optimal hip and foot width
    Looking for spine "hinges"
    Poor control in torsional tasks
    Stable patterns during challenged breathing
    Endurance Testing
    Specific movement screens
A philosophical approach for selecting specific tests, and designing the program
    Step 1. What are the demands of the sport/activity?
    Step 2. What are the capabilities of the athlete – together with current deficits
    Step 3. Designing the program
A final note on qualifying the athlete for specific training exercises
References

Part III Building the ultimate performer – Putting it all together

Some preliminary matters
    Some notes for the chronic back
        Keeping a journal of daily activities
        Ensure continual improvement
        How long should each stage be?
        Training with labile surfaces underneath the athlete
        Training harder and longer is not always better
        Some final thoughts on reps, sets and sessions
        Stages of athlete progression
References

    A note on the training environment
    Awareness of spine position and muscle contraction
        Lumbar spine proprioception training
        Corrective standing approaches
        Corrective walking approaches
        A convincing demonstration of the influence of posture on strength
        Distinguishing hip flexion from lumbar flexion – Teaching the motion pattern
        Perfecting the "hip hinge"
        A note on spine stability, spine motion and control
        Locking the rib cage onto the pelvis
    Mental imagery
        Steps of mental imagery
        Other imagery exercises to develop motion/motor awareness

Important abdominal patterns
    Abdominal hollowing is dysfunctional – Abdominal brace instead
    Teaching abdominal bracing
    A note on fascial raking
Building squat patterns
    Re-training the gluteal complex
        1. Learning to activate gluteus medius
        2. Learning to activate gluteus maximus
        3. Beginning basic squat patterns
Star exercises
Active flexibility and stretching for back performance
    Active flexibility for the back
    Sparing the back while stretching the hips and knees

The washed-up baseball catcher
The CEO who had painful "midnight movement"
Building the power lifter
The misguided football lineman
Training a sprinter
Back troubles in the long distance runner
The Rock Climber
The champion squash player
The dancer building to the arabesque
Two former gymnasts and the spine instability legacy
Sciatic case-flossing
The "Strongman" competitor unable to conquer the sticking points
Blending speed, stiffness, strength and compliance for the martial artist
A Squat "Clinic"
A comment on forensic cases

Acknowledgments

When I wrote my first book for a clinical audience I dedicated the work to all of my teachers. Nothing has changed. Any contribution that I have been able to make has been directly influenced by these special people in my life:

My parents John and Elizabeth, I thank them for their courage to start a new life in a new country and "make it" with hard work. Professor Robert Norman, my PhD supervisor and mentor, who continued the molding. The many great academic personalities in the spine world with whom I have had discussions and debate, and studied their writings, that enhanced my education and perspective – Harry Farfan, Bill Kirkaldy-Willis, Don Chaffin, Bill Marras, Nik Bogduk, Manohar Panjabi, Lance Twomey and Mike Adams. And the academic clinicians who have stimulated me with their written and spoken thoughts – Vlad Janda, Shirley Sahrmann, Dick Erhart, Rick Jemmett, Paul Hodges, Andry Vleeming, Craig Liebenson, Peter O'Sullivan and Clayton Skaggs. My many research colleagues from around the world, too numerous to mention here, who have taught me the many perspectives needed to temper the arrogance that comes so naturally when one is the only person privy to new research results. Wonderful graduate students—Jacek Cholewicki, Vanessa Yingling, Jack Callaghan, Sylvain Grenier, Lina Santaguida, Crisanto Sutarno, John Peach, Craig Axler, Lisa Brereton, Greg Lehman, Jennifer Gunning, Richard Preuss, Joan Scannell, David Bereznick, Kim Ross, Natasa Kavcic, Kelly Walker, Simon Wang, John Gray, Steve Brown, Janice Moreside, Sam Howarth, Leigh Marshall, Justin Yates, Stephanie Freeman, Rupesh Patel, David Frost, Drs Doug Richards and Claudio Tampier. Our lab technicians - Amy Karpowicz and Chad Fenwick, and Post-docs – Francisco Vera Garcia. The old dog has learned a few of your new tricks. The many patients and athletes referred to me for consultation – I know I have been able to help a number of you but in our experimental work to prevent, rehabilitate and train, you have taught me immensely. Too often I am away from home giving a course in back rehabilitation and training. Many of the clinicians who have attended these courses and with whom I have shared ideas have given me direction in knowing the next issue to study and attempt to solve. I thank all of them. And finally, the many performance gurus with whom I have had discussions – these have assisted me in knowing what important aspects to test. While it is difficult to pick out a few I will mention in particular, people like the late Mel Siff, Juan Carlos Santana, Al Vermeil, Jerzy Gregorek, Pavel Tsatsouline, Mark McCoy, Art McDermott, John Chaimberg and Bill Kazmaier – all immensely clever, and generous, men. For this fourth edition I also wish to thank many of you who have emailed me with your kind and encouraging words.

Finally, I thank my wife Kathryn and children, John, and Sarah, from whom I stole time to complete this book.

Preface

A great variety of books, videos and manuals are available which show low back exercises and promote "instructions" with the claim that they reduce low back pain, enhance low back performance and protect against low back injury. In a similar vein, brief pamphlets are available showing sets of "recommended exercises". This is problematic. In fact no pamphlet illustrating recommended back exercises will ever help many people. This is because each person is an individual. Some may do well with one approach while others may be further exacerbated, or made worse. A clear illustration of this is found among those who try the latest fad of the day – perhaps "pilates training" or yoga. While these approaches may help a few they will make many others worse – it depends on variables such as their back trouble history, age, and exercise objectives, to name just a few.

No clinician, or therapy approach, will be entirely successful without removing the cause of the back troubles. Integrated prevention efforts are supremely important for success. It is problematic that very few of the available books/manuals are based on documented spine function and injury mechanisms. This has resulted in many "recommendations" for prevention, rehabilitation and training that are unworkable and impractical. In some cases "accepted" guidelines actually replicate known mechanical causes of back damage! This is why it is essential to provide some scientific evidence so that individuals are able to determine which approach is best for them. There will be no single best solution for all – the best individual solutions require familiarity of the issues which form the foundation upon which decisions are based. Basic knowledge of injury mechanisms is introduced here for better selection of training approaches. A variety of prevention solutions and training progressions are provided to guide the reader in making the most effective choice. This book was written to educate, prevent low back disorders and enhance efforts for performance training.

During 2001, I wrote a book for health professionals on evidence-based low back injury prevention and rehabilitation (*Low Back Disorders: Evidence Based Prevention and Rehabilitation, with a second edition 2007*). It quickly became a best seller in several bookstores and on-line vendors with many lay individuals purchasing the book as well. In the last chapter, I had mentioned that I would be writing a book on performance training once I had more data and evidence. I received email daily asking if that book was finished. These messages certainly motivated me to continue working on it. For the clinicians, health/exercise or prevention professionals, who are seeing this book for the first time, you are encouraged to see the original book, written specifically for you providing the full scientific foundation and explanations for person/patient testing, exercise design and prevention approaches.

Training backs, and in fact the "whole" athlete, requires an understanding of the demands that they are being trained to perform. Obviously, I have poor expertise and understanding of the techniques of many sports. However, I use an algorithmic approach to determine the vital components needed for optimal performance. This approach is explained in this book to enable the reader to prepare an athlete for virtually any form of physical competition. This is essential.

The intention of this book is to briefly introduce controversial issues, and introduce the best available scientific evidence to enhance low back performance in the safest manner possible. Rather than perpetuate clinical and training myths, this book will challenge them and propose valid and justifiable alternatives. It is designed to assist those who work to train the back – either their own, or those of others. Not only will athletes benefit, but also workers performing demanding work who may be considered "occupational athletes". The book forms a perfect synergy with my first book "*Low Back Disorders*" in that extensive background information and evidence was provided in that volume – the interested reader is encouraged to obtain a copy of that resource. I hope that this book will foster a better process resulting in fewer troubled backs. I have no interest in being "average", nor in researching or teaching "average" material – I am an elitist! My intention, stated arrogantly without apology, is to assist elite clinicians, trainers, coaches, athletes and lay people who are interested in building ultimate back performance.

Finally, this is a self-published book which results in two advantages for the reader: it makes it cheaper to buy and I am able to incorporate new information more quickly with each print run. The disadvantage is that the book lacks polish regarding layout as titles and figure captions sometimes "flow" onto the next page. C'est la vie!

A Note of Caution to Lay Readers

I wrote my first book for clinicians but quickly found that many lay people were buying it. They would write to me reporting that they had found many self-help approaches. While it was gratifying to hear about their successful self-treatment, the approach removes one of the safeguards in the rehabilitation and training process. Thus, I encouraged lay people who bought my first book to always consult a physician at the outset to rule out any possible existence of a condition that would contraindicate exercise. I must repeat the recommendation here. Also, whether you are a lay individual with a bad back and wish to partake in more activity, or are an athlete training for world class performance, continue to work with a qualified professional to ensure that you are making the wisest choices.

Fourth Edition

The second edition added the new concept of "superstiffness" to assist in developing the optimal transitional exercise program, The third edition created a better synergy with "*Low Back Disorders*". More of the background material was moved to *Low Back Disorders*. More facts were presented in bullet lists to enhance reading and implementation. Now, the fourth edition is an update of the science that our team has been able to significantly develop over the last couple of years. Our studies of elite strongman competitors together with some of the top MMA fighters in the world, added unique insights into performance that we had to get into this book. More quantified training exercises are also included in this edition. Our journey continues. Thanks for the encouragement.

Accompanying DVD's

1. The Ultimate Back: Assessment and therapeutic exercise

A great number of you, who have attended my clinical courses, asked for a companion DVD showing some of the clinical assessment techniques and therapeutic exercise progression methods. The material in my textbooks is essential for making the most appropriate clinical decisions. This DVD illustrates techniques that are best shown "live" – see www.backfitpro.com.

2. The Ultimate Back: Enhancing Performance

Attaining the highest level of performance from each individual requires a blend of science and clinical technique. The trick is to train to the highest level without injury. In this DVD many specific exercises are shown. Footage from actual training sessions are included with athletes you may recognise as some are the best in the world. What they do works. It is our honour to work with them.

Part I   Scientific Foundation

This section is designed to lay a scientific foundation that will enable back professionals to design better back training programs.

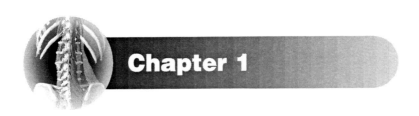

Chapter 1

Laying the Foundation: Why We Need a Different Approach

"Isolate the muscle at a joint and challenge it through its range of motion". "Get out the gym balls to train spine stability". "Learn to activate transverse abdominis". "Exhale when raising a weight and inhale when lowering it'. "This really worked for me, it will work for you" – the list goes on and on. These are examples of frequently heard suggestions that have either a thin, or non-existent, scientific foundation. In contrast, some evidence suggests that they could retard the development of performance! Worse yet, they may compromise the safety of training. Years ago, as I began to develop scientific investigations into various aspects of low back function, I would ask my graduate students to find the scientific foundation for many of the "common sense" recommendations I was hearing in scientific, clinical and training settings. To my surprise, they often reported that the literature yielded no, or very thin, evidence. Body building principles specifically designed to hypertrophy muscle have become widespread in both rehabilitation and in performance training yet they are often a detriment for achieving optimal health and athletic performance.

Many manuals promote "recommended" programs without considering the individual, their capabilities, their objectives, their injury history and age. This will only ensure that those who follow these progressions will obtain mediocre results at best. A regimen that builds one athlete may be ill-prescribed for another resulting in them breaking down to an injured state. Understanding the science of training, when blended together with experience is the only way optimal performance can be achieved while remaining injury free. As you read this book, be prepared to challenge current thoughts and rethink currently accepted practices of training the back for ultimate performance.

Throughout the book I refer to low back "tissues". Tissues include bone (e.g. vertebrae), cartilage (e.g. vertebral end plates), ligaments and muscle/tendons. All tissues respond to load - either they will weaken if the load is excessive, or they will atrophy and weaken if the load is too little. Optimal load defines the stimulus or exposure that results in tissue strengthening without breakdown – it is a moving target. "Load" refers to the cumulative forces that are imposed on the tissues that result from daily activity and training sessions.

The ultimate approach

The approach described in this book shows you how to measure the capabilities of the athlete, understand the demands of the sport, and then devise a program to best prepare them to be ultimate performers within that sport. Many urban myths abound regarding how the best athletes train. Speed and power, when executed with precise control, produce winning performances. Strength without control is useless. Building the ultimate back follows a five stage process that ensures a foundation for eventual strength, speed and power training. In this book you will learn the details to enable the five stages to build the ultimate back:

Stage 1. Groove motion patterns, motor patterns and develop appropriate corrective exercise
- identify perturbed patterns together with their cause
- progress basic movement patterns through to complex activity specific patterns
- design basic balance challenges through to complex balance specific environments

Stage 2. Build whole body and joint stability
- build stability while sparing the joints
- ensure sufficient stability commensurate for the demands of the task
- stability for one joint may require mobility at another

Stage 3. Increase endurance
- build endurance without becoming tired
- perform basic endurance training to build the foundation for eventual strength
- transition to activity specific endurance (duration, intensity)

Stage 4. Build strength
- spare the joints while maximizing neuromuscular compartment challenge
- enhance and utilize speed strength and multi-articular functional strength
- develop optimal timing and "steering" of strength

Stage 5. Develop speed, power, agility
- develop ultimate performance with the foundation laid in stages 1-4
- optimize neuromuscular efficiency

Overlay for all stages: The position of performance
The balance environment

We are not in the business of seeing the average bad back, and most go to conventional clinics. We are referred the special cases at the extremes of the spectrum, from the disabled to the ultimate performers. Thus, I do not work with the average "bad back", I only work with the worst of the "basket case" bad backs that have failed other therapies and some of the best athletic performers in the world. These two populations are similar in that the margin of safety is often razor thin. For a bad back, the exercise dosage needed to stimulate adaptation is very close to the load that will make them worse. The exercise type and dosage must be perfectly selected. As the client/athlete progresses with rehabilitation, the margin of safety increases as they are able to tolerate more loading. However, as an athlete approaches competitive levels the training dosage increases and approaches the tolerance, which when crossed, results in injury (see figure 1.1). An injured athlete cannot perform. Average approaches, and average clinicians and coaches can have success when dealing with the middle stages of training or rehabilitation. Having success at the extremes (dealing with the extreme tender backs or with the "hard gainers" at world record level) requires the ultimate expertise. This book will provide insights for you to achieve this level.

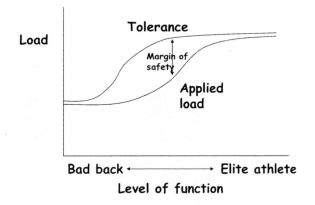

Figure 1.1 Exercise is called "therapy" when used in rehabilitation, and "training" for performance athletes. The dose of exercise must be sufficient to produce adaptation yet too much results in injury. The difference between the dose and the tolerance is the margin of safety. The margin of safety is smallest when dealing with intransigent bad backs or elite performers. Success with these "end of the spectrum" individuals needs the highest clinical expertise.

The concept of tolerance and capacity

The concepts of *tolerance* and *capacity* are the key for successful training of the back. Each individual has a tolerance for work. The tissues will break if the load tolerance is exceeded. If the tissues are already weakened with injury, the tolerance is lower. One must never cross the tolerance line. Understanding the tolerance of each individual will assist in choosing the appropriate dosage-load for each stage of training.

In a similar way, each individual has a capacity for work. Capacity is the sum total of all activities over a period of time – perhaps over a training session, a day, or a week. Capacity is a finite commodity as it has a definite limit. People use up a portion of the daily capacity with every task that they do. For example, some use up too much capacity in warmup activities, causing them to break form in the actual activity. Others stupidly use capacity by adopting poor standing and sitting posture, setting up their backs for pain and dysfunction during the actual training session, and afterwards in the restoration phase.

Ideal training occurs when both tolerance and capacity are increased, together with perfecting form and ultimately performance.

Current low back disorder myths

Many "wisdoms" abound regarding back training - here are a few.

The myths associated with stretching

Name a study that has shown that working to increase back flexibility has increased performance. I have not been able to find one despite people claiming this is so. Studies of weightlifters have shown those with more flexibility tend to be the better performers but this is specific to the shoulders and hips – not the back. Power, as in most sports, comes from the hips and legs, not the back. Cross-sectional studies of some team sports have shown that the higher performing athletes are, in many cases, the "tighter" ones! For example, despite the widely held notion that many athletes should be lengthening hamstrings, it is curious that the better performers (such as basketballers) appear to be the ones with "tight" hamstrings. They are "wound like springs" and take full advantage of this. Further, hamstrings contribute shearing stability to the knee such that lengthening them has been reported to be associated with elevated disruption of the anterior cruciate ligament. No wonder the bulk of the literature has shown no link between hamstring tightness and back pain, either current pain or predicting future pain (eg Biering-Sorenson, 1984, Hellsing,

1988). There is some evidence to suggest that asymmetry of hamstring flexibility is linked to back pain (Ashmen et al, 1996). The point to be made here is that each such notion must be considered within context of the individual, safety, health and performance. Rather than simply stretching – stretching to correct asymmetry has a foundation. Some longitudinal studies have shown that the more flexibility one has in the back, the greater the risk is of having future back troubles, at least in "normal people". Is stretching a good "warm-up" or should a warm-up precede a stretching session? Some data suggests that pre-stretching modulates the stretch receptors to inhibit subsequent performance – at least in children. Stretching to increase range of motion is often the goal. Yet stretching modulates all sorts of neuromuscular processes so that more consideration regarding the stretching exercise prescription is often needed. Remember that high performance is not a stretching contest. Mobility is a requirement, but loose joints without precisely controlled strength are unstable. This decreases performance and increases the risk of subsequent injury.

Many demanding sports require a very strong and stable torso to transmit forces developed in the upper body, through the torso, for optimal projections through the legs to the floor. Some world class athletes have almost total disability according to the American Medical Association definition for low back disability – based on loss of spine range of motion. Our research on workers has shown that spine range of motion has little to do with function at work (Parks et al, 2003) – Olympic weightlifters have proven they are functional using minimal spine motion when setting world records! However, they have wonderful range of motion ability in the shoulders, hips, knees and ankles which they can control with incredible strength. A spine must first be stable before moments and forces are produced to enhance performance, and arranged in a way that spares the spine from a potentially injurious load.

Stretching of the low back is perceived by many to "feel good", yet very few with bad backs actually qualify to train with this approach. Flexion and rotational stretching overloads the annulus fibers often exacerbating the spinal tissues which can occur unbeknownst to the individual. Yet they continue the practice, reporting that it "feels good". They are perceiving stretch, probably via the muscle based stretch receptors, which provides the illusion of something helpful. Generally they are ensuring that they remain chronic and will not make advances until stretching is stopped! Solomonow's group (2003, 2008) have shown that static stretching of the spine ligaments can cause muscle spasms and diminishes the stretch reflex. The reflex is a protective mechanism! Should stretching be incorporated into a warm-up routine? Not always. Do all athletes need stretching? Some do and some don't. Do some mobilizing exercise approaches such as "yoga" and "pilates" work? They help some and hurt others. Flexibility without strength and motor control is useless. Two principles guide our approach to stretching: One, each athlete must be pre-qualified to perform a specific stretch, and if a stretch is indicated, to ensure no exacerbation of pain or injury risk. Two, we look for opportunities to train the motion and develop an appropriate motor pattern to ensure ultimate performance throughout the range, as opposed to blindly stretching at joint end range. Stretching is about training the neuromuscular processes. "Active" flexibility is a concept developed by others, but explained in this book along with approaches to train it to enhance performance.

A special note is needed here regarding "perceived" hamstring tightness and pain. Too many of the patients referred to me have been prescribed hamstring stretches; apparently this is routine in many clinics. Yet when we perform provocative testing the pain is exacerbated by neural tension. This type of pain and tension cannot be stretched away. Ceasing this stretching allows the nerves to desensitize and a greater range of pain-free motion returns. The moral of the story is that there needs to be a rationale for stretching.

Stabilize what needs to be stabilized, mobilize what needs to be mobilized, know the difference, the consequences and the symbiosis.

The myths associated with strengthening: rehabilitation vs. training for performance

When rehabilitating bad backs, there is often a clinical emphasis on increasing back muscle strength. Interestingly, several studies have shown that muscle strength cannot predict who will have future back troubles (Biering-Sorenson, 1984). On the other hand, Luoto and colleagues (1995) have shown that muscular endurance (as opposed to strength) is protective. Further, many studies that have attempted to trial strengthening approaches have chosen exercises designed to injure the back – for example, including sit-ups to strengthen the abdominal muscles. No wonder they reported that a positive health effect was not achieved or worse – more bad backs were created! Of course back and abdominal strength are important for performance but different rules apply for the back than for other body parts. Power (force times velocity) should come from the hips. The risk rises when power is developed in the spine. The implication is that when high spine torques are developed, the velocity of spine motion must be low. Conversely, high spine velocity is safe only when the torques are low. Weightlifters develop enormous hip power but virtually no spine power (high force and low velocity) because the spine is locked into a static position while the high velocity angular motion is provided by the hips.

What is so interesting is that when the technique of workers or athletes is examined, generally those who have bad backs are the ones who load their backs to higher levels performing the same task. Evidence on rowers has documented those with the "hard catch" tend to be the ones with symptomatic backs. Workers with back troubles tend to lift using their back extensors and hamstring muscles. They tend not to use their hip extensors. A study of national class powerlifters has shown that those with lower back moments, but higher hip moments, lifted closer to the world record. Similar findings have been made in Olympic weightlifters. A healthy back, and a high performance back, depends on highly functional hips, and other parts of the body – these are also addressed in this book.

There is no question that strength is important for performance. But if muscle strength cannot be directed through the skeletal linkage so that weaker joints are not forced to absorb some energy, so that the force projections ultimately have the maximal effect elsewhere in the body, it is of little value. The training approaches justified in this book develop multiarticular strength to optimize performance. They are not designed to hypertrophy muscle. Further, there are several prerequisites that form a foundation of back function prior to efforts to seriously strengthen the back, another major theme of this book.

Motion and motor changes from back injury: Pain inhibits optimal motor patterns

The old body building axiom "no pain, no gain" does not hold for backs. Those with back troubles develop aberrant motor patterns that remain as both a detriment to performance and an impediment to recovery. The presence of pain prevents the re-establishment of "healthy" motor patterns that will be required to conduct subsequent training regimens for performance. Training with pain will ensure the establishment of perturbed motor patterns – for rehabilitation objectives; exercises must be painfree. Training for performance involves discomfort and pain. The best coaches/clinicians never confuse rehabilitation objectives with performance objectives.

Just as motor patterns are perturbed from having injury, inappropriate motor patterns can also cause injury. Some injuries just happen as the result of motor control errors. (This interesting mechanism is introduced in chapter four, where we describe witnessing an injury using videoflouroscopy to view the spine.) These may be considered random events and their occurrence may be more likely in people with poor motor control systems (Brereton and McGill, 1999).

Perturbed motor control systems both cause, and are a consequence of, injury. Top level rehabilitation and training programs must address them.

What distinguishes the best athletes?

Think of the superstars of any sport. Are they the ones with the largest muscles? Rarely. Are they the ones who spend hours in the gym lifting weights? Rarely. Typically they perform poorly when compared to their teammates and peers in pre-season testing of specific tasks such as bench press and barbell squats (bench pressing power lifters excepted since this is their event). Instead their distinguishing qualities are motor control. The ability to exert strength quickly, deactivate muscle quickly, and optimally project forces throughout the body linkage, is characteristic of this skill. The techniques described in this book are directed towards enhancing this fundamental neuromuscular skill in addition to the "traditional" focus of athletic performance training.

Focusing on multifidus, or transverse abdominis or any other single muscle: misdirected clinical effort

Over the last few years, there has been enormous effort directed towards enhancing the function of single muscles, such as transverse abdominis. This was motivated by the research from Australia showing perturbed motor patterns in the transverse in some people with back troubles. However, athletes focusing on single muscles are creating dysfunction in spines! Newer studies have shown that virtually all muscles demonstrate perturbed patterns of activation following back troubles in athletic populations (eg. Cholewicki et al, 2002) and in workers (McGill et al, 2003). Muscles create joint torque but also most importantly ensure stability for optimal health and performance. Data is provided to prove that muscles work as teams to optimize these objectives across several joints during many complex tasks. The task and motion must be trained – not a specific muscle.

The confusion between rehabilitation and performance training

Rehabilitating a bad back is for pain reduction and health enhancement – period. Establishing motor and motion patterns with no pain, and building function for daily activity (although what constitutes daily activity will be different in each individual), while building tissues and avoiding further injury are the objectives. In contrast, performance training demands that risks be taken, that the body systems be overloaded into the razor-thin zone brinking on failure. These two objectives and approaches must be separated if optimal rehabilitation and performance are to be achieved, yet too often, they are confused.

The pollution of body building approaches in low back training

Many body building principles such as isolating a muscle during training, the basic design of reps and sets and so forth, have little place when training the back for performance. They were simply intended to hypertrophy muscle. Strength development depends on the stimulation of motor units which are more fully trained by different joint configurations, using different speeds and different force projections. Training a whole-body motion involves balance of force throughout the linkage. Too much force, or too little at a joint, or force applied at an incorrect time results in poor performance and injury. Motor control is what separates the best athletes from the poorer competitors even though the poorer performers may have larger muscles. This book describes techniques to maximize performance – which is almost always at odds with conventional body building approaches.

Athletic bad backs: Dealing with the cause and the role of prevention

No good doctor, clinician, or specific therapy will heal a bad back if the causes of the problems are not removed. Understanding the cause of low back disorders is necessary since these specific factors must be identified and removed from the program of each athlete – at least for the initial stages. This book provides information to assist in identifying the causes and guidelines for preventing them (what could be called rehabilitation/athletic Ergonomics) to assist you in becoming an elite expert.

The mind and performance

Several elite coaches and former athletes have mentioned to me that training is more about training the mind. This may seem astounding to some. They mean this in a few ways. Aspects of sports psychology are critical. Anyone who has worked with a group of athletes has observed those who withhold from supreme effort. In another way the mind is the controller of movement and the ability to activate and deactivate muscle is a neuromuscular skill. The skilled mind can create a neurokinetic swirl of motor unit firing resulting in strength far beyond the reach of the untrained and unskilled.

The Russian approach to systematically develop discipline in all aspects of the athlete's life is part of the parcel to positively direct the mind. Those without an ego have too much respect for their opponent. They will not give full performance out of respect or because they believe that they can't. The opponent may be a bar, it may be a person. The supreme performer simply knows that they will not be defeated. I have no expertise in the psychology of performance, but I am keenly aware of its influence. This book will assist in developing the physical aspects of back performance. A sports psychologist may assist with the mental aspects.

Consider the thoughts of Vasili Alexeyev during the height of his world dominance in super-heavyweight Olympic lifting, expressed to Dmitri Ivanov: "You see, the question is not one of strength, not one of talent. It's a matter of what's in the head. In the physical sense you should, you need to work very hard, but with the nerves".

The strength and skill of the body, when combined with the strength and the skill of the mind, make for a third strength and skill far in excess of the sum of the two. Techniques used by some top athletes to achieve this "third strength" are described in this book.

The doctor says the pain is in your head: Don't believe it!

Among those with chronic bad backs, athletes included, too many are accused of being psychosocial cases. The pain is in the head – just toughen up! Many physicians using inappropriate approaches get frustrated with the lack of positive progress and begin to blame the owner of the bad back – suggesting that they are not trying hard enough or they are mentally weak and therefore succumb to pain. The evidence shows that psychosocial components are involved in influencing how an individual will express pain behaviour. But only biomechanical overload can cause tissue damage; psychosocial factors do not directly damage tissue. However, once the damage has occurred, pain behaviour is modulated by psychosocial factors. But how can these factors be addressed? Teasell (1997) argued quite convincingly that while psychological factors have been cited as being causative of pain and disability, in fact, psychological difficulties arise as the consequence of chronic pain (See also Gatchel et al., 1995; Radanov et al., 1994) and disappear upon its resolution (see also Wallis et al., 1997). He uses the example of the highly paid and intrinsically motivated athlete who is unable to play due to back troubles. The inability to play is costing him millions. The evidence is compelling—real back disorders, pain and psychological variables appear to be linked, but simply addressing the psychosocial issues will fail. Pain during the rehabilitation process impedes the establishment of healthy motion and motor patterns and pain is usually the result of a poor program. It appears that too many of those with back troubles who have failed to respond to conventional rehabilitation approaches or traditional training approaches are accused of not trying and worse yet, being mentally weak. My opinion is that the medical personnel simply reached the end of their expertise – the failure more often being theirs, not the patients or the athletes.

Address the chronic pain, and the psychosocial issues will nearly always resolve. Any of us who consider ourselves tough-minded lose the mental will when deprived of sleep through chronic pain. This book will describe exercise approaches that can be pain-free for patients, and spine sparing for performance training.

Each person is an Individual: There are no approaches that work with all

As people, we have personal differences in our capabilities. Some of us are more endurable and suited for "lighter" but prolonged work while others are stronger and capable of heavier work. Some can tolerate sitting and others not. A few can even survive the rigours of playing the linebacker's position in the NFL. Could a St. Bernard tolerate the training or work exposure at a racetrack, or conversely a Greyhound carry a heavy load? This would be a poor bet. Matching the current capabilities of an individual with the loading demands of a task is important. Choosing optimal loading, rest periods, and controlling the duration of exposure is both an art and a science. Evaluating each athlete and identifying the appropriate challenge is critical for success. The best practicioners are those with clinical wisdom based on experience but who also have a well developed understanding of the science. Several approaches to matching a training load with an individual are documented in this book.

Are back troubles a life sentence?

What if you currently have back troubles - can these back troubles linger for a lifetime? In this context, it is interesting that elderly people appear to complain less about bad backs than younger people. Valkenburg and Haanen (1982) showed that back troubles are more frequent during the younger years. Weber (1983) provided further insight by reporting on patients who were 10 years post disc herniations (some of them had had surgery while others had not) and were engaged in strenuous daily activity—while still receiving total disability benefits! It would appear that the cascade of changes resulting from some forms of tissue damage can take years but generally not longer than 10 years. Although the bad news is that the affected joints stiffen during the cascade of change, the good news is that eventually the pain is gone. Troublesome backs are generally not a life sentence.

For athletes, once a back injury has occurred, generally they will not be "healed" even though the symptoms have resolved. It is interesting to consider the comments of those who have several world records to their credit in weightlifting following back injury. They state that a back injury forced them to maintain perfect lifting form because they realized that if they lost the "locked" spine they would become re-injured in an instant. Thus, at least during their competitive careers, they had to utilize stabilizing technique for their backs. They competed successfully. It is interesting to consider those I have seen as patients several years after their competitive days who became symptomatic after they lost their fitness and ability to stabilize. The original tissue damage was still there and became troublesome.

Food for thought

Resist the urge to assume that conventional wisdom is correct – it is often not. First consider the evidence and then form your own opinions.

How we obtain the evidence to improve back training: Our unique approach

I have been exposed to many schools of thought regarding training, and how the spine functions. Initially, some make sense and sound convincing. But after study and investigation, opinions change. This book contains many non-traditional viewpoints on how the spine functions, becomes damaged and can be trained. While some of these viewpoints have been obtained with field studies of real people, most of these perspectives have emerged from a unique biomechanically based approach. A brief introduction to the approach is provided here.

I sometimes joke that I will perform investigations on back-related controversies with anyone, anytime, anywhere, using any technique – a spine nymphomaniac! I am not married to a single approach but am willing to try several approaches and even develop new ones, if I can obtain more insight. Having stated this, our usual approach is to begin the process as engineers, and then morph into clinicians. The following example illustrates this general approach. A civil engineer needs three types of information to design and build a bridge:

- The amount and type of traffic to be accommodated, or the applied load
- The type of structure to be used (e.g., space truss or roman arch), as each architecture possesses specific mechanical traits and features
- Characteristics of proposed materials that will affect strength, endurance, stability, resistance to structural fatigue, etc.

We approach back investigations in the same way where performance is assessed with an eye towards predicting the risk of tissue damage. When the applied load is greater than the tissue strength, tissue failure (injury) occurs. Analyzing tissue failure in this way requires two distinct methodological approaches requiring us to develop two quite distinct laboratories. Our first lab ("in-vitro") is equipped for testing actual spines, in which we purposefully try to create herniated discs, damaged end plates, and other tissue-specific injuries. The second lab ("in vivo") is equipped to examine living people for their response to stress and loading. Individual tissue loads (vertebra, muscles, discs, etc.) are obtained from sophisticated modeling procedures. Finally, we test and perfect techniques and trial efficacy in the research clinic. Examples are provided below.

The *In-Vitro* lab

The harvested spine lab is equipped with loading machines, an acceleration rack, tissue sectioning equipment and an X-ray suite to document progressive tissue damage. For example, by performing discograms (as performed on people at the hospital) with radio opaque contrast liquids, we can document the mechanics of progressive disc herniation in a way not possible on real people. We can create loading scenarios to replicate heavy lifting where a lifter may employ different lumbar-hip movement strategies, or we may examine how some simultaneous twisting would change spine stresses. This offers insights, available for the first time, on how disc herniation progresses and how the progression can be halted - or the herniation prevented. We investigate any other injury mechanisms in the same way — that is, by applying physiological loads and motion patterns and then documenting the damage with appropriate technology (see figure 1.2).

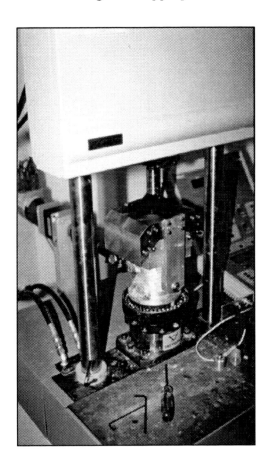

Figure 1.2 This is our disc herniation machine where motion segments and discs (wrapped in plastic film here to preserve hydration) are repeatedly flexed/extended.

Since many technical issues can affect the experimental results, the decision to use one approach over another is governed by the specific research question. In many cases animal models allow us to exercise control over genetic homogeneity, diet, physical activity, and so forth to contrast an experimental cohort with a matched set of control spines. Of course, we must validate and interpret the results for them to be relevant to humans.

The *In Vivo* lab

In the other "living people" lab we document the loads on the many lumbar tissues. This knowledge lends powerful insight into spine mechanics, both of normal functioning and of failure mechanics. Since we cannot routinely implant transducers in the tissues to measure force, we must use non-invasive methods. The intention of the basic approach is to create a virtual spine. This virtual model must accurately represent the anatomy that responds dynamically to the three-dimensional motion patterns of each test subject/patient, and must mimic the muscle activation patterns chosen by the individual. In so doing, it enables us to evaluate subjects' unique motor patterns and the consequences of their choices and skill.

How the Virtual Spine Works: Briefly, a computerized representation of the person's anatomy with a focus on their low back is generated. Then as the person moves and activates their muscles, we measure these events with sophisticated sensors and drive the virtual spine to move, mimicking the motions of the person and their muscles that are used to "turn on" their virtual spine muscles in the computer (see figure 1.3).

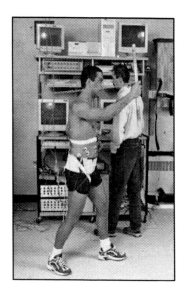 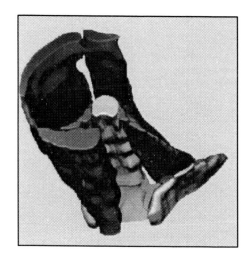

Figure 1.3 (a) Subject monitored with EMG electrodes and electromagnetic instrumentation to directly measure three-dimensional lumbar kinematics and muscle activity. (b) The modelled spine (partially reconstructed for illustration purposes, although for the purposes of analysis it remains in mathematical form) moves in accordance with the subject's spine. The virtual muscles are activated by the EMG signals recorded from the subject's muscles.

Using biological signals in this fashion helps us assess the wisdom of the many ways that we choose to move and support loads. The output consists of muscle and passive tissue forces, spine joint loads and quantified spine stability. Such an assessment is necessary for evaluating injury mechanisms, formulating injury-avoidance initiatives and obtaining insight into performance potential. A large number of associated research papers have documented the evolution of this process over the past 20 years. They are listed on my University website (http://www.ahs.uwaterloo.ca/kin/people/StuMcGill.html).

The Research Clinic: The third component to the triad of investigation is the research clinic where we see patients and athletes on a consultancy basis. This is where we find out if our work has value. While the lab work reveals mechanisms to help us understand what, how and why, this final testing ground is where we confirm what works for who, and when.

References for the modelling process

Cholewicki, J., and McGill, S.M. (1996). Mechanical stability of the in vivo lumbar spine: Implications for injury and chronic low back pain. *Clin. Biomech.,* 11 (1): 1-15.

Howarth, S. J., Allison A.E., Grenier, S., Cholewicki, J., and McGill, S.M. (2004) On the implications of interpreting the stability index: A spine example. J. Biomech. 37(8):1147-1154.

McGill, S.M. (1992). A myoelectrically based dynamic 3-D model to predict loads on lumbar spine tissues during lateral bending. *J. Biomech.,* 25 (4): 395-414.

McGill, S.M., and Norman, R.W. (1986). The Volvo Award for 1986: Partitioning of the L4/L5 dynamic moment into disc, ligamentous and muscular components during lifting. *Spine,* 11 (7): 666-678.

References pertaining to the finer details of the modelling process

Brown, S., McGill, S.M. (2009) Transmission of muscularly generated force and stiffness between layers of the rat abdominal wall. SPINE, 34(2): E70-E75.

Brown, S., McGill, S.M. (2008) How the inherent stiffness of the in-vivo human trunk varies with changing magnitude of muscular activation. Clin. Biomech., 23(1): 15-22.

Brown, S., McGill, S.M. (2008) Co-activation alters the linear versus non-linear impression of the EMG-Torque relationship of trunk muscles. J. Biomech., 41: 491-497.

Brown, S.H. and McGill, S.M. (2005) Muscle force-stiffness characteristics influence joint stability. Clin. Biomech. 20(9):917-922.

Cholewicki, J., and McGill, S.M. (1994). EMG Assisted Optimization: A hybrid approach for estimating muscle forces in an indeterminate biomechanical model. *J. Biomech.,* 27 (10): 1287-1289.

Cholewicki, J., and McGill, S.M. (1995). Relationship between muscle force and stiffness in the whole mammalian muscle: A simulation study. *J. Biomech. Engng.,* 117: 339-342.

Cholewicki, J., McGill, S.M., and Norman, R.W. (1995). Comparison of muscle forces and joint load from an optimization and EMG assisted lumbar spine model: Towards development of a hybrid approach. *J. Biomech.*, 28 (3): 321-331.

Grenier, S.G., and McGill, S.M. (2007) Quantification of lumbar stability using two different abdominal activation strategies. Arch. Phys. Med. & Rehab., 88(1):54-62.

Kavcic, N., Grenier, S.G., and McGill, S.M. (2004) Quantifying tissue loads and spine stability while performing commonly prescribed stabilization exercises. Spine. 29(20):2319-2329.

Kavcic, N., Grenier, S., and McGill, S. (2004) Determining the stabilizing role of individual torso muscles during rehabilitation exercises. Spine. 29(11):1254-1265.

McGill, S.M. (1988). Estimation of force and extensor moment contributions of the disc and ligaments at L4/L5. *Spine*, 12: 1395-1402.

McGill, S.M. (1996). A revised anatomical model of the abdominal musculature for torso flexion efforts. *J. Biomech.*, 29 (7): 973-977.

McGill, S.M., Juker, D., and Axler, C. (1996). Correcting trunk muscle geometry obtained from MRI and CT scans of supine postures for use in standing postures. *J. Biomech.*, 29 (5): 643-646.

McGill, S.M., Juker, D., and Kropf., P. (1996). Appropriately placed surface EMG electrodes reflect deep muscle activity (psoas, quadratus lumborum, abdominal wall) in the lumbar spine. *J. Biomech.*, 29 (11): 1503-1507.

McGill, S.M., and Norman, R.W. (1985). Dynamically and statically determined low back moments during lifting. *J. Biomech.*, 18 (12): 877-885.

McGill, S.M., and Norman, R.W. (1987a). Effects of an anatomically detailed erector spinae model on L4/L5 disc compression and shear. *J. Biomech.*, 20 (6): 591-600.

McGill, S.M., and Norman, R.W. (1987b). An assessment of intra-abdominal pressure as a viable mechanism to reduce spinal compression. *Ergonomics*, 30 (11): 1565-1588.

McGill, S.M., and Norman, R.W. (1988). The potential of lumbodorsal fascia forces to generate back extension moments during squat lifts. *J. Biomed. Engng.*, 10: 312-318.

McGill, S.M., Patt, N., and Norman, R.W. (1988). Measurement of the trunk musculature of active males using CT scan radiography: Implications for force and moment generating capacity about the L4/L5 joint. *J. Biomech.*, 21 (4): 329-341.

McGill, S.M., Santaguida, L., and Stevens, J. (1993) Measurement of the trunk musculature from T6 to L5 using MRI scans of 15 young males corrected for muscle fibre orientation. *Clin. Biomech.*, 8: 171-178.

McGill, S.M., Seguin, J., and Bennett, G. (1994). Passive stiffness of the lumbar torso about the flexion-extension, lateral bend and axial twist axes: The effect of belt wearing and breath holding. *Spine*, 19 (6): 696-704.

McGill, S.M., Thorstensson, A., and Norman, R.W. (1989). Non-rigid response of the trunk to dynamic axial loading: An evaluation of current modelling assumptions. *Clin. Biomech.*, 4: 45-50.

McGill, S.M. (2004) Linking latest knowledge of injury mechanisms and spine function to the prevention of low back disorders. J. Electromyography and Kines.14(1):43-47.

McGill, S.M., Grenier, S., Kavcic, N., Cholewicki, J. (2003) Coordination of muscle activity to assure stability of the lumbar spine. Journal of Electromyography and Kines. 13:353-359.

Santaguida*, L., and McGill, S.M. (1995). The psoas major muscle: A three-dimensional mechanical modelling study with respect to the spine based on MRI measurement. *J. Biomech.*, 28 (3): 339-345.

Sutarno*, C., and McGill, S.M. (1995). Iso-velocity investigation of the lengthening behaviour of the erector spinae muscles. *Eur. J. Appl. Physiol. Occup. Physiol.*, 70 (2): 146-153.

References for the chapter

Ashmen, K.J., Swanik, C.B., Lephart, S.M., (1996) Strength and flexibility characteristics of Athletes with chronic low back pain, J. Sport Rehab., 5:275-286.

Biering-Sorensen, F. (1984) Physical measurements as risk indicators for low-back trouble over a one-year period. *Spine*, 9: 106-119.

Brereton, L., and McGill, S.M. (1999) Effects of physical fatigue and cognitive challenges on the potential for low back injury. Human Movement Science 18: 839-857.

Cholewicki, J., Greene, H.S., Polzhofer, G.K., Galloway, M.T., Shah, R.A., Radebold, A., (2002) Neuromuscular function in athletes following recovery from a recent acute low back injury. J. Orthop. Sports Phys. Ther. 32:568-575.

Gatchel, R.J., Polatin, P.B., Mayer, T.G., (1995) The dominant role of psychosocial risk factors in the development of chronic low back pain disability, Spine 20:2702-2709.

Hellsing A.L., (1988) Tightness of hamstring and psoas muscles: A prospective study of back pain in young men during their military service, Upsala J. Med. Sci., 93:267-276.

Luoto, S., Heliovaara, M., Hurri, H., et al. (1995) Static back endurance and the risk of low back pain. *Clin Biomech*, 10: 323-324.

McGill, S.M., Grenier, S., Bluhm, M., Preuss, R., Brown, S., and Russell, C. (2003) Previous history of LBP with work loss is related to lingering effects in biomechanical physiological, personal, and psychosocial characteristics. Ergonomics, 46(7): 731-746.

Nachemson, A.L. (1992) Newest knowledge of low back pain: A critical look. *Clinical Orthopaedics and Related Research,* 279: 8-20.

Parks, K.A., Crichton, K.S. Goldford, R.J. and McGill, S.M. (2003) On the validity of ratings of impairment for low back disorders. SPINE. 28(4):380-384.

Radanov, B.P., Sturzenegger, M., DeStefano, G., and Schinrig, A. (1994) Relationship between early somatic, radiological, cognitive and psychosocial findings and outcome during a one-year follow up in 117 patients suffering from common whiplash. *Br. J. Rheumatol.*, 33: 442-448.

Solomonow, D., Davidson, B., Zhou, B.H., Lu, Y., Patel, V., Solomonow, M., (2008) Neuromuscular neutral zones response to cyclic lumbar flexion. J. Biomech. 41:2821-2828.

Solomonow, M., Zhou, B-H., Bratta, R.V., Burger, E, (2003) Biomechanics and electromyography of a cumulative lumbar disorder: response to static stretching, Clinical Biomechanics, 18:890-898.

Teasell, R.W. (1997) The denial of chronic pain. *J. Pain Res. Management,* 2: 89-91.

Valkenburg, H.A., and Haanen, H.C.M. (1982) The epidemiology of low back pain. In: White, A.A., and Gordon, S.L. (Eds.), *Symposium on idiopathic low back pain*. St. Louis: Mosby.

Wallis, B.J., Lord, S.M., Bogduk, N., (1997) Resolution of psychological distress of whiplash patients following treatment by radiofrequency neurotomy: A randomized double-blind placebo controlled study, Pain, 73:15-22.

Weber, H. (1983) Lumbar disk herniation: A controlled prospective study with ten years of observation. *Spine,* 8: 131.

Chapter 2

Exercise Science and the Back: Removing the Confusion

Introduction

A general foundation in exercise science is required for those interested in back development and performance. This chapter is intended to introduce and discuss some of the more salient elements of this foundation to justify the general approaches to training that are documented in later chapters. Some readers will find this chapter long, while others will find it brief in places. For those readers wanting the highest level of background expertise in general exercise science, I wish to recommend some excellent sources. For general neuromuscular function with relevance to training, it is hard to beat Dr. Roger Enoka's book *Neuromechanical Basis of Kinesiology*. Some of the introduction into the Russian systems of training presented here can be found in more detail in Dr. Mel Siff's excellent book entitled *Supertraining*, a "must read".

There is a notable contrast in developments within exercise science between the West (North America and Western Europe) and the East (the former Soviet Union and the Eastern Bloc), particularly since WWII. The East continued to perform scientific investigations into performance development in what we would consider today the fundamental understanding of motion and motor patterns. In contrast, the West increasingly focused on cardiovascular components, with the Swedish influence and the publishing and promotion of very popular fitness books such as Dr. Cooper's "Aerobics". To be "fit" in the West required a high MVO2 score. We have measured many people with high MVO2 scores who do not have command of some simple motor patterns, and while they could run a distance, they literally would have trouble running with another simultaneous challenge – be it carrying a load or chewing gum! As a consequence, the exercise physiologists became fitness experts – many of whom had little or no expertise beyond cardiac and muscle hypertrophy issues. Their general ignorance of musculoskeletal function has led to the proliferation of exercises which replicate injury mechanisms. Many machines have been developed to isolate muscle and enhance hypertrophy to the detriment of performance. In contrast, the East continued to develop science on all aspects of fitness and with application, produced enviable results in international competition during this period. Certainly over the last decade, the "Western" science has broadened and has created a place for an approach contained in this book.

Too much effort is directed towards training the "muscle" in many performance programs. Isolating a muscle about a joint and training it with progressive overload is purely a body building hypertrophy approach. Functional training incorporates the goal of enhancing strength throughout the body segment linkage. This ensures that strength is generated quickly, throughout complex motions and postures, in an environment that preserves balance and joint stability while avoiding injury risks. Specifically, functional training involves:

1. *Intramuscular coordination of fibers within a muscle.* Muscles contain varying ratios of fast twitch and slow twitch fibers that have distinctive recruitment and firing patterns based on speed of force production, direction, etc. This means that different training approaches are needed for different muscles within the body and also different approaches are needed between people to recognize different fiber type distributions in the population.

2. *Intermuscular coordination between muscle groups.* Many muscles assist one another to create moments (or torque) about a joint – these are typically called synergists. Muscles contracting to create moments on the other side of the joint are called the antagonists. This distinction is acceptable for only the most rudimentary discussion of function but is problematic for discussions directed towards developing true high level functional training. Each muscle, in a group of synergists, has a different architecture in that they are performing different functions – they are not synergists at all. Take the example of the "hip flexors" of rectus femoris, psoas and iliacus. Each plays a different role in its function to protect the joint and stabilize adjacent joints. This would have profound effects when designing a stretching routine for the hip flexors – calling them synergists ignores the majority of their function, and ensures poor functional exercise design. Likewise, with the antagonists – while they may be moment antagonists, these muscles are serving functions to stabilize the joint, balance joint shearing forces and motions, and contribute functional roles to adjacent joints linked with the associated tendons.

3. *Facilitory and inhibitory reflexive pathways.* These pathways act to modify muscle contraction throughout the body linkage. These are often perturbed by the existence of both chronic and acute pain. They are

affected by posture and the balance environment. These are also highly adaptive and trainable.

4.   *Motor learning.* Motor learning involves the programming and encoding of motion/motor patterns together with training the ability to react and modify patterns for optimal performance in an ever changing environment. Massive gains in performance early in training programs are a consequence of the motor learning accomplished at the muscular level, and the motor program level.

Summary message:

The motor control system is not organized to isolate and control single muscles but rather is designed to control movements. Train movement – not muscle.

Training affects all systems

Neuromuscular stimulation is fundamental for all training programs due to the plasticity of the human system at all levels – from the nerve and muscle cell, through the hierarchy of involved systems, to the movement produced. Not only are neural systems highly trainable but the consequences of muscle activity, namely loads on the skeletal components, stimulate adaptation in the tissues to bear more load. Joint proprioception is also critically important in enhancing both the rehabilitation process and ultimate performance. Monkeys who have had surgical rhizotomies (the severing of sensory nerves as they outlet the various spinal levels) to remove joint sensory perception in one arm will not use that arm even though all motor ability is intact. Not until the good arm is tied behind their back will they use the arm with joint sensory deficits (Taub, 1976). Now consider the challenge to the rehabilitation professional who must assist a back patient who has undergone a surgical rhizotomy (these are performed in an attempt to reduce pain in the back extensor muscles). The motor nerves remain intact. The belief that rhyzotomized muscles are only minimally compromised is misguided – the muscles need both motor stimulation and the stimulation supplied from the joint receptors. More evidence to support the importance of considering the proprioceptive system is contained in the injury prevention literature where proprioceptive training at the ankle has been proven to reduce subsequent injury rates among soccer teams (Tropp et al, 1984). Optimal functional training must involve loading the entire musculoskeletal system even when training the back. "Isolating the joint" is a misguided wisdom from the muscle physiology and body building culture. The implications of this are:

1.   Training should be designed to stimulate optimal adaptation in the muscle and cardiovascular systems, the neural systems and in the tissues themselves.

2.   The use of machines that buttress joints and restrict range of motion at specific joints not only retard the various levels of motor learning required for optimal functional performance, but can encode patterns that are directly detrimental to both performance and the avoidance of injury.

3.   The encoding of patterns by repeated stimuli means that even brief periods of inappropriate patterns (poor form, poor balance, use of non-related aids) can be detrimental to performance. Interestingly, many of the top teams develop training facilities so that all training exercises are performed in the position of play.

4.   Using aids such as belts, joint bandages, shoe wedges and elastic training suits, for example, can inappropriately modify the control system.

5.   For injured athletes, return to competitive performance levels is possible with the development of compensatory motor patterns – several examples in his book prove this to be true.

6.   Each person has different proportions of body segment lengths, muscle insertion lengths, muscle to tendon length ratios, nerve conduction velocities, intrinsic tissue tolerance, etc. Their personal style and skill in many cases have evolved based on some level of optimization of these variables. Imposing a stereotyped "ideal" technique will often prevent an athlete from reaching their full potential.

7.   Subtle technique can be very important. Many examples are provided in this book about things like intentional hip activation profiles that can enhance performance.

Preliminary issues for designing a program

A major theme of this book is the progressive and systematic development of challenge for the athlete. Specifically, first establish the motor and motion patterns, then develop endurance all of which occurs prior to specific efforts to build strength. Once strength training has begun in earnest, the commencement of a program is characterized by the extensification phase typified with a greater volume of work but with low intensity (lower load and strength challenge). The basic periodization model progresses towards decreasing volume and increasing intensity (resistance). Several variables assist in this progression and can include:

1. Type of strength (speed strength, ultimate strength etc)
2. Types of muscle contractions (concentric, eccentric, isometric)
3. Changing speeds of contraction throughout a task (critical point acceleration)
4. Rest intervals (reps, sets, training days)
5. Method of recovery (active or passive)
6. Sequencing of exercises
7. Relative strength and control of stabilizers, joint antagonists, agonists etc
8. Training history of the individual – have they "been there" before?
9. Injury history of the individual
10. Proficiency level of the athlete

Strength

There are many types of strength – at least in terms of deficits to performance or limiting performance. Ultimate one time strength is rarely limiting – rather performance limits are almost always speed strength and endurance strength. Specifically, the rate at which force is produced together with the rate of deactivation and the ability to continually produce force is important for developing a program. It is interesting that strength training is considered synonymous with weight training for most people. However, this belief limits the potential of too many athletes. Furthermore, "slow" strength at the level of the muscle is quite often the easiest to develop of all necessary attributes – perhaps those seeking rapid results gravitate to strength training. Speed strength is another matter.

Factors that limit training outcome

Identifying the variables associated with training that can limit ultimate performance is a process that assists in overcoming them. Some of the main factors include:

1. *Trainability* – the ability to progress depends on many genetic factors ranging from chemical and cellular function through to anatomical variables. In addition, many previously trained adaptations can be re-obtained much more quickly.
2. *Neuromuscular efficiency* – Dr. Roger Enoka (eg Enoka, 1994) has documented extensively the science in understanding the enormous contribution of factors such as the ability to recruit/de-recruit muscle fibers, sections of muscles etc.
3. *Biomechanical efficiency and suitability* – leverage characteristics are determined by body segment length proportions to one another, muscle connection areas and architectural features such as muscle to tendon length ratios. Of course, control factors overlay the biomechanical factors and influence joint stability and loading, and ultimately safety and performance.
4. *Psychological factors* – factors such as aggression, motivation, concentration, pain tolerance, perception of spectator behaviour, adherence to programs, ability to deal with the pressure of an event, general mental toughness and the ability to relax are just a few variables that constrain performance.
5. *Social factors* – societal influences and expectations impose perceived limits and define acceptable behaviour often to the detriment of performance and in some cases, safety.

6. *Pain and fear of pain* – distinguishing between the pain of injury and the pain of effort is very important. Pain prevents injury when utilized effectively and limits performance when utilized ineffectively. Further, the presence of pain inhibits specific muscle and motor patterns that may be essential to both injury avoidance and ultimate performance.

7. *Fatigue* – mental and physical fatigue inhibit performance over a workout session but can also build throughout a poorly designed, and poorly periodized, training schedule so that the athlete remains continually fatigued.

Biomechanics and training

Ligaments and other joint passive tissues generate force when they are stretched as the joint reaches its end-range of motion. Likewise muscular forces contribute to movement by acting on the skeletal system. The ability of a muscle or ligament to create joint torque or moment of force is a function of the magnitude of the force multiplied by the distance to the mechanical fulcrum of the joint. This may be the center of rotation of the joint or it may be the balance point of linear forces around the joint.

The concept of the moment

Muscles and ligaments create forces which are applied to the bones that articulate around a joint. Their force working through a moment arm (the perpendicular distance from the force line to the fulcrum in the joint) creates the moment. Thus the moment may be increased by increasing the force, or by increasing the moment arm. The moment arm changes as a function of the joint angle since the attachment points of tendons are fixed on the bone that arcs through rotational motion.

This concept of the moment has implications on both the risk of injury and performance. Imagine holding five pounds in the hand. Because the elbow flexors work through a moment arm of about $1/15^{th}$ that of the load, they must contract with 15 times the five-pound hand load to support the posture – or 75 pounds in this example. This 75 pounds of force directed via the muscle spans the joint, causing 75 pounds of joint load at the bone-on-bone interface. Thus the joint pays dearly for supporting the load. This same analogy occurs in the back. Awkward loads that produce a large moment arm distance to the spine can result in tons of muscular force to be imposed on the spine. In this way technique either places the spine in peril or spares it when performing a given task. (see figure 2.1)

In summary, the concept of the moment incorporates two parts – the external moment, or the reaction moment, and the internal moment, or the support moment. The external moment results from external forces placed on the body, and the effects of gravity and motion of the body segments. This is affected by body mass and acceleration, the distance of hand-held objects to the joint center, and body posture. The support moment created by the muscles, ligaments and bony stops acting around a joint are influenced by muscle or ligament force magnitude, the moment arm (which is a function of the muscle line of action), joint position and size of the muscle (a bulkier muscle increases the distance to the joint fulcrum), just to name a few.

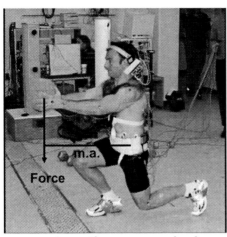 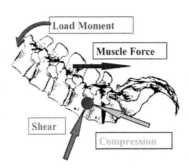

Figure 2.1. The moment is the product of the line of force and its perpendicular distance (moment arm) to the axis or lumbar spine in this case (left panel). The extensor muscles, in this example, have a moment arm of just a few centimeters (right panel). This means the muscle must contract at a force magnitude many times that of the hand-load to maintain the posture. The hand-load creates a reaction moment and the muscles create the support moment.

The concept of the moment of force just illustrated is based on a single joint, making it flawed for performance. Many muscles span several joints, requiring an analysis over the full length of the muscle-tendon complex.

Muscle mechanics

The ability of a muscle to produce force depends on several features – its size or physiological cross-sectional area, its ability to develop stress (or force per unit of cross-sectional area) and its neural drive. The force developed by these factors is further modified by the instantaneous length of the muscle and its velocity of either shortening or lengthening.

The modulating influence of velocity is depicted in the force-velocity relationship. Essentially, when a muscle is required to shorten at faster velocities it is compromised in its ability to produce force. At higher levels of activation (there are more motor units and muscle fibers contracting), more force is developed as the muscle is forced to lengthen in an eccentric contraction. But at lower levels of activation, the lengthening muscle "yields", greatly compromising the ability to produce force (Sutarno and McGill, 1995). The back extensors exhibit "yielding" during rapid torso flexion motions. Specifically, the faster a muscle is forced to lengthen, and when its activation is low, the more easily it gives way. This appears to be due to the inability of the sarcomere cross-bridges to obtain a foothold on an available binding site. In contrast, under conditions of full activation to the muscle, the lengthening motions cause higher forces – the cross-bridges are able to obtain and maintain footholds. Paradoxically, this is a situation where muscle and tendon injuries occur. Watching a rugby game the other night on television, a player sustained an achilles tendon tear. In slow motion replay the mechanism was shown so clearly. As the player was landing on the ball of his foot lengthening the achilles, he simultaneously began accelerating through the hips and knees to drive forward. This produced the high activation to the muscles under a lengthening condition and the resultant destructive force.

Interestingly, the force-velocity relationship is not only dependent upon individual muscle architecture and other anatomical variables – it is trainable. Zatsiorsky (1995) demonstrated the positive shift in strength at lower velocities with heavy strength training ("strength-speed training") and the shift to producing strength at higher velocities with lower load, higher velocity training ("speed-strength"). Training was specific and enhanced the trained variable. But Zatsiorsky's work has shown that the ability to produce ultimate strength is not related to sporting speed. They are two different motor abilities. Those who simplistically believe that increasing strength (or worse yet simply hypertrophying muscle) will enhance performance have neglected the skill components required to produce the required strength at the precise instant in time – to quote Dr. Mel Siff "just the right amount at the right time". This has been lost in too many of the "Western" programs when compared with the "Eastern" ones.

Muscle length also influences a muscle's ability to produce force and is of much greater concern in those muscles that span more than a single joint. Skill and technique take advantage of this relationship. Specifically, joints have optimal configurations to achieve optimal muscle lengths to produce force. Compromise of force development in muscle as a function of length is most extreme in two joint muscles like the hamstring group that span both the knee and the hip. With full hip extension and simultaneous knee flexion, the muscle is so short it cannot produce force. Yet in the opposite conformation (full hip flexion and knee extension) the stretch in the muscle can increase to levels that cause tearing.

No discussion of biomechanical influences would be complete without introducing mechanics and the governance of Newton's laws. Understanding them is required to achieve optimal technique for training and performance. However, they have been explained in a later chapter where they are used to assist in the design of training programs.

The Russian philosophy of training

The science of training developed by the Russians was years ahead of Western progress. The data in this book confirms this. Collectively, this research lead to eight interrelated principles for scientific training (much more completely documented by Yessis, 1987, Matveyev, 1981 and Siff, 2002) which will be introduced here:

1. **The principle of awareness** – The athlete must complete formal education to understand their own mind and body from several perspectives. These include basic function of the organ systems, physiology, biomechanics, psychology etc, all of which the athlete utilizes in an attempt to optimally control and gauge work.

2. **The principle of all-round development** – Effort is directed towards developing a wide variety of qualities including physical strength, speed, coordination, and endurance together with will-power, mental toughness, group influence and exemplary moral conduct – to name a few.

3. **The principle of consecutiveness** – This principle is operationalized at two levels. The first recognizes the systematic increments in challenge (of all variables noted in the previous principle) as the training program progresses. The second level recognizes the pacing within a training session to ramp up intensity and correspondingly ramp down intensity at the conclusion. Certainly these qualitative descriptions are supported by science, showing the beneficial biochemical consequences of this regimen. In addition, injury prevention approaches utilize this principle to reduce tissue stress. During static postures, tissues at the joint interface accumulate micro deformations. A well designed warm-up slowly introduces motion as these tissues regain their "normal" confirmation, preventing destructive stress concentrations.

4. **The principle of repetition** – This is based on Pavlov's three-stage theory for development of conditioned reflexes. The first stage requires the athlete to understand what must be learned; the athlete directs full concentration on the repeated performance, perfecting the motor and skill ability. The final stage is characterized by the athlete no longer needing to concentrate on the task since the task is automatic. Perfect practice technique together with repetition, rest and recovery are vital for optimizing this principle.

5. **The principle of visualization** – The athlete must be able to visualize the movement at many levels. They must be familiar with kinematic patterns at different joints, in motor patterns in different areas in the body. One technique that we employ to optimize this principle is to have the athlete draw the motion and motor patterns of the task following his/her analysis of the components. This obviously is an "academic" session away from the competition arena. We are often made aware of major misperceptions

or misunderstandings on the part of the athlete through this principle. It can be extremely valuable for progressing to optimal performance.

6. **The principle of specialization** – Two levels of specialized training are recognized as vital. The first is usually well incorporated in various specificity training principles of the physical variables, while the second is not as well recognized and practiced – namely the practice of elements that are experienced only in competition. This may include distractions of audiences or other athletes, or challenges from unpredicted weather, for example.

7. **The principle of individualization** – Every athlete is an individual from many perspectives. This implies that no single training regimen will suit all in a sport or all members of a particular team.

8. **The principle of structured training** – Again this principle operates at two levels. The first level pertains to the design of a single workout. The session typically begins with a warm-up with specific effort directed to tissue-joint and physiological systems warm-up, and for creating conditions for skill learning. The main component of the workout typically begins with activity to perfect technical and tactical skill, and then progresses to speed and agility training, then to strength training, and finally to endurance training. This is followed by a concluding phase to enhance eventual recovery and enhance retention of motor skills. The second level of this principle deals once again with progression from one session to the next. Athletes cannot maintain peak performance levels. If they are truly peak, they will breakdown the person. Periodization consists of planned cycles of training that may incorporate many mini-cycles within the larger cycles. Obviously, this varies widely between sports and events.

Consideration of these principles and how they may be incorporated into a training program is a key component when I design programs. The implication is that the athlete is a thinking, working, entire human who must develop their understanding of their body to fully master control over it.

A note on plyometrics

Developed by the Russians to enhance "speed-strength", plyometrics combines active muscle dynamics and motor control with elastic stretch-shortening of the muscle-tendon complex. Also known as "shock training", rapid eccentric contraction is immediately followed by rapid concentric contraction. It is intended to increase speed by enhancing muscle contraction dynamics together with enhancing the connective tissues associated with the contractile components of the muscle to better store and recover elastic energy. When performed well, it also trains rapid activation/deactivation of motor units needed for ultimate speed, yet this is rarely discussed. Typically this approach is associated with jumping and bounding – perhaps from a box onto the floor with subsequent leaps to train forward or upward projection of the ensuing rebound. Extreme caution and vigilance is required for successful plyometric training to optimize the performance enhancement effect while avoiding injury through the extraordinary ballistic forces developed and imposed on the body. Any plyometric training is preceded by a core conditioning program. Focus is on landing position so that the projection of the upper body mass is directed through the low back to minimize loading in this vulnerable area. Of course, simple jumping and bounding exercises would precede any box jumps. Focus is directed towards foot landing dynamics, relative heel and body position, arm use, torso posture, and general balance to achieve the blend of performance enhancement and safety. Examples are described in the later chapters.

Strength and posture

Many features determine the ability to create functional strength – those listed include the internal biomechanics (muscle and joint architecture, and body segment variables) together with external biomechanical variables (such as projected force vectors from the floor through various joints, distances from external loads to various joints, etc). Posture affects all of these. For example, the lumbar extensors change function as a function of lordosis (see the next chapter). Lifting strength is affected by spine, neck and shoulder posture. For example, the back extensors "hang" from the neck. Strong men and women cannot have a "slouched" posture.

Proprioception training

One method of enhancing proprioceptive efficiency is to block input from other sensory systems, such as the visual system. Hence, many proprio progressions that involve balance and strength incorporate a blindfold. In fact, Roman (1986) has shown that many exercises are performed with more precision and stability when the eyes are closed. Focus is directed towards kinematic motion patterns. The intention is that they are enhanced once the eyes are reopened.

The science of flexibility

The word *flexibility* may be often misunderstood and misused, thus requiring a short general discussion here. Blindly increasing the range of motion rationalized by the belief that it is beneficial is problematic. In fact, there is no relationship between static joint flexibility and dynamic performance. Further, there is a documented negative correlation with more flexibility in the back and higher subsequent back troubles, at least in occupational athletes. Our work confirmed that low back range of motion capabilities of an injured worker had little relationship with their return to work and ability to perform their job. This relationship exists in other joints as well. Many great athletes run or lift skillfully employing their springs (read passive tissues). If this is the case, never stretch these athletes beyond the range of motion required in their event. On the other side of the coin, obviously some "tight" athletes cannot achieve optimal motion patterning nor the economy of motion required for many events. But be very careful, as many athletes are great because of their ability to employ passive tissues for force production and recoil. Decisions must be made for each individual. No two athletes should be trained exactly the same way.

Joint range of motion is a function of several variables - muscles about a joint (the key being the recognition that more than one muscle will have influence), passive tissue restrictions (bony stops and ligamentous structures), neuromuscular modulation of length and tension, non-functional tension in other multiarticular muscles and the pain threshold of the individual, to name a few. Stretching, to many individuals, is done to lengthen muscle in a passive sense yet there is little evidence that this occurs or is even a potent mechanism. Rather more evidence favours stretching to modify the neuromuscular processes. Further, this premise demands that the neuromuscular processes be continually challenged as an ongoing part of training, and in a functional way where "stretching" is performed simultaneously with tension challenge. The evidence suggests that modifying the neuromuscular processes has the most effect on the functional range of motion, but that these changes are short lived, and must be challenged daily. Such is the basis for PNF approaches to stretching. Next, stretching of the muscles and fascia (increasing their length) can be attempted but any results are slow to appear. Evidence where joint resistance to motion was quantified has confirmed that in many cases increases in joint range of motion were not achieved by stretching the passive tissues. It was achieved by the athlete training their tolerance to stretch thus allowing them to take the joint to further positions, the passive tissue stiffnesses and loads did not change at a specific joint angle (eg. Magnussen et al, 1998). Then, finally, in terms of importance, joint passive tissues can be lengthened and these effects tend to be longer lasting. Yet once again, there may be a price to pay for stretching tissue in terms of joint stability and risk of injury. A joint that has lost some passive stiffness requires more muscular contraction to maintain stability.

The neuromuscular processes involved with length and tension are described in detail in texts such as Kandel, Schwartz and Jessell (2000) for the interested reader. Briefly, a variety of reflex-related structures are contained in the muscle to sense length (muscle spindles) and tension (golgi tendon organs). These modulate the stretch reflex and when integrated with the proprioceptive system, form complex responses that facilitate and inhibit different muscles. All responses can be justified as appropriate, in specific situations, and attempts to modify them may result in unforeseen troubles. The goal of the athlete is to tune the system.

Thus, the concept of "active flexibility" is more important for performance, where muscular force is produced throughout a range of motion. Optimization of this concept is enhanced with knowledge of injury mechanisms. In our approach, active flexibility about the spine is emphasized (shoulders, knees and hips) but is not always justifiable in the spine itself – it depends heavily on the person and the demands of the task.

Implementing what is known scientifically assists in drawing these general guidelines for stretching technique:

1. **Specificity:** Several studies have shown the effect of specificity of repeated activities and the subsequent range of motion. For example, for athletes who require range of motion about the hips, and who may have a history of back troubles, cycling would not be a wise choice for aerobic activity training. Not only is the hip trained in a restricted range (thus becoming trained not to perform outside the range), but cyclists often show the hamstring dominant patterns during hip extension termed the "crossed pelvis syndrome" by Janda. The evidence once again suggests that while passive tissues are influenced, the proprioceptive component requires focused attention. Training with machines, where the motion pattern is specific is not addressing this important aspect of performance.

2. **Several approaches are needed:** Different methods and approaches for training range of motion are required to target passive tissues together with the neuromuscular components.

3. **Fibre type considerations:** Slow twitch muscles tend to have heavier connective tissue when compared to predominantly fast twitch muscles consistent with their function. Stretching of these tissues may or may not be important for a specific athlete – but if they are, they may require longer stretches.

4. **Static and ballistic stretching:** Both static and ballistic stretching techniques affect tissue properties and the neuromuscular components. But static stretching tends to focus on the passive elastic components of muscle while ballistic stretching tends to train the series elastic component. This is critical for the athlete who employs techniques to store and recover elastic energy to enhance muscle efficiency (jumpers, sprinters, lifters, throwers, etc).

5. **Functional directional stretching:** Stretching (active flexibility approaches) in all directions is important to train the tissues from a structural perspective and also from a neuromuscular perspective.

6. **Caution based on injury mechanism:** Tissue failure mechanics reveal that the weakest link during slow loading is the tendon/ligament junction with the bone periosteum. Rapid loading of these structures shifts the failure site to the collagenous or mid-substance of these structures. Consider the injury mechanism – if any.

7. **Sport specificity:** Evidence from different sports suggests the link between performance and flexibility is sport specific. While some studies of basketball players, for example, have shown that the better performers may have lower passive range of motion at a joint, Soviet data has shown that weightlifters with larger ranges of motion (but not the spine) tend to

be the better performers (Iashvili, 1982). Not surprisingly, active flexibility correlated with performance more strongly than passive flexibility. Active flexibility is enhanced with training the joints under load throughout the range of motion, and that mimic the sporting range of motion throughout the linkage, if possible.

8. **Does a warmup always include stretching?** Stretching is not a "warmup". In fact, there is evidence (Drabek, 1996) showing that initial static stretches can decrease subsequent coordination by resetting some of the organs involved in joint and muscle proprioception. Solomonow's work (2003) confirms this negative effect of back stretches. Once again, there are no rules, only guidelines for you to consider and apply when appropriate.

In summary:

* For athletes who use their "springs" (the runners, lifters, throwers, etc), generally don't stretch them beyond their competitive range of motion.
* Generally, bias your efforts towards facilitation of the neuromuscular system rather than dampening with stretching. Stretching is generally a cooling down activity.

Progression of a program with younger athletes

First and foremost, the younger athlete needs to develop motion and motor patterns in a safe way that will ultimately lead to high performance levels. Children are not miniature adults. Motor skills are best developed in the early years between the ages of three to nine, as observed by Piscopo and Baley, (1981) who documented the effectiveness of gross movements rather than focusing on the fine motor skills. Strength comes much later. The emphasis at this stage is on handling body weight and general training. Competition is limited and restricted to playful interaction. Brook (1985) documented progression guidelines as the younger athletes develop further (generally ages 13-14 years for most, but not all, sports) where more specific training is incorporated as are the numbers and intensity of training sessions. Specific skill, time spent and training intensity increase, together with strength development which becomes more focused following puberty.

Training balance

What separates those athletes who dominate their sport from their peers? Think of Jordan, Ali, Pele, and Gretzky and their ability to perform "in balance". None were muscle bound men who could impress with their bench press ability! Strength cannot be directed to enhance performance if the athlete is off-balance, unable to direct their strength in optimal directions at the right time and with the optimal region of the body. Furthermore, balance is a dynamic variable in which inertial forces developed during movement add to the challenge of optimizing performance. There is a sophisticated system involved in functional force development that depends on feedback from the visual and auditory systems, vestibular system, and the proprioceptive system. All aspects must be challenged and conditioned to achieve optimal performance. Not only are we seeking to control the center of gravity within the base of support, but also to optimize the ability to develop supreme muscular force and then create force projections that maximize performance. Methods to train balance are outlined in the third section of this book.

The popularity of the Olympic lifts: justifiable or misdirected

Many strength coaches, ranging from high school through to collegiate levels believe in building their programs around the Olympics lifts – in particular the first phase of the clean and jerk or the "power clean". There is no question that this will build strength, but at what cost and with what utility? Too many young athletes ruin their backs with this exercise.

In the former Soviet system, athletes were carefully selected for the Olympic lifts based on their body segment proportions, natural speed and flexibility. Very few North American men possess these attributes to even obtain the initial "set" at the beginning of the lift where the bar is pulled, to minimize back loading for safety. Further, very few can withstand the cumulative toll on the body of this very demanding event to survive for a necessary amount of time. Our data (Cholewicki and McGill, 1991) from national level powerlifting competition (not Olympic lifting) showed that better lifters actually sustained lower back loads than their less skilled competitors (less skilled meaning poorer performance and less weight lifted). They were able to obtain a body posture that spared their joints but the posture demands joint positions that are at the extreme range of the population continuum. Without question, there is merit for Olympic lifts when training some athletes, but with using much lighter loads and modified starting positions and postures. Greg Wilson and colleagues (1993) noted that optimal power development occurs with much lower load and much higher speed than is conventionally practiced. Finally, the Olympic lifts are sagittal plane challenges. Many athletes trained this way are strong in this plane but fail our screens for matching torsional strength. A pull on their sleeve reveals this imbalance and weakness for general athleticism.

Given the potential assets and liabilities of training athletes with the Olympic lifts, on balance, they are overemphasized in many programs. Certainly for team training programs where there is an interest in these lifts, a qualification procedure is absolutely necessary to identify those athletes who are candidates for low risk training, and to restrict those who do not possess the hip, knee, ankle and shoulder flexibility to perform the lifts with impeccable technique. A final consideration must be given to recovery. Many coaches do not realize the lengthy recovery time needed by some athletes following an Olympic lifting session. Only some athletes will be able to withstand the rigours of an intense Olympic program; others will need much greater recovery time compromising the training intensity.

Training with machines: a discussion

What is a machine? Machines are intended to offer resistance to the musculoskeletal linkage that many consider to be in a non-functional way, or as some commercial advocates will argue, in a functional way. Free weights on the other hand are considered more "functional" given the need to stabilize the body linkage and project internal forces through the linkage to the floor. But even within traditional free weight training, comparison between the use of dumbbells vs barbells is interesting. How often in a sporting situation are the hands tied through a linkage like a bar (barbell)? I can't think of one other than some specific competitions that use a barbell (eg powerlifting). Performing a military press with a dumbell produces an entirely different response through the torso than with a two-handed barbell. This example points to the continuum of "functionality" with the use of virtually any device that offers resistance. Using the body weight itself, enhanced with cables etc, certainly has a place in complete functional training.

Machines can regulate the magnitude of the resistance, the speed of joint motion and the motion in adjacent joints. Some have the potential for graphical output of performance. However, some constrain centers of rotation and set up unnatural stress concentrations and/or diminish the need to balance, stabilize and coordinate multi-joint motion. Safety is sometimes claimed to be a feature of machines primarily through various mechanisms to stop a load from falling on the person. This notion may be misguided. Training in a proprioceptively starved environment does not challenge the system needed to ensure that no single tissue experiences damaging overload.

While not all machines require a sitting posture, too many of them do. The professional teams with whom I consult are very conscious to train their athletes in "playing position". Performance simply cannot be trained in a sitting posture – yet count the number of machines that require sitting in your local gym (see figure 2.2). Further, the sitting posture required of many machines results in increased bending loading to the back – for example, many seated leg press machines force the lumbar spine into flexion with the application of combined shear and compression. Atypical muscle activation patterns result. I would very rarely recommend this approach except in some very particular cases. While this approach is popular with some body builders who are interested in training particular muscles we are interested in training the squat mechanism (notice I did not state the muscles involved). **Train the motion, not the muscle.**

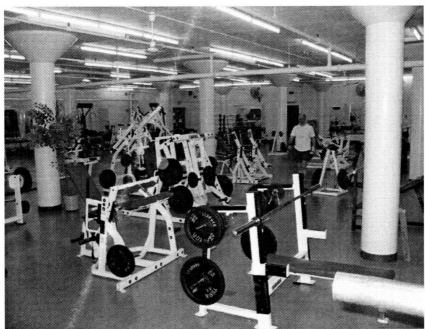

Figure 2.2 Look at the modern gym and notice the number of machines that require the person to sit. In this gym every machine requires sitting or lying. And unfortunate as this is, this gym was designed for training performance athletes!

For the purposes of this discussion, cables to weight stacks are not considered machines since they do not isolate joint motion and add resistance to whole-body motion patterns. As we will see in a subsequent section, these types of exercises form part of a performance-based program. Exercises like the cable overhead pull and woodchop require directed hand forces through a stable body linkage with a projection to the ground. The way the forces are transmitted through the body linkage will determine the level of performance resulting from a given strength exertion.

There are many other examples of machines that require consideration for optimizing performance and safety:

- Various squat machines which can constrain load trajectory and produce high knee shear loads, and lumbar loads.
- Some spinal extension machines, in particular twisting machines.
- Some leg machines that produce shear and unnatural patellar loading and tracking.
- Any machine that requires a sitting posture.
- Any machine which place joints into weak and vulnerable biomechanical position (eg. seated military press).

Subsequent chapters will introduce devices (although not classed as "machines") to enhance lability underneath the athlete, or to add lability to the load. The benefits to enhancement of both spine and whole body stability will be demonstrated.

The principle of dynamic correspondence

Mel Siff wrote about this principle in terms of matching the method of training with the specific demands of the sporting activity. Specific motor qualities that were considered included: matching the motion, accentuated region of force production, dynamics of effort, rates of force production and regimen of muscular work. There is much more to this list than meets the average eye. For example, a sprinter may train hip extension. In contrast, a sprinter understanding the implications of this principle will simultaneously train hip extension with corresponding hip flexion about the other hip. In this case the principle would operationalize with one-legged squats, performed at a high rate of acceleration, with simultaneous high acceleration hip flexion, eventually driving into a takeoff from the ground. Obviously this high performance exercise would be preceded by the hierarchy of training progression (ensuring the existence of stabilizing motor patterns etc). Dynamic correspondence is a component of optimal performance exercise.

Safety issues: a generic discussion

Injury may result from three generalized situations: accident (improper or unexpected technique or execution) during training or during a sporting event, undertraining (insufficient preparation of tissues and the way that forces are controlled), and overtraining (cumulative trauma in tissues). Since perfection in each of these components will never be achieved, injury will occur. While a summary of injury is provided elsewhere in this book, some elements are worthy of discussion here. Violation of any of the qualitative motion analysis principles noted in chapter seven could result in overload of a specific tissue. Certainly, continual movement or technique errors will cause cumulative trauma. Inadequate rest, perturbed motor patterns, inappropriate sleep and nutrition, inappropriate breathing, development of muscle imbalance in terms of both strength and endurance, and even personality characteristics have all been shown to modulate the risk of injury through modulation of tissue loading. The implication is that injury avoidance results from activity design based on the deepest understanding.

Principles for designing a good warm-up

Warm-up is important prior to any training or competition. This is a graduated process of taking the body from rest to ultimate performance. Several systems are involved. Prolonged loads on the joints cause small deformations at the joint interface or area of contact. When standing, for example, a dent is created in the knee cartilage. If an athlete were to perform rapid motion and loading, enormous stress concentrations would develop along the edge of the deformation in the cartilage causing wear and even micro-tearing. In the spine, viscose behaviour in the annulus causes similar stress concentrations until gentle motion removes the friction. This is why motion, with a low load is used to initiate the warm-up as this approach directly spares joints. Fuel consumption mechanisms and energy metabolism must be taken from a rested state to a higher level to achieve efficiencies needed for endurance and strength. A rushed warm-up does not allow for the vascular dilation, altered cardiac and liver output and other physiological systems to meet the higher demands. Muscle warm-up is necessary but rarely includes deliberate stretching, particularly when dealing with the back.

A well designed warm-up has two phases – general preparation and specific preparation. General preparation begins with easy walking, progressing into jogging and calisthenic exercise. Specific preparation is designed to enhance the specific physical and mental demands of the task. Range of motion exercises may enhance "active flexibility" and may or may not include specific stretches. For example, leapers, bounders and runners may progress to some acceleration runs. Lifters may begin the potentiation process for ultimate strength by lifting an unloaded bar with progression to some heavy exertions.

The objective of the warm-up is to prepare for performance and not to tire. Rough guidelines, which of course shall be considered for each individual, suggest that calisthenic exercises be repeated 8-10 times to achieve lower viscosity and neuromuscular preparation. A selection of exercises is used to develop a 10-15 minute warm-up regimen. Tempo and rhythm should be considered and matched to the athlete. The warm-up should involve all body parts to ensure that one does not "cool". Consider weather and the need to blend more active with less active exercise.

While notes on mobilization and "active flexibility" were provided throughout this book, a few often overlooked approaches are noted here. Spine mobilization may be achieved in the most spine sparing way with the cat-camel exercise performed on all fours (see chapter 10). After this, spine mobilizing progressions are highly sport specific and cannot be generalized here. But hip mobility is the key to sparing the spine in many tasks together with enhancing performance. Lunge walks both in the sagittal and frontal planes are excellent "active flexibility" warm-up exercises. Some other hip progressions that are not common include transverse plane mobilization combined with balance and strength such as the transverse plane "airplane". Wall squats are another excellent facilitator of the hips with controlled torso stability (chapter 10).

In summary, consider the three overarching components of a general warmup that will result in performance enhancement:

1. First, think "Biomechanically" and mobilize the joints.
2. Second, think "Physiologically" and activate the various systems.
3. Third, think "Neurologically" and potentiate the neuromuscular system for rapid activation/deactivation in desirable patterns.

Specific considerations for rehabilitative back exercise

Training for rehabilitation objectives forms a continuum with training for performance. However, there is a distinction that rehabilitation must constitute low risk while performance training naturally involves more risk due to higher overload. The discussion in this section is directed to the rehabilitation end of the continuum. *Low Back Disorders* focussed on rehab and the interested reader is directed to read it for much more detail – a brief outline of the issues is provided here.

Back flexibility

Whether or not to train for optimization of spine flexibility depends on the person's injury history and exercise goal. Further, given the many features of "flexibility science" outlined in the previous pages, athlete and activity specific considerations are necessary. Generally, for the injured back, spine flexibility should not be emphasized until the spine has stabilized and has undergone strength and endurance conditioning—and some may never reach this stage! The most successful rehab programs appear to emphasize trunk stabilization through exercise with a neutral spine (e.g., Hides et al., 2001; Saal and Saal, 1989) while stressing mobility at the hips and knees (Bridger et al., 1992, and Scannell and McGill, 2003 demonstrate advantages for sitting and standing, while McGill and Norman, 1992, outline advantages for lifting).

Interestingly, many patients present with regions of their backs that are stiff, and locked in either an extended posture or a flexed posture. Another region of their back is very mobile creating a spinal "hinge". The hinge point is, not surprisingly, often the site of pain. This can be difficult to address. Soft tissue work and mobilization at a specific site may have merit together with developing control and stiffness at the mobile hinge.

For these reasons, torso flexibility exercises during rehabilitation phases must be considered carefully often resulting in limited unloaded flexion and extension for those concerned with safety. With symptom alleviation, those interested in specific athletic activities may begin performance training and incorporate "active" flexibility into their routines. (Of course, spine flexibility may be more desirable in certain types of athletes who have never suffered back injury.)

Strength and endurance

In general, cross-sectional studies of strength seems to have little to do with low back pain status even though increasing torso muscle strength is a popular objective of low back rehabilitation protocols. Leino et al (1987) found that neither isometric nor dynamic trunk strength predicted the development of low back troubles over a 10-year follow-up period. The Biering-Sorensen (1984) study previously noted found that isometric back strength did not predict the appearance of low back trouble in previously healthy subjects over a one-year follow-up. Holmstrom and Moritz (1992) recorded reduced isometric trunk extensor endurance times in male workers with low back disorders compared to those without, but found no differences in isometric flexion or extension strengths. Both Biering-Sorensen (1984) and Luoto and colleagues (1995) suggested that while isometric strength was not associated with the onset of back troubles, poor static back endurance scores are. Strength appears to have little, or a very weak, relationship with low back troubles. In contrast, muscle endurance, when separated from strength, appears to be linked with better back health.

Perhaps it is the inactivity in the back patients that causes their muscles to adopt an anaerobic metabolism characteristic of fast twitch motor units. However, the back muscles are designed, and better suited, for endurance capacity. Certainly, a stable spine requires endurable muscles, not necessarily strong muscles. A recent study (McGill et al., 2003) has suggested that having a history of low back troubles is associated with a different flexion-to-extension endurance ratio, with the extensors having less endurance and the flexors having more endurance. This imbalance in endurance also appeared between the right and left side lateral musculature as evidenced by the asymmetry in right and left endurance holding times (e.g., (Right side bridge)/(Left side bridge) ratio that differed by more than 5% was linked to those who had a history of low back troubles). The next issue addressed the question of whether strength and endurance are related. Interestingly, the flexor strength (N.m) to endurance (sec) ratio was between 3 and 3.5 for the flexors in both "normal" backs and in those with a history of troubles, and for the extensors of the normals. The ratio was much larger for the extensors (5.3, $p = .033$) in those with a history of LBD. But what was so interesting was when the workers were observed lifting, those who had back troubles lifted in a way to load their backs to higher levels. They did not use their hip capacity. In fact they used more back strength capacity! Programs designed to build hip extension capacity to spare the back are outlined in section 2 of this book. The point is that strength is important, but that several precursors for building ultimate strength must be addressed first. Graduated, progressive exercise programs (i.e., of longer duration and lower effort), should emphasize endurance first, then progress to strengthening exercises.

In summary, "bad backs" generally use their backs more and their hips less – consider this in the rehabilitation plan.

Spine power: integration of flexibility and strength discussions

Power equals force times velocity. Power generated in the spine is therefore specific to angular motion of the vertebrae (and spine muscle length change and the muscular torque). Generating power in the back increases the risk of injury and generally decreases performance. Spine velocity has been shown to identify occupations with high risk of back troubles (Marras et al, 1993). Low spine power must not be confused with poor strength or poor range of motion. Generating high strength (or force) is much safer with a back that is not bending (i.e. low power). Undergoing rapid spine motion is much safer when the forces are lower. Thus the object of most movement technique to spare the back, both in rehabilitation and during performance tasks, is to maintain low spine power. Generally good technique requires power to be developed about the hips.

Motor patterns

As previously noted, those with a history of back troubles "forget" how to use their gluteal muscles. Similarly for a challenged breathing task, those with a history were unable to maintain constant abdominal muscle stiffness to maintain sufficient spine stability. These are just two of the examples of the widespread changes in motor control that occur with chronic back pain. Without addressing these fundamental motion and motor patterns, back troubles will continue with repeated episodes of troubles.

Eliciting volitional movement: Given the motor deficits mentioned above, approaches for facilitating movement and teaching muscular responses have been developed and utilized over many years. Quick stretch techniques have been used in athletic and rehabilitation situations as have vibration and light touch and brushing techniques. While quick stretch will evoke monosynaptic reflexes that can augment a rapidly sequenced motor command, there is also a potentiation process augmenting subsequent activation. Potentiation also has a brief time window for which it could be of help. While vibration has been used, mostly to invoke the tonic vibration reflex, it also produces movement and body segment position illusions. We would not use this approach with athletes. Finally, light touch and brushing of skin overlaying muscles that are to be facilitated can be very helpful. While actual increases in range of joint motion have been documented in post-stroke patients, the athlete can benefit from brushing techniques when learning motor patterns in stage one of the program outlined in section two of this book. For example, when teaching gluteal activation patterns, those athletes that have trouble reducing hamstring dominance can be assisted with brushing of the quadriceps into mild activation, reducing hamstring activation as a consequence. "Fascial raking" techniques, particularly for abdominal contraction, are also introduced later in this book.

Aerobic exercise

Mounting evidence supporting the role of aerobic exercise in both reducing the incidence of low back injury (Cady et al., 1979) and treating low back patients (Juker at al., 1998) is compelling. Recent investigation into loads sustained by the low back tissues during walking (Nutter, 1988) confirm very low levels of supporting passive tissue load coupled with mild, but prolonged, activation of the supporting musculature. A study we performed a few years ago demonstrated why slow walking tends to aggravate many backs while fast walking is relieving. Of particular note is the role of arm swing which reduces loads on the spine. The moral of the story is that fast walking with arm swing is often advocated. We even recommend wearing a backpack to help some specific types of bad backs! More on this later.

Studies on the connection between fitness and injury disability

It is fruitful to discuss briefly the role of fitness in the link between injury and disability. Although several studies have shown links between various fitness factors and the incidence of LBD (e.g., Suni et al., 1998, who showed that higher maximum oxygen consumption scores were linked to LBDs), these cross-sectional studies cannot infer causation.

Probably the most widely cited longitudinal study was reported by Cady and colleagues (1979), who assessed the fitness of Los Angeles firefighters and noted that those who were rated "more fit" had fewer subsequent back injuries. However, what is not widely quoted by those citing this study is that when the more fit did become injured, the injury was more severe. Perhaps the more fit were willing to experience higher physical loads. Several studies have suggested that a psychological profile is associated with being fit (e.g., Hughes, 1984; Ross and Hayes, 1988; Young, 1979) and that the unfit may complain more about the more minor aches. Along those lines, some athletes have demonstrated the ability to compete despite injury. Burnett and colleagues (1996) reported cricket bowlers with pars fractures who were still able to compete. Is this due to their supreme fitness and ability to achieve spine stability or their mental toughness? Perhaps it is both. The issue remains unresolved. Further, low back pain patients assigned to exercise programs that involved strengthening the back musculature experienced lower psychosocial dysfunction (Kisch et al., 1993).

Order of exercises within a session

Because the spine has a loading memory, a prior activity can modulate the biomechanics of the spine in a subsequent activity. For example, if a person sat in a slouched posture for a period of time sufficient to cause ligamentous and disc creep, they would have residual ligament laxity for a period of time (we have measured laxity of over a half hour in some cases (McGill and Brown, 1992). The nucleus volume appears to redistribute upon adopting a standing posture (Krag et al., 1987). This redistribution takes time. If the spine is flexed in one maneuver, then it probably should return to neutral or extension for the next.

Viscosity is another property of biological tissues—in this case a frictional resistance to motion within the spine and torso tissues. This is why motion exercises are usually performed first as part of a well-designed warm-up. Once the viscous friction has been reduced, subsequent motion can be accomplished with less stress.

A final consideration is the need to continually groove healthy, joint-conserving, and stabilizing motor patterns. Depending on the exercise objectives, we often begin an exercise/training session with some spine-stabilization exercises to groove the patterns that will continue over to other exercises in the program.

Establishing grooved patterns

We have found that people are best served when we establish the grooved motion/motor patterns at the beginning of the session. In a performance-oriented training program, this is called neuromuscular activation by some. Further, the session may also conclude with various motion and motor patterning exercises.

Breathing

Debate continues regarding the entrainment of breathing during exertion. Should one exhale or inhale during a particular phase of movement or exertion? Research has not adequately addressed this issue.

In the rare cases of very heavy lifting or maximal exertions (which would not be part of a rehabilitation program), high levels of intra-abdominal pressure are produced by breath holding using the Valsalva maneuver (eg maximum lifting or sprinting efforts). This elevated IAP, when combined with high levels of abdominal wall co-contraction (ie abdominal bracing), ensures spine stiffness and stability during these extraordinary demands. Another motivation given for striving to achieve higher IAP is the need to reduce the transmural gradient in the cranium, which may lessen the risk of blackout or stroke (McGill et al., 1995). The explanation for this risk reduction is as follows: Building IAP is associated with a rise in the CNS (Central Nervous System) fluid pressure in the spine, which forms an open vessel to the CNS and brain. But upon exertion, enormous elevation in blood pressure occurs (documented in weightlifters to be well over 400 mmHg). This pressure in the cranial vessels creates a large transmural pressure gradient that would be reduced if the CNS fluid pressure were elevated, reducing the load on the vascular vessels. This mechanism should be considered only for extreme weightlifting challenges—not for rehabilitation and performance training exercise.

When designing rehabilitation exercise, a major objective is to establish spine-stabilization patterns. An important feature of stable and functional backs is the ability to co-contract the abdominal wall independently of any lung ventilation patterns. Good spine stabilizers maintain the critical symmetric muscle stiffness during any combination of torque demands and breathing patterns (such as when playing a basketball game, for example). Training a breathing pattern to an exertion cycle may not be helpful. For example, exhaling while raising a load and inhaling while lowering it is for body building, not athletic performance. This would be of little carryover value to other activities; in fact, it could be counterproductive.

Time of day for exercise

As will be pointed out in part II, the intervertebral discs are highly hydrated upon rising from bed; the annulus is subjected to much higher stresses during bending under these conditions. The end plates fail at lower compressive loads as well. Thus, performing spine-bending maneuvers at this time of day is unwise. Because the discs generally lose 90% of the fluid they will lose over the course of a day within the first hour after rising from bed, we suggest simply avoiding this period for exercise (that is, bending exercise) either for rehabilitation or performance training. While there hasn't been a study on the enhancements obtained during exercise routines as a function of time of day, Snook and colleagues (1998) did prove that the conscious avoidance of forward spine flexion in the morning improved their patients' back troubles.

Clinical relevance for rehabilitation exercise

Exercise professionals face the challenge of designing exercise programs that consider a wide variety of objectives. Consider these guidelines for those with back troubles; performance training guidelines are later in this book:

1. **Exercise daily**. While some experts believe that exercise sessions should be performed at least three times per week, low back exercises appear to be most beneficial when performed daily (e.g., Mayer et al., 1985).
2. **Exercise must not exacerbate back pain**. The no pain-no gain axiom does not apply when exercising the low back, particularly when applied to weight training. Scientific and clinical wisdom would suggest the opposite is true. If the exercise causes back pain, you are doing something wrong.

3. **Add walking to the routine**. Research has shown that general low back exercise programs that combine cardiovascular components (such as walking) are more effective in both rehabilitation and injury prevention (e.g., Nutter, 1988). In particular, fast walking with an upright torso and arm swing reduces aggravating spine loading.

4. **Avoid spine bending after rising from bed**. Diurnal variation in the fluid level of the intervertebral discs (discs are more hydrated early in the morning after rising from bed) changes the stresses on the disc throughout the day. People should not perform full-range spine motion under load shortly after rising from bed (e.g., Adams and Dolan, 1995, McGill and Axler, 1996).

5. **More repetitions of less demanding exercises will enhance endurance and strength**. Low back exercises performed for health maintenance need not emphasize strength with high-load, low-repetition tasks. Given that endurance has more protective value than strength (Luoto et al., 1995), strength gains should not be overemphasized at the expense of endurance, at least during the first three stages of training detailed in this book. Of course, serious strength training demands far fewer repetitions.

6. **No set of exercises is ideal for all individuals**. An appropriate exercise regimen should consider an individual's training objectives, be they rehabilitation, reducing the risk of injury, optimizing general health and fitness or maximizing athletic performance. While science cannot evaluate the optimal exercises for each situation, the combination of science and clinical experiential wisdom will result in enhanced low back health.

7. **Be patient and stick with the program**. While many people report almost immediate benefits, others with the intransigent bad back will occasionally need patience. For example, success with earlier stages of training to increase function and reduce pain may not be experienced for up to three months (e.g., Manniche et al., 1988). The good news is that this approach is successful at preventing recurrent acute episodes and disability (Suni et al, 2006). The corollary to this approach is that when training for performance, gains must be continuous or a program change is necessary.

The process of injury: tissue response to mechanical load

Exercise design, whether for rehabilitation, general fitness or for performance, must consider mechanisms for injury. This section is intended to begin discussion of back injury from a load-dose response perspective of a biological system. Specific tissue injury mechanisms are discussed in the next chapter.

Any clinician completing a worker/patient compensation form is required to identify the event that caused the injury. Many players and coaches attribute an injury to an "event". This is mythical as very few back injuries result from a single event or episode. This section documents the more common cumulative trauma pathway leading to the culminating event of a back injury. The cumulative trauma may arise from poor training design, or may occur from faulty motion/motor patterns. Because the culminating event is falsely presumed to be the cause, prevention efforts are then focused on that event. This misdirection of efforts fails to deal with the real cause of the cumulative trauma.

Having stated that few injuries occur from a single event, it is curious that some patients/athletes report that their acute instigating episode was a sneeze, or they "threw their back out tying their shoe" or "when picking a pencil off the floor". These are real injuries. The mechanism is buckling. However, a series of events led to the conditions that allowed buckling to occur. This issue is more fully explained in a subsequent chapter dedicated to the science of spine stability.

Obviously, an excessive load larger than the failure tolerance of the tissue, applied once, produces injury. More commonly, injury during occupational and athletic endeavors involves cumulative trauma from repetitive subfailure magnitude loads. Here, injury results by either the repeated application of relatively low load or the application of a sustained load for a long duration. An athlete such as a rower who repeatedly loads the tissues of the low back (several tissues could be at risk) to a subfailure level (see figure 2.3) experiences a slow degradation of failure tolerance (e.g., for vertebrae, Adams and Hutton, 1985; Brinckmann et al.,1989). As tissues fatigue and weaken with each cycle of load, the margin of safety eventually approaches zero, at which point this individual will experience low back injury. Obviously, the accumulation of trauma is more rapid with higher loads. The avoidance approach would include reconsidering the exercise program design and interval training, together with a change in technique.

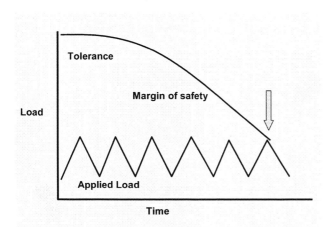
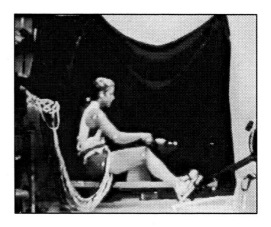

Figure 2.3 Repeated subfailure loads lead to tissue fatigue, reducing the failure tolerance, leading to failure on the Nth repetition of load (or cycle of rowing in this case – the image is poor having been taken from a data screen from an elite rower in the lab).

Yet another way to produce injury with a subfailure load is to sustain stresses constantly over a period of time. The cyclist shown in figure 2.4, with his lumbar spine fully flexed for a prolonged period of time, is loading the posterior passive tissues and is initiating time-dependent changes in disc mechanics. Under sustained loads these viscoelastic tissues slowly deform and creep. The sustained load and resultant creep causes a progressive reduction in the tissue strength. Correspondingly, the margin of safety also declines until injury occurs at a specific percent of tissue strain (i.e., at the breaking strain of that particular tissue). Note that this cyclist is not lifting a heavy load; simply staying in this posture long enough will elevate the risk of injurious damage. Of course, these athletes do not have ordinary spines as they has been "self-selected" and have trained – the average back could not tolerate this extreme posture and loading for lengthy periods. The injury may involve a single tissue, or a complex picture may emerge in which several tissues become involved.

Understanding the process of tissue damage in this way emphasizes why simple injury prevention approaches often fail. More effective injury intervention strategies recognize and address the complexities of tissue overload.

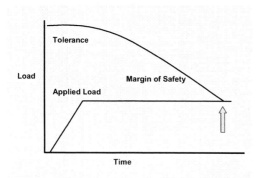
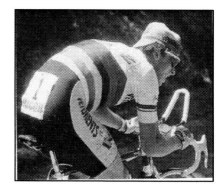

Figure 2.4 The typical road cyclist with a fully flexed lumbar spine is loading posterior passive tissues for long durations, reducing the failure tolerance leading to failure at the Nth% of tissue strain (arrow indicates where the margin of safety has been reduced to zero and the injury occurs).

In summary, avoidance of loading altogether is undesirable. The objective of injury prevention and training strategies is to ensure that tissue adaptation stimulated from exposure to load keeps pace with, and ideally exceeds, the accumulated tissue damage. Thus, exposure to load is necessary, but in the process of accumulating microtrauma, rest periods allow the healing/adaptation process to gradually increase the failure tolerance to a higher level. Many studies have documented the concept that links tissue loading and injury risk. Typically a U-shaped relationship emerges of not too much and not too little load (see figure

2.5), thus determining the optimal load for health encompasses both the art and science of medicine and tissue biomechanics. Too little loading will not stimulate adaptation – too much will overly damage the tissue. Figure 2.6 presents a final load-time history to demonstrate the links among loading, rest, and adaptive tissue tolerance. What this means to the coach/athlete is that more than casual thought should be given to the design of interval training regimens, work/rest/recovery schedules, and movement technique.

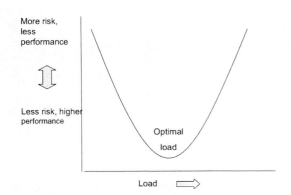

Figure 2.5 Optimal training and selection of the training load results from defining the U-shaped function. Too little load will not stimulate adaptation while too much load will overload tissue and lead to injury. The variables defining the U function continually change with rehabilitation and training.

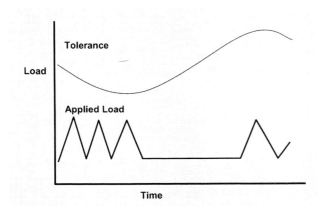

Figure 2.6 Loading is necessary for optimal tissue health. When loading and the subsequent degradation of tolerance is wisely followed by a period of rest, an adaptive tissue response increases tolerance. Tissue "training" results from the optimal blend of art and science in medicine and tissue biomechanics.

References

Adams MA, Hutton WC, Gradual disc prolapse. Spine 10: 524, 1985

Adams, M.A., and Dolan, P. (1995) Recent advances in lumbar spine mechanics and their clinical significance. *Clin Biomech*, 10: 3-19.

Biering-Sorensen, F. (1984) Physical measurements as risk indicators for low back trouble over a one year period. *Spine*, 9: 106-109.

Bridger, R.S., Orkin, D., and Henneberg, M. (1992) A quantitative investigation of lumbar and pelvic postures in standing and sitting: Interrelationships with body position and hip muscle length. *Int J Ind Ergonom*, 9: 235-244.

Brinckmann, P., Biggemann, M., Hilweg, D. (1989) Prediction of the compressive strength of human lumbar vertebrae. *Clin. Biomech*. 4: Suppl. 2, S1-S27.

Brook, N.D., (1985) Conditioning and the growing athlete, Athletics Coach, 19(4):31-35.

Burnett, A.F., Khangure, M., Elliot, B.C., Foster, D.H., Marshall, R.N., and Hardcastle, P, (1996) Thoracolumbar disc degeneration in young fast bowlers in cricket: A follow-up study, Clin. Biomech. 11, 305-310.

Cady, L.D., Bischoff, D.P., O'Connell, E.R., et al. (1979) Strength and fitness and subsequent back injuries in firefighters. *J Occup Med*, 21 (4): 269-272.

Cholewicki, J., and McGill, S.M., (1991) Lumbar spine loads during the lifting of extremely heavy weights, Med. Sci. Sports and Exerc. 23(10):1179-1186.

Cholewicki, J., McGill, S.M. (1996) Mechanical stability of the in vivo lumbar spine:Implications for injury and chronic low back pain. *Clin. Biomech*. 11(1): 1-15.

Drabek, J., (1996) Children and sports training, Island Pond, Vermont.

Enoka, R., (1994) Neuromechanical basis of Kinesiology, Human Kinetics Publishers, Champaign.

Holmstrom, E., Moritz, U., (1992) Effect of lumbar belts on trunk muscle strength and endurance: a follow up study of construction workers, J. Spinal Disorders 5(3):260-266.

Hides, J.A., Jull, G.A., and Richardson, C.A. (2001) Long-term effects of specific stabilizing exercises for first-episode low back pain. *Spine*, 26: E243-248.

Hughes, J.R. (1984) Psychological effects of habitual aerobic exercise: A critical review. *Prev. Med*. 13: 66-78.

Iashvili, A., (1982) Active and passive flexibility in athletes specializing in different sports, Toeriya I Praktika Fizischeskoi Kultury, 7:51-52 (translated by M. Yessis).

Juker, D., McGill, S.M., Kropf, P., and Steffen, T. (1998) Quantitative intramuscular myoelectric activity of lumbar portions of psoas and the abdominal wall during a wide variety of tasks. *Med Sci Sports Exerc*, 30 (2): 301-310.

Kandel, E.R., Schwartz, J.H., Jessell, T.M., Principles of Neural Science, Fourth edition, McGraw-Hill, New York, 2000.

Koes, B.W., Bouter, L.M., Beckerman, H., et al. (1991) Physiotherapy exercises and back pain: A blinded review. *Br Med J*, 302: 1572-1576.

Krag, M.H., Seroussi, R.E., Wilder, D.G., and Pope M.H. (1987) Internal displacement distribution from in vitro loading of human thoracic and lumbar spinal motion segments: experimental results and theoretical predictions. *Spine*, 12 (10): 1001.

Leino, P., Aro, S., and Hasan, J. (1987) Trunk muscle function and low back disorders, *J. Chron. Dis.*, 40: 289-296.

Luoto, S., Heliovaara, M., Hurri, H., et al. (1995) Static back endurance and the risk of low back pain. *Clin Biomech*, 10: 323-324.

Manniche, C., Hesselsoe, G., Bentzen, L., et al. (1988) Clinical trial of intensive muscle training for chronic low back pain. *Lancet*, 24: 1473-1476.

Magnusseon, S.P., Aagard P., Simonsen, E., Bojen-Moller, F., (1998) A biomechanical evaluation of cyclic and static stretch in human skeletal muscle, Int. J. Sports Med., 19(5):310-316.

Marras, W.S., Lavender, S.A., Leurgans, S.E., et al, (1993) The role of dynamic three dimensional trunk motion in occupationally related low back disorders: The effects of workplace factors, trunk position and trunk motion characteristics on the risk of injury. Spine, 18:617-628.

Matveyev, L., (1981) Fundamentals of sports training, Progress Publ. Moscow (English).

Mayer, T.G., Gatchel, R.J., Kishino, N., et al. (1985) Objective assessment of spine function following industrial injury: A prospective study with comparison group and one-year follow up. *Spine*, 10: 482-493.

McGill, S.M. (1995) The mechanics of torso flexion: Situps and standing dynamic flexion manoeuvres. *Clin Biomech*, 10 (4): 184-192.

McGill, S.M., and Brown, S. (1992) Creep response of the lumbar spine to prolonged full flexion. *Clin. Biomech.*, 7: 43-46.

McGill, S.M. (1997). Invited Paper: Biomechanics of Low Back Injury: Implications on current practice and the clinic. J. Biomech. 30(5): 465-475.

McGill, S.M., Grenier, S., Bluhm, M., Preuss, R., and Brown, S., Russell, C., (2003) Previous history of LBP with work loss is related to lingering affects in biomechanical, physiological, personal, and psychosocial characteristics. Ergonomics, 46(7):731-746.

McGill, S.M., and Norman, R.W. (1992) Low back biomechanics in industry—The prevention of injury. In: Grabiner, M.D. (Ed.), *Current issues of biomechanics*. Champaign, IL: Human Kinetics.

McGill, S.M., and Axler, C.T. (1996). Changes in spine height throughout 32 hours of bedrest: Implications for bedrest and space travel on the low back, Arch. Phys.Med.Rehab. 38(9): 925-927.

McGill, S.M., Sharratt, M.T., and Seguin, J.P. (1995) Loads on spinal tissues during simultaneous lifting and ventilatory challenge. *Ergonomics,* 38: 1772-1792.

Nutter, P. (1988) Aerobic exercise in the treatment and prevention of low back pain. *Occup Med*, 3: 137-145.

Pavlov, I., (1927) Conditioned reflexes, Oxford University Press, London.

Piscopo, J. and Baley, J. A., (1981) Kinesiology – the science of movement. John Wiley and sons, New York.

Roman, R., (1986) Trenirovka Tyazheloatleta (Training of the weightlifter), Fizultura I Sport Moscow.

Ross, C.E., Hayes, D. (1988) Exercise and psychologic well-being in the community. *Am. J. Epidemiol.* 127: 762-771.

Saal, J.A., and Saal, J.S. (1989) Nonoperative treatment of herniated lumbar intervertebral disc with radiculopathy: An outcome study. *Spine*, 14: 431-437.

Scannell, J.P., and McGill, S.M. (2003) Lumbar posture – should, and can, it be modified? A study of passive tissue stiffness and lumbar position in activities of daily living. Phys. Ther., 83(10): 907-917.

Siff, M., (2002) Supertraining, Sixth Edition, Supertraining Institute, Denver.

Snook, S.H., Webster, B.S., McGarry, R.W., Fogleman, M.T., and McCann, K.B. (1998) The reduction of chronic nonspecific low back pain through the control of early morning lumbar flexion: A randomized controlled trial. *Spine,* 23 (23): 2601-2607.

Solomonow, M., Zhou, B-H., Bratta, R.V., Burger, E, (2003) Biomechanics and electromyography of a cumulative lumbar disorder: response to static stretching, Clinical Biomechanics, 18:890-898.

Suni, J.H., Oja, P., Miilunpalo, S.I., Pasanen, M.E., Vuori, I.M., Bos, K., (1998) Health related fitness test battery for adults: association with perceived health, mobility and back function and symptoms, Arch. Phys. Med. Rehab. 79(5):559-569.

Suni, J., Rinne, M., Natri, A., Pasanen Statistisian, M., Parkkari, J., Alaranta, H., (2006) Control of the lumbar neutral zone decreases low back pain and improves self-evaluated work ability: A 12 month randomized controlled study. Spine, 31(18):E611-E620.

Sutarno, C., and McGill, S.M. (1995). Iso-velocity investigation of the lengthening behaviour of the erector spinae muscles. *Eur. J. Appl. Physiol. Occup. Physiol.,* 70 (2): 146-153.

Taub, E., Motor behavior following deafferentation in the developing and motorically mature monkey, In: Herman, S., Grillner, R., Ralston, H.J., et al eds, Neural control of locomotion, New York, Plenum Press, 1976, 675-705

Tropp, H., Ekstrand, J., Gillquist, J., (1984) Stabilometry in functional instability of the ankle and its value in predicting injury, Med. Sci. Sports and Exerc. 16:64-66.

Wilson, G.J., Newton, R., Murphy, A., Humphries, B., (1993) The optimal training load for the development of dynamic athletic performance, Med. Sci. Sports. Exerc. 25(1):1279-1286.

Yessis, M., (1987) Secrets of Soviet Sports Fitness and Training, Arbor House.

Young, R.J. (1979) The effect of regular exercise on cognitive functioning and personality. *Br. J. Sports Med.* 13

Zatsiorsky, V., (1995) Science and Practice of Strength Training, Human Kinetics, Champaign.

Chapter 3

Helpful facts: Anatomy, Injury Mechanisms and Effective Training

Low Back Disorders contains a detailed summary of clinically relevant anatomy, biomechanical features, and description of injury mechanisms. To be an expert, consider this essential reading. There is no need to repeat this detail here, rather, a listing of facts that will enable better program design will be introduced.

Sadly, many people injure their backs when the cause could have been avoided. Had they known the structure of their back and how it works, they could have consciously adopted a safer strategy and avoided the trauma. For example, what is a fractured end-plate? What is spondylolisthesis? What causes a herniated disc and how can it be prevented? The answers to these types of questions are found with an understanding of functional anatomy. Further, training regimens intended to meet specific objectives may be inappropriately applied and performed without an understanding of the architecture of musculoskeletal system. The Russian system recognized the value in an educated athlete regarding anatomy and function of their body. They realized the added potential for athletes who are able to image their own architecture when working to optimize muscle usage and movement in general. This section is helpful to build their "biomechanical" education to assist in making decisions needed for training the back for ultimate performance. The elite will delve further into *Low Back Disorders*.

Some anatomically based facts

Basic neural structure - activating back muscles:

The true strongmen I have encountered are very wise in understanding the process of activating muscles and groups of muscles. They are masters at using imagery to control the motor unit recruitment process. Here are the basics of what you need to know about neural integration for the back. Much better resources are available for more complete understanding (eg. Kandel, Schwartz, and Jessell, 1982). Motion may occur from a conscious thought in the brain which instigates muscle activation, or the activation may result from a more subconscious process involving an encoded pattern thought to reside in the spinal cord. Traumatic events can re-code these patterns to perturbed states as can chronic and acute pain. Re-coding these perturbed patterns back to normal is an issue addressed in *Low Back Disorders*.

Neural integration processes can be sub-categorized into two systems for study purposes only – training practices must consider the whole. There is the afferent side which sends signals to the muscles, while the efferent side involves sensors that reside in the muscles, ligaments and joints and produces signals that travel from the muscle to processing centres either in the cord or higher in the brain. Typically, reflexive responses are located in the cord while responses requiring more complex integration usually involve the brain.

The afferent system functional unit is the motor unit, comprising of a motor neuron and its associated muscle fibres. The number of muscle fibres in a motor unit (innervation ratio) is commensurate with its function. For example, ocular muscles (eye movement) may have only a few fibres controlled by a single neuron while larger muscles in the legs and back may have a few thousand fibres. A motor unit may be either a slow twitch unit or a form of fast twitch units (there are several categories for fast twitch units). Human muscles are made of a combination of fast and slow twitch units. Back muscles, on a relative scale with other muscles in the body, tend to be predominantly slow twitch. However, the ratio of fast to slow twitch, while largely pre-determined at birth, can be altered with specific training. This process is known as fibre plasticity. For example, there are many Olympic weight lifters who avoid aerobic activity such as even walking up a flight of stairs for fear of stimulating some adaptation of fast fibres into slower ones. While fast fibres utilize a glycolytic metabolism for rapid deployment, they rapidly fatigue. Slow fibres operate on an aerobic metabolism and are more fatigue resistant, but produce maximal twitch force more slowly and at a lower magnitude than their fast counterparts. Most functional tasks including sporting activity require both types of motor units. However, there are extreme event requirements at either end of the fibre type demand continuum – for example a weight lifter (fast twitch) versus a marathon swimmer (slow twitch).

The type of training activity influences the functional transformation of one fibre type into another. For example, inactivity results in a higher ratio of fast to slow twitch fibres – slow twitch fibres transform to use a glycolytic metabolism. Those with chronic low back pain lose their endurance capability as they have a higher proportion of fast twitch fibers than normal (Mannion et al, 1997). This is yet another reason why chronic back pain patients/athletes require an endurance approach to exercise prescription to establish more normal muscle metabolism and function. In another study by Mannion's group (Mannion et al, 1998) they suggested that back extensor strength was more a function of muscle fibre size and not a function of the fast/slow twitch ratio. This is almost correct. Think of the twitch response – the area under the force time curve is the impulse (see figure 3.1). While the fast twitch fibres reach their peak force sooner, they also extinguish their force sooner. In contrast the slow twitch fibre takes longer to reach the peak force but retains the tension longer. Even though the peak force is lower, the longer duration of the twitch results in an impulse that is almost equivalent to that of fast twitch fibres. Since the force that the whole muscle produces is a sum of all impulses, a sustained muscle force will not be overly affected by the fibre type ratio. On the other hand, if a fast ballistic force is optimal, then higher fast twitch ratios are beneficial. Incidentally, women tend to be predominantly more slow twitch than their male counterparts.

Grading force within a muscle is accomplished by organizing the recruitment of motor units and increasing the firing rate of those already recruited. Knowledge of this process has been propelled recently by technical advances to measure individual motor unit behaviour at higher levels of overall muscle activity. For example, while firing rate was thought for years to saturate at a rate of about 60Hz, Professor Deluca's team at Boston University has been able to document that firing rate continues beyond 60 Hz when higher levels of force are required – saturation does not occur. Furthermore, motor unit recruitment was thought for years to follow an orderly recruitment order. Specifically, the smallest, slow twitch units are recruited first as muscles begin to contract with the larger units progressively becoming recruited at higher levels of force (following the Henneman size principle). If this were true, designing training regimens would be much simpler. But it is not true. Many variables affect the motor unit recruitment order and firing rate. These include the rate at which muscle force develops, whether a muscle is increasing or decreasing force, and subtle direction changes in joint load, to name just a few. Dynamic motion greatly activates more motor units when compared to a static contraction of similar force level.

Machines cannot create the many variations of force development within a muscle to stimulate all motor units. In the torso, for example, the oblique muscles have many neuromuscular compartments that must be stimulated with demand. This is why ultimate strength training cannot be constrained with the slow and isolationist approaches typical of body building. Speed training is essential for functional strength as is a rich environment providing variable motion, balance and force projection direction challenges involving the full-linkage.

The efferent system utilizes sensors in the tissues as feedback to tune the control system. For example, signals of tendon force (golgi tendon organs), muscle length (muscle spindles), and many passive tissue organs that sense force, position, and pressure provide the motor control system with feedback on things like joint position and stress. They are essential for performance and for injury avoidance. They are also modulated by phenomena such as vibration. Vibration to tendon causes force registrations that result in position illusions in the motor cortex. Finally, the vestibular system transduces head position, and head linear and rotational acceleration mostly through apparatus located in the inner ear. Vestibular performance is highly trainable if not compromised with disease. The main implication of the efferent system is that if you expect to compete in a specific environment – then train it. If not, it may be silly to artificially create conditions that may de-tune the system such as involving vibration, unnatural joint pressure and odd balance positions such as hanging upside down on a roman chair.

In summary, the type of training regimen together with the sum of all activities that are part of a daily routine determine the fast/slow twitch ratio. While this may be important for short power events, ultimate training for the back and torso neural system extends far beyond the fibre type issue. Endurance can be trained with little compromise of strength. In addition, the way in which motor units are recruited is determined by the features of the task. Full stimulation and training of the motor units cannot be achieved with machines that prescribe motion profiles and that offer support and stability at some joints. An excellent training program recognizes the value of free motion, balance, velocity range, and eccentric and concentric contraction, just to name a few critical variables. Ultimate training results from a careful inventory of the tasks that have neural demand which are then incorporated into the regimen. Finally, many motion/motor patterns are encoded and can become perturbed with pain – addressing the perturbed patterns is an essential component in training the ultimate back.

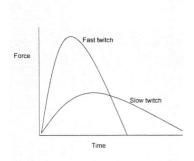

Figure 3.1. Fast twitch fibres reach their peak force sooner than slow twitch, but also extinguish their force sooner. The speed-strength athlete benefits from faster force production. The area under the force-time curve (impulse) tends to be more equivalent between the two. Thus for sustained contractions there is little difference between the force (impulse) contributions of the two fibre types. Endurance time is extended with trained slow twitch fibres.

Are you a master of your motor control domain?

Many tests exist to measure balance, force development, and acceleration in an attempt to master motor patterns. Many athletes visualize muscle contraction without actively contracting. Some evidence documents that performance increases and that the mechanism is through more efficient neural integration. Later in this book, when we begin to develop motor patterns, you will learn techniques to begin to activate muscle together with the fine perception this sometimes requires. If you have access to some quality EMG equipment try the following:

- Attach the electrodes on your cheeks (your face has fine motor control).
- Don't smile, but simply think about smiling. If you are a master you will see the first one or two motor units recruited which will fire at a rate of about 5-6 Hz. Better yet, play the output signal through an audio amplifier into speakers. Hearing the "orchestra" of motor units is a fantastic experience, and a premier way to appreciate fine motor control.

Actually smiling creates an electrical storm that obliterates individual motor units. Practice this recruitment discipline – some professional strongmen do.

The full spine

The spine has twelve thoracic and five lumber vertebrae (see figure 3.2). The natural curves (kyphosis in the thoracic region and lordosis in the lumbar region) are characterized by a range defined by natural variability. What we recently found was that those who tend to be at the hyper-lordotic end of the population spectrum stand in elastic extension while those at the hypo-lordotic end have more elastic stress when they sit (Scannell and McGill, 2003). An exercise intervention was able to reduce some of the standing stresses in the hyper lordotic spines!

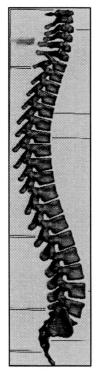 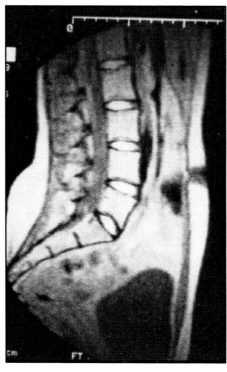

Figure 3.2 The 12 thoracic vertebrae connect to ribs and have less motion than their 5 lumbar counterparts. The thoracic region has a natural kyphotic curve and the lumbar region a natural lordotic curve. Position of the spine is about halfway between the front and the back of the torso (right panel).

The vertebrae

Athletes will be interested in the hydraulic aspects of vertebral/disc behaviour. The discs are avascular and receive nutrition from fluid flow across the vertebral end-plates (the top and bottom of the vertebral bodies). The plates are made of a deformable thin cartilage which is porous for the transport of nutrients such as oxygen and glucose. Under large compressive loads which result when training, fluids from the disc are squeezed out through the end plate. On one hand, this results in a narrower disc space yet when the load is removed, fluid flow restores the height and facilitates nutrient transport. When we measured the increase in spine length following a bout of inversion therapy (hanging upside down to load the spine in tension) the person grew in length. However, normal length and fluid balance was restored within 15 minutes of walking around. Our work with stadiometry (measuring spine length as a function of load exposure) suggests that the same time course of about 15 mintues is correct (McGill et al, 1996). Even relatively short rests have dramatic affects on spine mechanics.

The vertebral bodies have a shell of cortical bone which is filled with cancellous bone, which, for the most part, is hollow space with the struts of bone (called trabeculae) forming a lattice. The lattice becomes thin, with some struts even disappearing in conditions of inactivity, or in degenerative states such as osteoporosis. However, the trabeculae harvested from specimens who performed heavy work (in particular, weightlifters) is thick and dense. The transverse trabeculae appear to be crucial in determining compressive strength. The "wedge fracture" seen in the weight and power lifters is characterized with extensive trabecular damage. If the damage continues, the cortical shell finally fractures, causing the vertebrae to appear "wedge shaped".

Vertebral end-plate fractures:

Under compressive loading, our work has shown the end-plate to be the first tissue to injure. It fractures, or cracks. When compressing spines in the lab, we hear an audible "pop" at the instant of end-plate fracture—exactly what patients/athletes report when they describe details of the event that resulted in their pain. Surprisingly this may, or may not, be painful! Understandably, those with end-plate fractures will not tolerate compressive loading.

Posterior elements of the vertebrae and neural arch fracture:

The posterior elements of the vertebrae (pedicles, laminae, spinous processes and facet joints) can fracture under excessive one-time loading and when exposed to repeated bending. Spondylolisthesis (an anterior slipping of one vertebrae on another) results from fracture and is endemic among female gymnasts and cricket bowlers to name a few (see figure 3.3). Athletes with spondylolisthesis generally do not do well with therapeutic exercise that takes the spine through the range of motion, rather, control of the neutral zone is required followed by spine stabilization training.

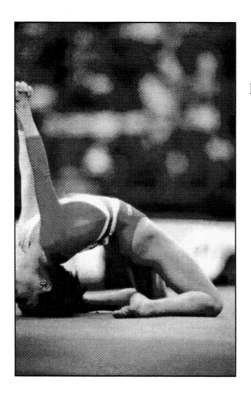

Figure 3.3 Repeated stress-strain reversals in the posterior elements of the vertebrae, such as what occurs during gymnastics moves, will eventually cause fatigue fracture—leading to spondylolisthesis. Interestingly, Michael Adams has measured deflections of the pars to 6 degrees in young women performing these tasks while the pars in the mature female only deflects about 1 degree. Coaching technique can increase or decrease this risk.

Optimizing health of the intervertebral disc

Disc health depends on many variables. Choosing your parents happens to be important but that is not your choice. All one can do is optimize the variables under their control. It is noteworthy that disc damage is most often accompanied by subdiscal bone damage (Gunning et al., 2001) so avoiding bone damage is important. In fact, Keller and colleagues (1993) noted the interdependence of bone status and disc health. Recent evidence also suggests that excessive compression can lead to altered cell metabolism within the nucleus and increased rates of cell death (apoptosis) (Lotz and Chin, 2000). Thus, the evidence suggests that compressive loading involving lower compressive loads stimulates healthy bone (noted as a correlate of disc health), but that excessive loading leads to tissue breakdown. The envelope of healthy loading moves up with training. Progressive training is the key to avoiding disc damage.

Avoiding disc herniation:

The science on disc herniation shows that:

1. Repeated flexion-bending of the spine is necessary to cause herniation (Adams and Hutton, 1982). In fact, herniation of the disc seems impossible without full flexion. This has implications for exercise prescription particularly for flexion stretching and sit-ups, or for activities such as prolonged sitting, all of which are characterized by a flexed spine. Some resistance exercise machines that take the spine to full flexion repeatedly must be reconsidered for those interested in sparing the posterior annulus portions of their discs. (While some appear to be helped by this approach, it is very problematic for others) (See figure 3.4)

2. Thousands of cycles of flexion are needed (Gordon et al., 1991; King, 1993; Callaghan and McGill, 2001) to herniate a healthy disc.

3. Prolonged sitting exacerbates the risk (Videman et al., 1990; Wilder et al, 1988).

4. Herniations tend to occur in younger spines (Adams and Hutton, 1985), because of the higher water content (Adams and Muir, 1976) and more hydraulic characteristics. Older spines do not appear to exhibit classic extrusion of nuclear material, but rather are characterized by delamination of the annulus layer and radial cracks that appear to progress with repeated loading (a nice review is provided by Goel et al., 1995).

5. The location of the herniation is a function of the dominant direction of loading. Our most recent work on disc herniation uncovered the dependency of the location of the herniating bulge on the axis of motion (Aultman et al, 2005). For example, flexing forward with some lateral bend to the right will most likely result in a bulge, posterior lateral to the left in the disc. This is powerful knowledge for exercise intervention since further motion about this axis would exacerbate the herniation. Look for a dominant motion pattern in a patient/athletes daily routine consistent with the bulge location, and eliminate it. If the causative motion pattern is part of the athletic event then major decisions will need to be made. More motion will only ensure the inevitable – can the technique be changed?

6. While we have not performed a lot of research on the effect of twisting on the discs, it appears that repeated twisting causes the annulus to slowly delaminate. This is evidenced by the tracking of the nucleus into the annulus in all directions. While we do not know the relationship between number of cycles and loads yet, we do know that added torsion to the twisting motion, reduces the compressive strength of the joint

(Aultman et al, 2004). For these reasons we do not recommend the spine twisting exercise machines.

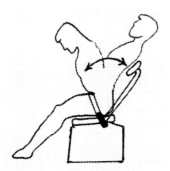

Figure 3.4 Some exercise devices are based on the approach to isolate lumbar motion. This creates stress concentrations in the lumbar discs. Replicating the range of motion (from neutral to full flexion), together with the compressive loads measured in some of these devices is one of the better ways we have found to produce disc herniation in the lab. On the other hand, it is possible that adjusting the range of motion (neutral into extension) may reduce some bulges (Scannell and McGill, 2009). This only appears to have potential for discs that have not lost more the 30% of their height.

Muscles

Training a system of muscles needs thought given to their activation control, endurance, strength, and inherent biomechanical advantages/disadvantages due to their architecture. Achieving optimal rehabilitation and optimal performance must embrace the trainable variables and architectural features – a few are briefly listed here.

Muscles of athletes vary greatly from the general population. Many are "gifted" in terms of muscle architectural variables that provide mechanical advantage, or speed, for example. An example is the transverse scan of the erector spinae from a seven-foot tall pro basketball player showing the enormous lumbar longissimus and iliocostalis muscles (and a relatively small multifidus) (See figure 3.5).

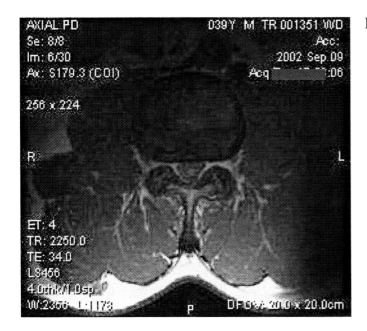

Figure 3.5 The enormous lumbar longissimus and iliocostalis muscles (and a relatively smaller multifidus) are shown in a seven-foot tall elite professional basketball player – he is suited for exceptional lumbar extensor torque development together with anterior shear support.

The proprioceptive function of the small Rotatores and Intertransversarii

These muscles are tiny and do not serve a major "force-development" function but are mentioned here for their importance in motor control (see figure 3.6). We now have data that indicates the rotatores and intertransversarii function as length transducers, and thereby position sensors, sensing the positioning of each spinal motion unit. These structures are likely affected during stretching and during various types of manual therapy with the joint at end range of motion (a posture used in chiropractic technique, for example).

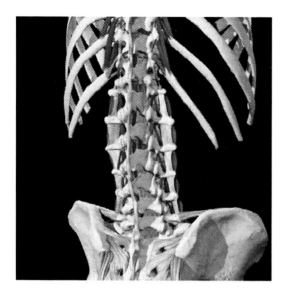

Figure 3.6 Short muscles of the spine claimed by anatomy texts to "rotate" the spine. Their small size and moment makes this impossible. Image courtesy of Primal Pictures, 2002.

The back extensors have several important roles - Longissimus, Iliocostalis, and Multifidus Groups:

Most anatomy books address the extensors in three groups although athletes are probably better served considering the thoracic group as one group and the lumbar portions as another group. The lumbar and thoracic portions are architecturally (Bogduk, 1980) and functionally different (McGill and Norman, 1987). First, in terms of fiber type, the thoracic sections contain approximately 75% slow-twitch fibers while lumbar sections are generally evenly mixed (Sirca and Kostevc, 1985). The thoracic components of longissimus and iliocostalis follow a line of action parallel to the compressive axis of the spine and just underneath the skin. This provides the greatest amount of extensor moment with a minimum of compressive penalty to the spine (see figure. 3.7). This means that these muscles extend the entire thoracic and lumbar spine. A wise lifter uses them – they would never isolate the lumbar muscles. The great ones have visible bulk in the extensors of the thoracic area (see figure 3.8).

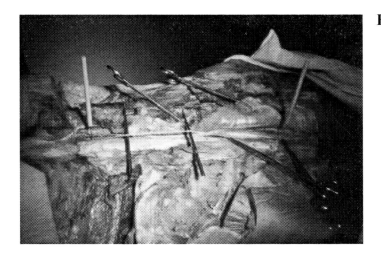

Figure 3.7 Longissimus thoracis pars thoracis (inserting on the ribs at T6) with its tendons lifted by probes course over the full lumbar spine to its sacral origins. They have a very large extensor moment arm (just underneath the skin) to provide the maximum mechanical advantage.

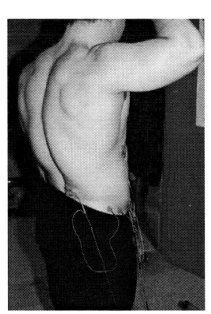

Figure 3.8 This world-class power lifter exemplifies the hypertrophied bulk of the iliocostalis and longissimus muscles seen in trained lifters. While this muscle bulk is in the thoracic region, it creates extensor torque over the entire thoracic and lumbar spine.

The lumbar components of these muscles (iliocostalis lumborum pars lumborum and longissimus thoracis pars lumborum) are very different from the thoracic portions and are special in their anatomy and function. Their line of action is not parallel to the compressive axis of the spine, but rather has a posterior shear component (see figure 3.9). These posterior shear forces support any anterior reaction shear forces of the upper vertebrae produced as the upper body is flexed forward in a typical lifting posture. This is critical for injury avoidance. This important line of action is modulated by posture. These muscles lose their shearing line of action and become more aligned to the compressive axis of the spine with lumbar flexion (McGill et al., 2000). In this way, lifters with a flexed spine are unable to resist damaging shear forces (see figure 3.10, a and b).

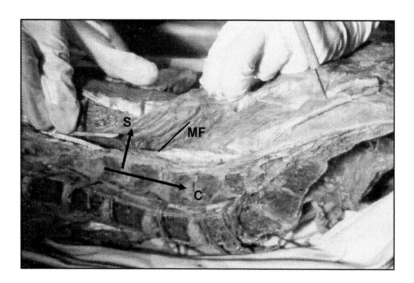

Figure 3.9 Iliocostalis lumborum pars lumborum and longissimus thoracis pars lumborum originate over the posterior surface of the sacrum, follow a line of action under the skin (muscle force (MF)) and then turn obliquely toward their vertebral attachments. This force pathway supports anterior shear (S) forces and extensor moments on each successive superior vertebrae. The compressive axis (C) is indicated.

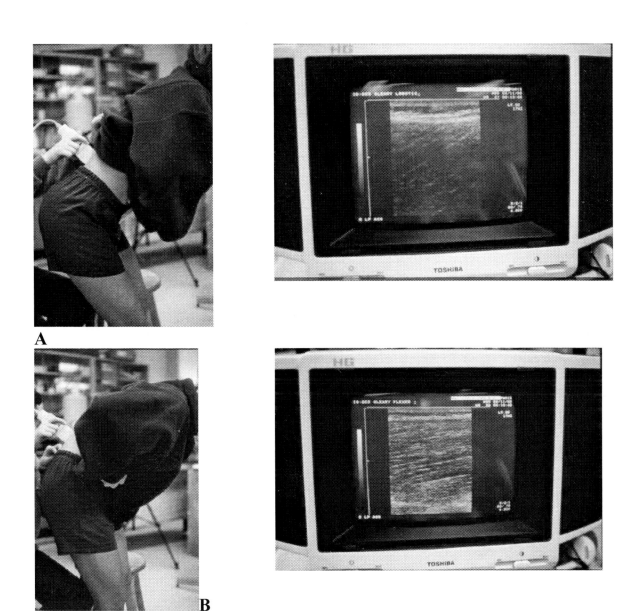

Figure 3.10 Posture determines the ability of the iliocostalis lumborum and longissimus thoracis to protect the spine against large anterior shear forces. When the spine is neutral the oblique angle of these muscles as viewed with an ultrasound imager is about 45 degrees (a). This means that about 70% of the force helps to support shear. When the spine is flexed this angle is reduced to about 10 degrees so that anterior shear forces cannot be supported (b). Thus the load bearing ability of the spine in shear is dependant upon posture – for many athletes a neutral spine is essential. Reprinted with permission *Clinical. Biomechanics,* McGill, S.M., Hughson, R.L., and Parks, K., 15 (1): 777-780, 2000.

The multifidus muscles span two or three segments (see figure 3.11) and perform a different function from those of the longissimus and iliocostalis groups. These shorter muscles tend to run parallel to the compressive axis. The multifidus muscles are involved in producing extensor torque (together with very small amounts of twisting and side-bending torque), but only provide the ability for corrections, or moment support, at specific joints that may be the foci of stresses. Being short, they have a different force-stiffness profile than their longer, more lateral, extensors which will come into play in the stability discussions. Interestingly, many people discuss multifidus when they actually mean the full erector spinae group. Further, we have not seen evidence for the ability of people to activate just multifidus. All muscles of the extensor group appear to activate together. Some therapy groups advocate trying to activate multifidus – in essence activating the extensors from medial to lateral in order. We do not think that this is possible. It is wiser to think about training the extensors up and down the spine (lumbar and thoracic), rather than from medial to lateral – or multifidus, then longissimus and iliocostalis. As will be shown in the third section of this book, this is how some of the strongest backs train.

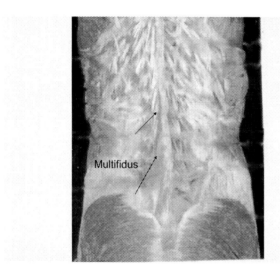 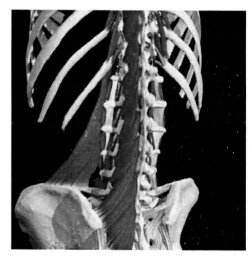

Figure 3.11 Multifidus is a relatively small lumbar extensor with shorter fibres that can span 1 to 3 vertebral segments. Its line of action does not support anterior shear of the superior vertebrae but actually contributes to it. Right panel courtesy of Primal Pictures.

Latissimus Dorsi is a critical performance muscle

Latissimus dorsi is a critical muscle for spine extension and enhancing overall strength via the "superstiffness" concept. It also assists in functioning as part of the "natural" back belt (see figure 3.12). When looking to enhance performance, this is one of the target muscles.

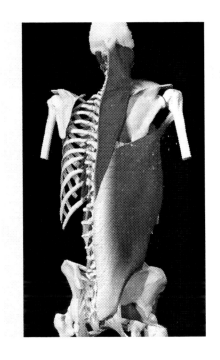

Figure 3.12 Latissimus dorsi originates from each lumbar spinous process via the lumbodorsal fascia and inserts on the humerus to perform both lumbar extension and stabilization roles. It is a key muscle for strength enhancing "superstiffness". It also helps in building the torso "corset". Image courtesy of Primal Pictures.

Abdominal muscles

The abdominal wall functions in most performance activities as a short-range stiff spring. This has major implications on training. It has both active muscle and important fascial components (see figure 3.13). The involved muscles function to: enhance torso stiffness to eliminate energy leaks for efficient transfer of hip generated power; efficiently store and recover elastic energy when the muscles are properly "tuned"; and generate moments about the three axes of torso motion.

Abdominal Fascia

The abdominal fascia surrounds the rectus abdominis and carries hoop stresses from one side of the torso around to the other. This fascial complex acts as an energy storage and recovery system used by athletes such as baseball pitchers in generating a whip-like action through the linkage to produce tremendous ball velocity.

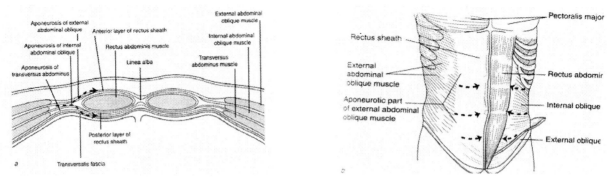

Figure 3.13 The abdominal fascia connects the obliques of the abdominal wall and surrounds the rectus abdominis to help to transmit hoop stresses around the abdomen. Adapted with permission from S. McGill, Low Back Disorders, 2002, Human Kinetics

Rectus Abdominis

The rectus abdominis is partitioned into sections with lateral tendons, rather than being a single long muscle. Rectus, by virtue of its beaded architecture, is not made to create force over a range in length – yet it is currently popular to perform curl-ups over a gym ball for example. This incorporates a potent injury mechanism for flexion intolerant or flexion provoked backs. For many athletes, training strength and power in the torso does not require the rectus to be challenged throughout the flexion/extension range of motion – but integration of the rectus with the other abdominal muscles is paramount. Instead train short-range stiffness to optimize the energy storage and recovery potential, particularly in throwers, punchers, kickers, and explosive athletes.

Some individuals believe in training the upper and lower rectus abdominis with separate exercises. This is usually not necessary as a distinct upper and lower rectus does not exist in most people (although some individuals may have the ability to preferentially activate one section slightly differently from the other in select activities). For example, we have measured the ability to activate upper and lower rectus separately in Middle-eastern belly dancers (Moreside et al, in press). However, this was only during very low levels of activation.

Abdominal Wall: Obliques and Transverse Abdominis

The three layers of the abdominal wall (external oblique, internal oblique and transverse abdominis) perform several functions. As a group they work together to flex, laterally bend and twist the torso. They are supremely important in spine stabilization given their criss-crossing architecture which cross-brace the lumbar spine. Much emphasis has been directed towards the transverse abdominis in training. Specifically, some think that it is an important spine stabilizer – but those who have quantified its stabilizing potential relative to other muscles have not found that it is particularly more important than any other abdominal muscle. Some have advocated abdominal hollowing to involve the transverse abdominis. The act of "hollowing" (drawing in the abdominal wall) should never be conducted for athletic performance – this is inhibiting to muscles necessary for performance (see figure 3.14). Evidence presented later in the stability chapter suggests that there is no justification for any special effort directed towards training transverse abdominis over any other muscle. In fact, our clinical experience suggests that efforts to isolate transverse is problematic - there is more important total muscle abdominal training that really matters for the athlete. As all three layers of the abdominal wall activate and stiffen together, a "superstiffness" is achieved – this enhances performance (Brown and McGill, 2009). Not surprisingly, many strength athletes who brace the abdominal wall consider every training exercise an abdominal exercise. They view abdominal stiffening as an essential aspect of their training.

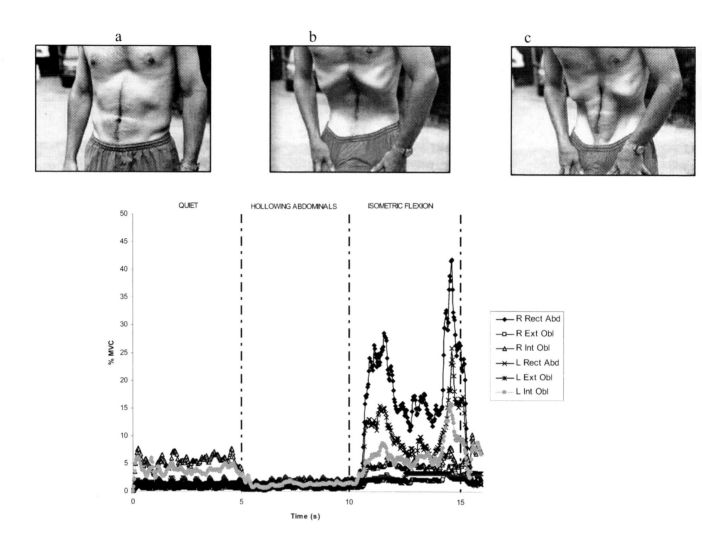

Figure 3.14 Some trained people have the ability to differentially activate specific portions of the abdominal musculature. This sequence shows an inactive abdominal wall and contraction of transverse abdominis(a), which draws and "hollows" the wall (b), and a flexor moment in which placing the hands on the thighs and pushing with good muscular control causes activation of just the rectus abdominis with the previously activated transverse and little oblique activity (c). The time history is shown (bottom panel). Note how "hollowing" can only occur as the abdominal muscles of rectus, and the obliques fall silent. This is not good for athletic performance.

Finally, the obliques are regionally activated, with several neuromuscular compartments. This means that several exercise techniques are required to fully challenge all components of the abdominal wall.

Psoas

The psoas, first and foremost, is a hip flexor. We know this from measuring its activation profile during all sorts of activities (see Juker et al., 1998a and b). However, upon activation it imposes substantial lumbar spine compression since it attaches to each lumbar vertebrae (see figure 3.15). Sprinters, and others who need to train hip flexion power know the risk due to the substantial spine compression penalty that is imposed on the spine when the psoas is activated. Use the guidelines later in this book to avoid injury while training effectively.

Psoas is also a stabilizer – think of it as a sock of concrete holding the lumbar column on the pelvis from each side. When the muscle is inactive (the concrete is wet) it plays little role but upon activation the muscle stiffens (the concrete sets) and buttresses the spine. Hip stiffening techniques described later add lumbar stability.

Referring to the iliacus-psoas group as iliopsoas is problematic and prevents the development of better training methods. For example, many stretch the "iliopsoas" with lunge movements and an upright torso. Unfortunately, the stretch performed in this way is only on the iliacus. Palpating the psoas tendon reveals more psoas tension from hip extension coupled with spine lateral bending. This means that different technique is needed to target these two different muscles – think of psoas and iliacus, not iliopsoas!

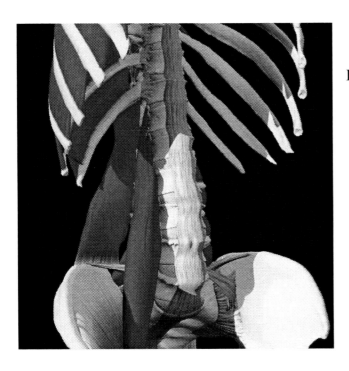

Figure 3.15 The psoas flexes the hip but also buttresses the spine to the pelvis. The quadratus lumborum attaches each transverse process with the ribs and iliac crest forming the guy wire support system. This is how hip stiffness can assist with spine stiffness. Courtesy of Primal Pictures, 2002.

Quadratus Lumborum

The quadratus lumborum (QL) is designed to be a stabilizer. In appearance, it looks like a guy wire system attaching every lumbar vertebrae to the rib cage and pelvis (see figure 3.15). The myoelectric evidence is more convincing in that the muscle is active in virtually every loading mode including flexion-dominant, extensor-dominant, and lateral bending tasks. It is even active when the individual stands upright and compresses the spine (McGill, Juker, and Kropf, 1996).

It is interesting that people with a paralyzed Quadratus cannot walk. The "strongmen" who compete in events such as the farmers' carry must bear compressive loads while walking. Interestingly, the QL is the muscle that most often gives them concern. During single leg stance of the gait cycle, the load up the support leg must traverse the pelvis and carry on up the spine. The pelvis must be lifted on the ipsilateral side to accomplish this – a task given to quadratus lumborum (McGill et al, 2009). This observation provides evidence for its role and also motivation to train this muscle to enhance this important athletic ability. It is an essential muscle to enable stepping and a critical component for athletic performance – it needs more attention in many training programs.

Ligaments

Spine ligaments check the end-range motion of the spine together with playing a significant proprioceptive role. Anatomical detail, together with histological features can be found in my "*Low Back Disorders*" book. Perhaps the most important feature relevant to exercise is the finding of a loss of the extensor muscle reflex with prolonged stretching of the spine ligaments together with aberrant muscle spasming (see Solomonow et al, 2000). Many athletes will need to rethink their current static stretching approaches.

The pelvis, hips, and related musculature are important considerations for the back

A healthy back depends on proper function in the pelvis and hips for several reasons. Power is usually generated at the hips and not the low back in most athletes.

Further, the pelvis acts as the platform for the spine. Psoas and iliacus have already been described for their role in hip flexion and stabilization. Gluteus maximus is primarily a hip extensor and external rotator while gluteus medius (and gluteus minimus) is primarily an abductor and thus tremendously important for any activity that requires single leg stance, or gait, with directional change. They assist the spine musculature (such as quadratus lumborum and the obliques) to help hold the pelvis up during single leg support and thus are key players in spine stability during gait. They also externally rotate the femur which is a functional feature we will use to full advantage in the design of squat exercises in section three of this book. There are other gluteal muscles known as the "deep six" (piriformis, obturator internus and externus, gemellus superior and inferior, and quadratus femoris) which together assist in controlling internal and external rotation.

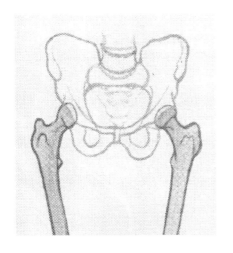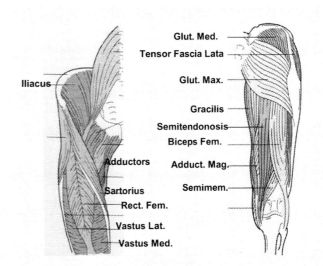

Figure 3.16 View of the pelvis and hips (left panel) with anterior muscles (middle panel) and posterior muscles (right panel). Together they function to stablilize and create hip power.

The hamstring group (biceps femoris, semitendinosus, semimembranosus) extend the thigh, flex the knee and perform stabilizing roles over each of these joints. In many situations their most important role is in "braking" with eccentric contraction. The medial thigh muscles adduct the thigh. The quadriceps extend the knee and provide a patellar tendon tracking function. One member of the "quads", rectus femoris, crosses the hip joint anteriorly to create hip flexion.

Many muscles cross the hip joint. Collectively, they are able to create significant power, and can direct force powerfully in many directions. In many cases, they are the major power source for athletic performance. Specifically they create and direct force while changing length at rapid speed. Many of them cross both the hip and knee joint indicating that functional training must involve tasks that challenge both joints moving independently and at different velocities. Further, this training must incorporate lateral motion, and rotational motion in the transverse plane.

The great ones train the hips

No single exercise can train all hip muscles although there are some particularly good ones. For example, the one legged squat is particularly functional since quadriceps are active for knee extension and patella control, hamstrings for knee stability and hip extension, the gluteals for hip extension and hip abduction and the adductors and gluteal deep six for hip stabilization. Another clinical issue is the peril in training hip flexion power as many sprinters know because of their resultant symptomatic backs. Hip flexion power (high flexion torque and velocity) is problematic since the psoas forces load the spine in compression and iliacus forces impose large flexion bending torques on the pelvis, which are transmitted to the spine. Wise athletes always build extensive spine stability prior to progressions into building hip power.

Finally

In this chapter, I have assumed that you have a rudimentary anatomical/biomechanical knowledge. I urge you to enhance your knowledge in this area. The challenge for athletes, superior coaches and sports clinicians alike is to become conversant with the functional implications of the anatomy, and use this information to develop the most appropriate training programs blending performance within the safest environment.

References

Adams M.A., and Hutton W.C. (1985) Gradual disc prolapse. *Spine,* 10: 524.

Adams M.A., and Hutton W.C. (1982) Prolapsed intervertebral disc: A hyperflexion injury. *Spine,* 7: 184.

Adams P., and Muir H. (1976) Qualitative changes with age of proteoglycans of human lumbar discs. *Ann Rheum Dis,* 35: 289.

Aultman, C.D., Scannell, J., and McGill, S.M. (2005) Predicting the direction of nucleus tracking in bovine spine motion segments subjected to repetitive flexion and simultaneous lateral bend, Clin. Biomech. 20:126-129.

Aultman, C.D., Drake, J., Callaghan, J.P. McGill, S.M. (2004) The effect of static torsion on the compression strength of the spine: An invitro analysis using a porcine spine model. SPINE 29(15):E304-309.

Bogduk, N. (1980) A reappraisal of the anatomy of the human lumbar erector spinae. *J Anat,* 131 (3): 525.

Brown, S., McGill, S.M. (2009) Transmission of muscularly generated force and stiffness between layers of the rat abdominal wall. SPINE, 34(2): E70-E75.

Callaghan, J.P., and McGill, S.M. (2001) Intervertebral disc herniation: Studies on a porcine model exposed to highly repetitive flexion/extension motion with compressive force. *Clin. Biom.,* 16 (1): 28-37.

Moreside, J.M., Vera-Garcia, F.J., McGill, S.M. Middle-eastern style dance motions give insight into neuromuscular independence and synchronizations of the abdominal wall. (in press).

Goel, V.K., Monroe, B.T., Gilbertson, L.G., and Brinckmann, P. (1995) Interlaminar shear stresses and laminae-separation in a disc: Finite element analysis of the L3-L4 motion segment subjected to axial compressive loads. *Spine,* 20 (6): 689.

Gordon, S.J. et al. (1991) Mechanism of disc rupture—A preliminary report. *Spine,* 16: 450.

Gunning, J.L., Callaghan, J.P., and McGill, S.M. (2001) The role of prior loading history and spinal posture on the compressive tolerance and type of failure in the spine using a porcine trauma model. *Clin. Biomech.,* 16 (6): 471-480.

Juker, D., McGill, S.M., and Kropf, P. (1998a) Quantitative intramuscular myoelectric activity of lumbar portions of psoas and the abdominal wall during cycling. *J. Appl. Biomech.,* 14 (4): 428-438.

Juker, D., McGill, S.M., Kropf, P., and Steffen, T. (1998b). Quantitative intramuscular myoelectric activity of lumbar portions of psoas and the abdominal wall during a wide variety of tasks. *Med. Sci. Sports Ex.,* 30 (2): 301-310.

Kandel, E.R., Schwartz, J.H., Jessell, T.M., (2000) Principles of neural science, 4th edition, McGraw-Hill, New York.

Keller, T.S., Ziv, I., Moeljanto, E., and Spengler, D.M. (1993) Interdependence of lumbar disc and subdiscal bone properties: A report of the normal and degenerated spine. *J. Spinal Dis.,* 6 (2): 106-113.

King, A.I. (1993) Injury to the thoraco-lumbar spine and pelvis. In: Nahum and Melvin (Eds.), *Accidental injury, Biomechanics and Prevention.* New York: Springer.

Lotz, J.C., and Chin, J.R. (2000) Intervertebral disc cell death is dependent on the magnitude and duration of spinal loading. *Spine,* 25 (12): 1477-1483.

Mannion, A.F., Weber, B.R., Dvorak, J., Grob, D., Muntener, M., (1997) Fibre type characteristics of the lumbar paraspinal muscles in normal healthy subjects and in patients with low back pain, J. Bone Jt. Surg., 15:881-887.

Mannion, A.F., Dumas, G.A., Stevenson, J.M., Cooper, R.G., (1998) The influence of muscle fibre size and type distribution on electromyographic measures of back muscle fatigability, Spine, 23 (5):576-584.

McGill, S.M., van Wijk, M., Axler, C.T., and Gletsu, M. (1996). Spinal shrinkage: Is it useful for evaluation of low back loads in the workplace. Ergonomics, 39(1): 92-102.

McGill, S.M., Juker, D., and Kropf., P. (1996). Quantitative intramuscular myoelectric activity of quadratus lumborum during a wide variety of tasks. *Clin. Biomech,* 11 (3): 170-172.

McGill, S.M., Hughson, R.L., and Parks, K. (2000) Changes in lumbar lordosis modify the role of the extensor muscles. *Clin. Biomech.,* 15 (1): 777-780.

McGill, S.M., and Norman, R.W. (1987) Effects of an anatomically detailed erector spinae model on L4/L5 disc compression and shear. *J Biomech,* 20 (6): 591.

McGill, S.M., (2002) Low back disorders: Evidence based prevention and rehabilitation, Human Kinetics Publishers, Champaign, Illinois.

McGill, S.M., McDermott, A., Fenwick, C. (in press 2009) Comparison of different strongman events: Trunk muscle activation and lumbar spine motion, load and stiffness, Journal of Strength and Conditioning Research.

Scannell, J.P., and McGill, S.M. (2003) Lumbar posture – should, and can, it be modified? A study of passive tissue stiffness and lumbar position in activities of daily living. Phys. Ther., 83(10): 907-917.

Scannell, J.P., McGill, S.M. (2009) Disc prolapse: Evidence of reversal with repeated extension. SPINE, 34(4): 344-350.

Sirca, A., and Kostevc, V. (1985) The fibre type composition of thoracic and lumbar paravertebral muscles in man. *J Anat,* 141: 131.

Solomonow, M., Zhou, B., Harris, M., Lu, Y., and Baratta, R.V. (2000) The ligamento-muscular stabilizing system of the spine. *Spine,* 23: 2552-2562.

Solomonow, M., Zhou, B.H., Baratta, R.V., Burger, E. (2003) Biomechanics and electromyography lumber disorder:response to static flexion. *Clinical Biomechanics,* 18:890-898

Videman, T., Nurminen, M., and Troup, J.D.G. (1990) Lumbar spinal pathology in cadaveric material in relation to history of back pain, occupation and physical loading. *Spine,* 15 (8): 728.

Wilder, D.G., Pope, M.H., and Frymoyer J.W. (1988) The biomechanics of lumbar disc herniation and the effect of overload and instability. *J Spine Disorders,* 1 (1): 16.

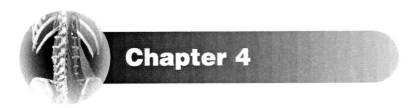

Chapter 4

Normal Back Function and Changes Following Injury

Once again, the detailed story of how the back works, together with extensive references, is in my textbook *Low Back Disorders*. Ultimate training for the back results from approaches that avoid injury mechanisms and address specific deficits in a systematic and progressive method. A brief outline about back function will assist in helping you design optimal programs. Also to assist you, a brief introduction to the changes that follow injury is provided.

How you stand is important: The concepts of tolerance and capacity were introduced in the first chapter of this book. Too many individuals with "back" issues waste precious capacity with poor standing posture. Commonly they may have a slightly flexed spinal posture, the chin "poking" forward, shoulders dropped and slouched. Strong men and women do not stand this way. It causes chronic contraction of the spine extensors, sapping strength, using capacity and reducing tolerance. Corrective standing exercises are found in section three.

Lumbo-Pelvic rhythm, bending, performance, and injury risk: Bending over typically involves both hip and spine flexion. Changes in muscle length were shown in McGill, (1991). It is interesting that nearly all muscles of the spine hardly change length compared to their counterparts in the limbs. As noted in the previous chapter some are not even designed for length change but for locking the torso. They require correspondingly different approaches to training. For example, Olympic weightlifters attempt to move entirely about the hips. They lock the lumbar spine close to the neutral position and rotate almost entirely about the hips. We call this fundamental pattern the "hip hinge". Learning to hip hinge (later in this book) is paramount for both injury avoidance and optimal performance.

Repeated spine flexion—even in the absence of moderate load—will lead to discogenic troubles. "Stretching it out" is not the solution since flexion stretching would only replicate the original injury mechanism. The number of individuals who begin to experience back discomfort training and believe that wearing a back belt will then help is tragic. This detracts focus on the real solution: change the training regimen. I am sent letters from these unfortunate individuals almost weekly.

Additional thoughts on spine bending: A simple experiment can be revealing. A number of years ago, we asked a group of athletes to stand with a barbell on their shoulders. We were measuring spinal micro shrinkage. Then we asked them to role their pelvis' anteriorly and posteriorly to impart some gentle motion to the lumbar region (see figure 4.1). They remained standing upright yet we had to stop the experiment due to the pain reported by the first few subjects. Training spine motion under load requires caution. No specific guidelines exist for determining training loads – however following the algorithmic approach in this book will assist in creating safer and more effective programs.

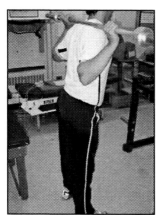 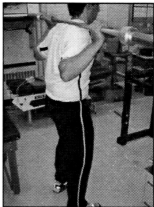

Figure 4.1 Standing with a bar on the shoulders while flexing and extending the lumbar spine is painful and disarming – proof that training the loading spine through a range of motion requires extreme caution.

General muscle activity magnitudes

Having a feel for the activation levels for a variety of torso muscles over a variety of activities is helpful (see Table 4.1 and Figure 4.2). These were obtained with surface and intramuscular EMG.

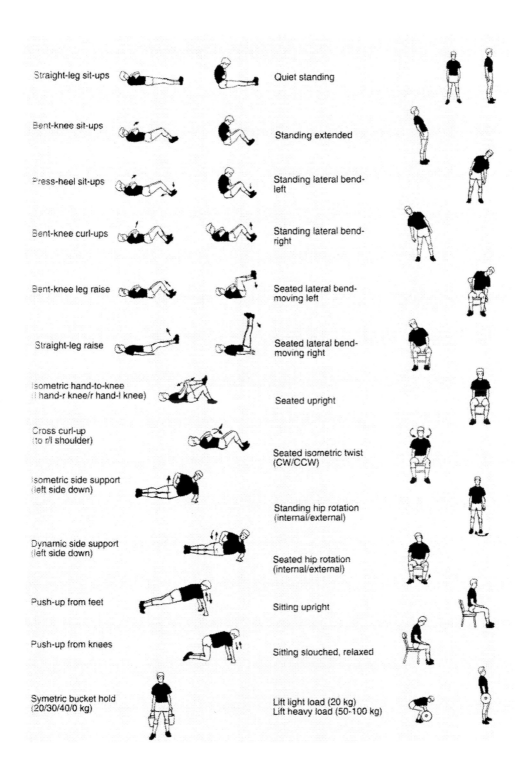

Figure 4.2 Schematic documenting various tasks during which EMG signals were obtained. They are listed in table 4.1. Reprinted with permission, Juker et al, Med. Sci. Sports Exerc. 30 (2): 301-310, 1998.

Table 4.1
Subject averages of EMG activation normalized to 100% MVC – mean and (Standard deviation).
Note: Psoas channels, external oblique, internal oblique and transverse abdominis are intramuscular electrodes while rectus abdominis, rectus femoris, erector spinae are surface electrodes.

Task	Psoas 1	Psoas 2	EOi	IOi	TAi	RAs	RFs	ESs
Straight-leg sit-ups	15(12)	24(7)	44(9)	15(15)	11(9)	48(18)	16(10)	4(3)
Bent-knee sit-ups	17(10)	28(7)	43(12)	16(14)	10(7)	55(16)	14(7)	6(9)
Press-heel sit-ups	28(23)	34(18)	51(14)	22(14)	20(13)	51(20)	15(12)	4(3)
Bent-knee curl-up	7(8)	10(14)	19(14)	14(10)	12(9)	62(22)	8(12)	6(10)
Bent-knee leg raise	24(15)	25(8)	22(7)	8(9)	7(6)	32(20)	8(5)	6(8)
Straight leg raise	35(20)	33(8)	26(9)	9(8)	6(4)	37(24)	23(12)	7(11)
Isom. hand-to-knee L. Hand → R. Knee	16(16)	16(8)	68(14)	30(28)	28(19)	69(18)	8(7)	6(4)
Right Hand → Left Knee	56(28)	58(16)	53(12)	48(23)	44(18)	74(25)	42(29)	5(4)
Cross curl-up Right Shoulder → across	5(3)	4(4)	23(20)	24(14)	20(11)	57(22)	10(19)	5(8)
Left Shoulder → across	5(3)	5(5)	24(17)	21(16)	15(13)	58(24)	12(24)	5(8)
Isom. Side support	21(17)	12(8)	43(13)	36(29)	39(24)	22(13)	11(11)	24(15)
Dyn. side support	26(18)	13(5)	44(16)	42(24)	44(33)	41(20)	9(7)	29(17)
Pushup from feet	24(19)	12(5)	29(12)	10(14)	9(9)	29(10)	10(7)	3(4)
Pushup from knees	14(11)	10(7)	19(10)	7(9)	8(8)	19(11)	5(3)	3(4)
Lift light load	9(10)	3(4)	3(3)	6(7)	6(5)	14(21)	6(5)	37(13)
Lift heavy load	16(18)	5(6)	5(4)	10(11)	10(9)	17(23)	6(5)	62(12)
Symmetric bucket hold 20 kg	2(4)	1(1)	7(4)	5(3)	5(1)	10(7)	3(3)	3(6)
30 kg	3(4)	1(1)	9(5)	6(4)	6(1)	10(8)	3(3)	4(7)

Task	Psoas 1	Psoas 2	EOi	IOi	TAi	RAs	RFs	ESs
40 kg	3(5)	1(1)	10(6)	8(6)	6(2)	10(8)	3(3)	3(2)
0 kg	1(2)	0(1)	2(1)	2(2)	2(1)	10(9)	2(1)	2(1)
Seated Isom. twist CCW	30(20)	17(15)	18(8)	43(25)	49(35)	17(22)	7(4)	14(6)
Seated Isom. twist CW	23(20)	11(8)	52(13)	15(11)	18(19)	13(10)	9(10)	13(8)
Standing hip internal rotation	21(18)	10(9)	18(12)	24(23)	33(20)	13(9)	9(7)	18(6)
Standing hip external rotation	27(20)	22(19)	17(13)	21(19)	31(17)	13(8)	19(11)	17(9)
Sitting hip internal rotation	19(15)	21(18)	36(31)	30(30)	31(29)	18(8)	20(19)	12(8)
Sitting hip external rotation	32(25)	25(20)	11(9)	15(17)	16(13)	15(9)	16(13)	8(8)
Sitting upright	12(7)	7(5)	3(6)	3(3)	4(2)	17(9)	4(2)	5(8)
Sitting slouched/relaxed	4(4)	3(3)	2(5)	2(2)	4(3)	17(11)	3(2)	5(8)
Quiet standing	2(1)	1(1)	3(4)	5(3)	4(2)	5(5)	3(3)	11(11)
Standing extended	3(2)	2(1)	12(9)	6(3)	5(3)	11(5)	4(3)	7(8)
Standing lateral bend Left	9(10)	1(2)	11(8)	18(14)	12(7)	13(7)	3(2)	11(13)
Right	6(5)	1(2)	19(18)	18(14)	25(20)	14(9)	3(1)	8(8)
Seated lateral bend moving left	2(3)	1(1)	21(19)	7(7)	7(11)	13(8)	4(3)	6(7)
Moving right	18(12)	12(2)	15(26)	10(7)	12(7)	17(20)	5(4)	5(8)
Upright	14(9)	8(4)	6(4)	5(3)	5(5)	19(23)	5(3)	6(8)

Note: Reprinted with permission Juker et al 1998 Copyright – Med. Sci. Sports Exerc.

Mechanics of specific activities

Loads on the low back during lifting: Low back tissue loads that develop during lifting result mainly from muscle and ligament tensions required to support the posture, and facilitate movement. This is why lifting technique is so important to reduce the risk of excessive loading. In extreme cases, we have measured compressive loads on the spines of competitive weightlifters that have safely exceeded 20 kN (4480 lb) (Cholewicki et al., 1991). The average tolerance for young men is about 12-15 kN (2688-3360 pounds) (Adams and Dolan, 1995).

While a lifting example is used here to provide a forum for discussion, similar situations for the spine exist in many athletic situations, such as the spine mechanics involved as a football lineman drives an opponent back. The lineman may elect to drive with the hip and a locked spine, or by flexing the spine. This strategy (spine flexion) has quite dramatic effects on shear loading of the intervertebral column and the resultant injury risk. Not only is the spine much stronger and better able to bear compressive load (about 25 to 45% stronger) when in a neutral posture (Gunning et al, 2001), but dangerous shear forces are also minimized (see figure 4.3). Cripton and colleagues (1995) found the shear tolerance of the spine to be in the neighborhood of 2000-2800 N in adult cadavers, for one-time loading. This example also illustrates the need for clinicians/coaches/athletes to consider other loading modes in addition to simple compression. In this example, the real risk is anterior/posterior shear load.

The lumbar/hip motion issue can also be applied to rowing technique for example – those who "over reach" on the catch (full lumbar flexion) have more back troubles than those who do not (or adopt a more neutral spine posture consistent with the squat posture).

The solution is to minimize spine flexion and move about the hips.

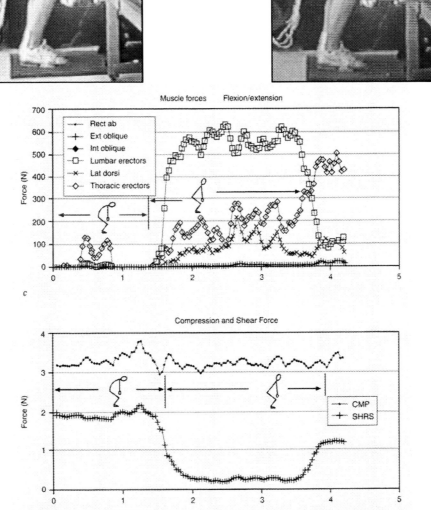

a

b

Muscle forces   Flexion/extension

- ···· Rect ab
- + Ext oblique
- ◆ Int oblique
- □ Lumbar erectors
- × Lat dorsi
- ◇ Thoracic erectors

Force (N)

c

Compression and Shear Force

Force (N)

- ─ CMP
- + SHRS

d

Figure 4.3 The fully flexed spine (a) is associated with myoelectric silence in the back extensors, strained posterior passive tissues and high shearing forces on the lumbar spine (from both reaction shear on the upper body and interspinous ligament strain, see previous chapter). A more neutral spine (b) posture recruits the pars lumborum muscle groups (c) to support the reaction shear and thus reduces total joint shear (d) (to approximately 200 N in this example). Reprinted with permission S.M. McGill, J. Biomech. 30 (5), 1997. Copyright by Elsevier Science.

Consider sitting to be a dynamic task: It is almost comical to hear the jokes about the school teacher deploring their students to sit upright. Our numerous studies on sitting have concluded that any single sitting posture causes static loads on the spinal tissues. This will eventually use capacity. Migrating the loads to different tissues is accomplished with posture change. Callaghan and McGill (2001b) showed that no single, ideal sitting posture exists; rather, they recommend a variable posture to minimize the risk of tissue overload. Having stated this, many troubled backs are flexion intolerant and are exacerbated by slouched sitting and unsupported upright sitting, which will eventually exceed the endurance capacity of the hip flexors and the back extensors (recall the higher Psoas activity when sitting upright from table 4.1). For these individuals, a lumbar support is essential to enhance tolerance and capacity needed for dedicated therapy and training exercise. This also has implications for athletes who sit on the bench between plays – see the chapter on injury prevention. Certainly athletes who resistance train in a seated position would be well advised to question their rationale.

The mechanics and implications of walking: Walking is, for many, wonderful therapy. As an activity it challenges the balance and proprioceptive system, provides gentle motion and imposes very low loading on the spine, when conducted with proper form. The concept of capacity, introduced earlier, can be extremely important. When I have to build capacity in an athlete, I start with correcting standing, walking, and squatting mechanics. Typical faults in walking patterns that use spine capacity are spine flexion, chin poking, no arm swing, and slow small steps. Our data shows that walking results in very tolerable spine loads, and gentle disc motion which they thrive upon. The data also shows how swinging the arms from the shoulders (not the elbows) also reduces spine loading (Callaghan et al., 1999). In fact, we have observed up to 10% reduction in spine loads from arm swinging in some individuals. This may be because swinging the arms facilitates efficient storage and recovery of elastic energy, reducing the need for concentric muscle contraction and the upper body accelerations associated with each step. Generally, to transform walking from an activity that wastes capacity into a training therapy, walk faster, with a more upright posture, while swinging the arms about the shoulders.

Pushing and pulling technique is critical: The way that pushing and pulling is conducted is critical. The magnitude of the hand forces is almost irrelevant until extremely high pushing/pulling forces are required. Specifically, when hand forces are directed through the low back they do not create a moment and in this way muscle forces are not required to support a moment. Poor technique causes the hand forces to be directed away from the spine causing excessive joint load. In other words, "steering" the force was the dominant technique factor. For athletes like rugby players or strongmen competitors pulling a bus, this same technique is used. Here the pushing/pulling force is driven as close through the feet as possible to enhance the foot grip together with ensuring minimal joint torque. These insights into the mechanics of pushing and pulling were obtained from our investigations comparing experienced firefighters with graduate students (Lett and McGill, 2006). The expert firefighters experienced much lower spine forces with higher performance. Technique was the dominant factor!

Loads on the low back during flexion exercises: A few studies have attempted to examine flexion exercises by simply reporting the activation of the abdominal muscles with EMG. This is problematic as the corresponding spine loads remain unknown. Many athletes with bad backs are prescribed back and abdominal exercises that exceed the tolerance of their compromised tissues. In fact, I believe that many commonly practiced flexion exercises result in so much spine compression that they will ensure that the athlete becomes a patient! Many institutions still hang on to the idea that speed situps somehow are a test of fitness – this is producing bad backs. Even the traditional slow-speed sit-up imposes approximately 3300 N (730 lbs) of compression on the spine (Axler and McGill, 1997), a criterion injury level set by some governments! It is a poorly designed exercise for many people. A few traditional abdominal/flexion exercises are quantified in table 4.2.

With this data, some traditional notions need re-examination. First, hanging with the arms from an overhead bar and flexing the hips to raise the legs is often thought to impose low spine loads because the body is hanging in tension—not compression. This is faulty logic. This hanging exercise generates well over 100 Nm of abdominal torque to a spine that is often flexed due to sloppy technique. Similar activation levels can be achieved with the side bridge (shown later and discussed in detail) with lower spine loads. Flexing and twisting is also risky for the discs.

This traditional approach to training of the abdominals will be replaced in section three of his book with regimens to enhance short-range stiffness and strength, both reducing injury risk and enhancing performance.

Table 4.2
Low back moments, abdominal muscle activity, and lumbar compressive load during several types of abdominal exercises.
Note: MVC contractions were isometric. Activation values higher than 100% are often seen during dynamic exercise. Reprinted with permission, Med.Sci.Sports.Ex., Axler and McGill, 29 (6): 804-811, 1997.

		Muscle Activation		
	Moment (Nm)	Rectus Abdominis (% MVC)	External Oblique	Compression (N)
Straight Leg Situp	148	121	70	3506
Bent Leg Situp	154	103	70	3350
Curlup feet Anchored	92	87	45	2009
Curlup Feet Free	81	67	38	1991
Quarter Situp	114	78	42	2392
Straight Leg Raise	102	57	35	2525
Bent Leg Raise	82	35	24	1767
Cross-knee Curlup	112	89	67	2964
Hanging Straight Leg	107	112	90	2805
Hanging Bent Leg	84	78	64	3313
Isometric Side Bridge	72	48	50	2585

Loads on the low back during various "pushup" exercises: Push-ups are another "abdominal exercise" but are interesting as muscles are challenged over a small motion range. Our work in quantifying the spine mechanics during traditional, plyometric, and labile load under the hands forms of the pushup revealed clues for clever exercise design (Freeman et al, 2006). While performing push-ups with the hands on labile surfaces has some effect on spine load, the one-armed and more ballistic forms of the exercise requiring the hands to move are much more spine demanding (see figure 4.4 and table 4.3) Those interested in challenging the abdominal obliques and "steering" the asymmetric force from staggered hand placement through the torso will be interested in the quite modest increase in spine compression demand.

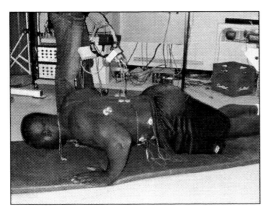

a

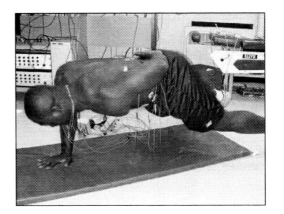

B

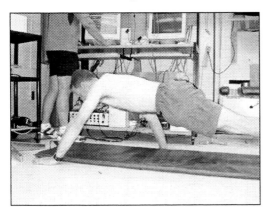

c

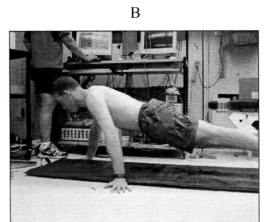

D

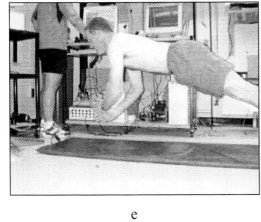

e

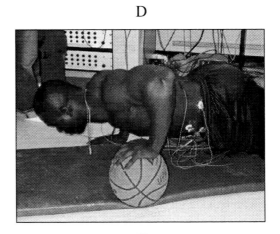

F

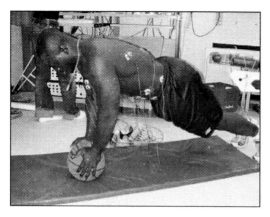
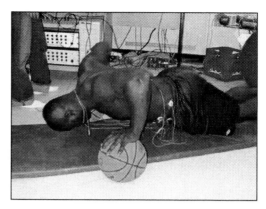

g   H

Figure 4.4 (a-i): The various forms of the push-up studied ranged from a standard push-up (a), a single arm (b), uneven hand placement: left forward(c), uneven hand placement: right forward (d), clapping (e), one hand on ball (f), and both hands on ball (g), and 2 hands on 2 balls (h).

Table 4.3 EMG amplitudes, (mean and standard deviation in % MVC) for muscles on the right side of the body for the styles of pushup shown in figure 4.4.

	RA	EO	IO	LD	ES	Pec	Delt	Tri	Bi
Standard	25 11	23 11	22 13	11 07	05 05	61 38	42 14	66 18	04 02
One arm	52 18	51 13	47 23	21 13	08 06	81 54	70 21	79 18	06 02
Left hand forward	39 16	32 17	29 22	16 09	08 11	58 45	53 22	53 22	09 05
Right hand forward	30 15	20 08	21 14	24 22	06 07	57 33	45 20	66 15	06 03
Clapping	57 27	56 31	56 43	27 14	09 07	89 49	61 20	89 21	31 17
One hand on ball	42 24	23 15	32 27	10 06	05 05	61 52	36 15	52 28	07 03
Both hands on ball	46 34	32 18	34 36	17 13	07 07	69 40	51 22	69 16	07 03
Two hand on two balls	61 31	34 17	45 33	15 13	05 03	81 54	44 17	66 25	08 03

Loads on the low back during extension exercises: There are plenty of EMG-based studies on extension exercises, but only one attempted to quantify the resulting tissue loads (Callaghan and colleagues, 1998). The following data illustrates how it is important to match the correct exercise with the individual (see figure 4.5 and tables 4.4 and 4.5). The common extension task of performing torso extension with the legs braced and the cantilevered upper body extending over the end of a bench or Roman chair activates all four extensor groups and typically imposes over 4000 N (about 1000 lbs) of compression on the spine. Even worse is the commonly prescribed back extension task in clinics, in which the patient lies prone and extends the legs and outstretched arms (superman); this again activates all four extensor sections but imposes up to 6000 N (about 1400 lbs) on a hyper-extended spine. This is not justifiable for any patient and is a poor method for athletes as well! The birddog is a superior stabilization exercise given the stabilizing motor patterns and the neutral spine posture. Additional quantification of more progressive extensor exercises are in the third section of this book.

Table 4.4
    Mean activation levels (+/- 1 SD) of 14 EMG channels, for 13 subjects performing a variety of extensor dominant exercises expressed as a percentage of MVC. Reprinted with permission, *Physical Therapy*, Callaghan, J.P., Gunning, J.L., and McGill, S.M., 78 (1): 8-18, 1998.

EMG Channel	Extension						
	Right Leg	Left Leg	Right Leg and Left Arm	Left Leg and Right Arm	Trunk and Legs	Trunk	Calibration Posture
Right RA							
$\overline{x}$	3.3	2,7	4.0	3.5	4.7	3.1	1.4
SD	2.4	1.9	2.0	2.0	2.2	1.8	1.0
Right EO							
$\overline{x}$	8.4	4.9	16.2	5.2	4.3	3.7	1.0
SD	4.9	1.5	6.0	2.3	2.5	1.7	0.6
Right IO							
$\overline{x}$	12.0	8.2	15.6	12.0	12.1	12.7	1.9
SD	6.8	2.5	8.2	4.2	10.1	10.8	1.2
Right LD							
$\overline{x}$	8.1	5.8	12.0	12.5	11.2	6.5	5.9
SD	5.4	3.5	9.6	6.2	4.3	4.0	8.5
Right TES							
$\overline{x}$	5.7	13.7	11.5	46.8	66.1	45.4	21.0
SD	2.0	7.5	6.6	29.3	18.8	10.6	9.0
Right LES							
$\overline{x}$	19.7	11.7	28.4	19.4	59.2	57.8	21.3
SD	9.1	4.9	10.2	11.0	11.7	8.5	4.6
Right MF							
$\overline{x}$	21.9	10.8	31.5	16.1	51.9	47.5	16.4
SD	6.3	6.0	8.2	12.0	14.7	12.3	5.6
Left RA							
$\overline{x}$	4.3	3.6	4.4	4.2	6.5	3.7	2.2

EMG Channel	Extension						
	Right Leg	Left Leg	Right Leg and Left Arm	Left Leg and Right Arm	Trunk and Legs	Trunk	Calibration Posture
SD	3.4	3.6	3.8	3.9	3.4	2.4	2.1
Left EO							
$\bar{x}$	5.4	9.0	6.2	15.9	6.3	5.2	1.8
SD	2.0	3.8	2.5	6.6	3.2	5.2	1.0
Left IO							
$\bar{x}$	16.0	11.3	22.6	15.2	11.0	12.5	1.6
SD	8.6	7.0	9.2	6.7	5.9	6.1	1.3
Left LD							
$\bar{x}$	4.5	5.0	10.7	6.2	9.2	5.1	6.1
SD	4.3	4.5	18.2	4.4	5.1	4.1	8.5
Left TES							
$\bar{x}$	15.0	4.5	42.9	10.5	63.6	41.6	21.2
SD	7.5	2.0	20.5	5.9	22.7	10.0	9.8
Left LES							
$\bar{x}$	11.3	16.8	19.5	25.5	56.8	57.0	23.3
SD	6.6	4.5	7.4	7.3	14.5	14.7	8.4
Left MF							
$\bar{x}$	11.9	22.3	16.6	33.8	57.3	53.3	18.7
SD	7.0	6.1	7.2	6.7	11.4	12.0	4.3

Electromyographic channel: RA = rectus abdominis muscle, EO = external oblique muscle, IO = internal oblique muscle, LD = latissimus dorsi muscle, TES = thoracic erector spinae muscle, LES = lumbar erector spinae muscle, MF = multifidus muscle. The calibration posture – standing, trunk flexed 60 degrees, neutral lumbar posture, 10 kg held in hands with arms hanging straight down.

Table 4.5

Activation magnitudes of some important muscles during the birddog ("d" in figure 4.5) and the roman chair extensor exercise ("a" in figure 4.5).

Muscle	Birddog	Roman Chair
Lumbar ES	30%	53%
Thoracic ES	47	45
Lat. Dorsi	12	7
Ext. Oblique	16	4

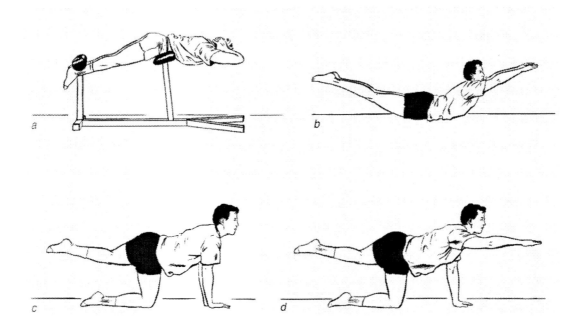

Figure 4.5 Specific extension exercises quantified for muscle activation and the resultant spine load (shown in Table 4.4): (a) trunk extension, (b) prone leg and trunk extension, (c) single-leg extension, (d) single-leg and contralateral arm extension (birddog). Reprinted with permission, McGill, Low Back Disorders, Human Kinetics, 2007.

Pulling patterns for the posterior chain: Objectives for general program design include pull, push, lift and carry exercises. Our recent work (Fenwick et al, in press) quantified the activation patterns of several pulling (or rowing) type challenges (see figure 4.6).

Sled drag and mini bands – Integrating the hips: Focusing on the hips is sometimes desirable as therapeutic exercise. Our recent study (Frost et al, in press) was designed to obtain the activation of gluteus medius and maximus while subjects pulled and dragged three loads together with "monster walks" with mini bands around the ankles of three stiffnesses (see figure 4.7) . We were surprised at the general equivalence of spine load and gluteal activation magnitudes, although the activation patterns were different within the stepping cycle. These are very appropriate exercise tools for the individual looking for more hip work.

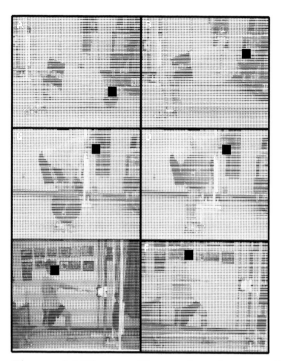
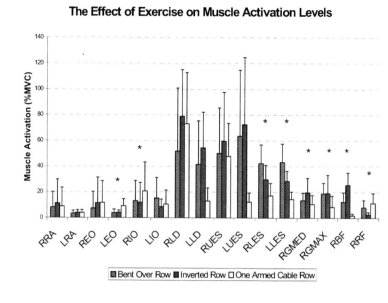

Figure 4.6 These pulling and rowing exercises emphasize the upper back erectors and latissimus dorsi.

On backpack carriage and training: Backpacks come in various designs which affect low back loading. Generally, if rough terrain is anticipated, the load should be placed low in the pack to minimize the moment arm or distance to the low back. As the load is carried over rough ground, it accelerates and decelerates. The load placed closer to the low back reduces the torso forces needed to move the backpack load. On the other hand, if smooth ground is anticipated, carrying the load high in the pack and over the fulcrum of the low back and hips means smaller torso muscle forces are needed – and lower lumbar spine loads result.

Now for the curious situation where backpacks can reduce spine loads. If an individual is flexion intolerant and exacerbated by prolonged sitting, generally they have difficulty standing up. Upon standing, a forward torso angle (antalgic posture) remains. For this type of individual, we prescribe to wear a backpack with about 10kg placed in it and go for a walk over uneven ground. Wearing the backpack acts to generate torso extensor moment, bringing the torso into an upright posture. This alleviates the spine extensors which were previously contracted in the standing, but flexed, posture. Given their larger moment arm, this reduces the compressive load on the spine. The compression reduction from the muscles shutting down is larger than the extra compression from the load in the pack resulting in a net reduction in total compression on the back. Walking over uneven ground provides gentle motion to the lumbar spine which is

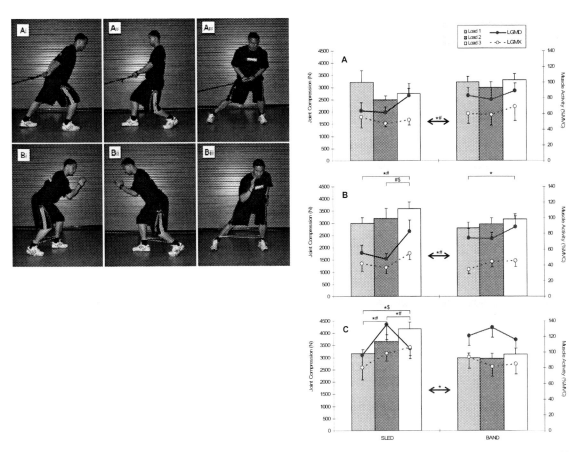

Figure 4.7 Sled dragging and monster walks with mini bands produced surprisingly similar back loads and activation of the gluteus medius and maximus.

therapeutic to the type of discogenic person we are describing here. Typically the patient returns saying, "thanks – that was amazing".

Bottom line: Backpacks are superior to weight vests for those with back troubles. The weight is behind the spine rather than on "top" of it with a vest. Try wearing a backpack with about 10 kg placed low in the backpack, about the level of the lumbar spine, and go for a walk over undulating ground.

Bed rest, back pain, and exercise: The spine needs bed rest. Bed rest reduces the applied (hydrostatic) load below the disc osmotic pressure, resulting in a net inflow of fluid (McGill et al., 1996). This is how the disc receives nutrients. Normally, the fluids are squeezed out over the day resulting in lower disc stresses (mostly over the first hour after rising). McGill and Axler (1996) documented the growth in spine length over the usual eight hours of bed rest and then over continued bed rest for another 32 hours. These unusual sustained pressure cause "swollen discs" and will usually cause backache. It also means that training, and particularly spine bending results in elevated risk when conducted in the first hour after rising from bed. Do not pull knees to chest, perform situps etc.

Other facts that assist performance

Spinal memory: The spine has a biomechanical memory. This is because the tissues deform to prolonged or repeated stresses but take further time to relax when the stress is removed. The current activity of an individual influences the biomechanics of the spine later, meaning that the order of training exercises, rests, and type of exercise matters. Sitting prior to exertion is an example where "spinal memory" can increase injury risk and decrease performance.

Confusion over twisting: Is twisting as troublesome as some state? The problem lies in the back injury literature in that a distinction is not usually made between the kinematic variable of twisting and the kinetic variable of generating twisting torque. Either single variable (the kinematic act of twisting or generating the kinetic variable of twist torque while not twisting) seems less dangerous than epidemiological surveys suggest. However, elevated risk from very high tissue loading may occur when the spine is fully twisted and there is a need to generate high twisting torque (McGill, 1991). In other words generating twisting torque, while twisting away from neutral, appears to be problematic. Now consider the torso twisting machines found in various fitness and training facilities. While there are always individuals who are able to tolerate specific modes of loading, here is a machine that will lead to troubles in many athletes. Even some of the best discus throwers, (a torsional task), cannot train with these types of exercises without exacerbating their back troubles. Athletes must be qualified for twisting, and twisting torque, training.

What about back belts: The average person must be confused when they observe both Olympic lifters and back-injured people wearing back belts. Several years ago, I conducted a review of the documented effects of belt wearing in occupational settings (an up-to-date review is in *Low Back Disorders*) since scientific investigations of athletic use were scarce. I summarized my findings as follows:

- Those who have never had a previous back injury appear to have no

additional protective benefit from wearing a belt.
- Those who are injured while wearing a belt seem to risk a more severe injury.
- Belts appear to give people the perception they can lift more and may in fact enable them to lift more.
- Belts appear to increase intra-abdominal pressure and blood pressure.
- Belts appear to change the lifting styles of some people to either decrease the loads on the spine or increase the loads on the spine.
- But, for athletes there is no question that belts add stiffness, elastic recoil and assist to lift more.

In summary, given the assets and liabilities of belt wearing, I do not recommend them for healthy individuals in routine work or exercise participation. However, the temporary prescription of belts may help some individual workers return to work. The exception to this recommendation is for extreme athletic lifting. Here, belts are not used to enhance health but instead to lift more weight.

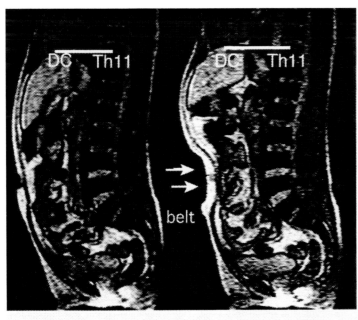

without-belt   with-belt

Figure 4.8 A lifter with a cinched belt shows how the visceral contents are compressed and the liver elevated in this MRI image. Courtesy of my friend Dr. Kei Miyamoto, Gifu University Medical School.

Guidelines for serious lifting athletes: There is no question that belts assist in generating a few more Newton-meters (or foot-pounds) of torque in the torso through elastic recoil of a bent torso. However, if a neutral spine is preserved throughout the lift this effect is minimal. In other words, to obtain the maximal effect from a belt, the lifter must lift poorly and in a way that exposes the back to a much higher risk of injury! There is no question that belts assist in generating torso stiffness to reduce the risk of spine buckling in extreme heavy lifts. Many athletes working at this edge of the envelope will receive this assist. However, other techniques are employed to maximize the torso stiffness – the lungs are filled to almost the top of tidal volume and the breath is then held. In some tasks, an athlete will only "sip" the air, never allowing much air to leave the lungs that would reduce torso stiffness. Belts also increase intra-abdominal pressure (see figure 4.9) which increases the CNS fluid pressure in the spine and in turn, the brain. This appears to decrease the transmural gradient (the pressure difference between the arterial blood pressure in the brain vessels and the brain itself) which in turn may reduce the risk of aneurysm, or stroke. But now for counter considerations: evidence suggests that people change their motor patterns, together with their motion patterns when using a belt. The evidence suggests that these motor control changes can elevate the risk of injury should a belt not be worn in a belt-training athlete. The severity of a back injury may be greater if a belt is worn.

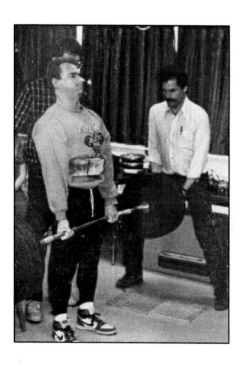

Figure 4.9 This world class lifter produced intra-abdominal pressure exceeding 340mmHg for the duration of the lift (over 500 pounds). Many elite lifters state that they perceive the belt assisting to stiffen their spine to prevent buckling.

Many adopt belts in training for one of three reasons:

- They have observed others wearing them and have assumed that it will be a good idea for them to do so.
- Their backs are becoming sore and they believe that a back belt will help.
- They want to lift a few more pounds.

None of these reasons are consistent with either the literature or the objective of good health. If one must lift a few more pounds, wear a belt. If one wants to groove motor patterns to train for other athletic tasks that demand a stable torso, it is probably better not to wear one.

Nature's back belt - the abdominal hoop and the Lumbodorsal Fascia: We all have a back belt, if we care to develop it! Anatomical/biomechanical study, together with examination of the activation of the latissimus dorsi and the deep abdominal obliques confirm the presence of the abdominal hoop. Specifically, it consists of the LDF posteriorly, the abdominal fascia anteriorly, and the active abdominal muscles laterally (see figure 4.10). As noted earlier, this also appears to be an important elastic energy storage-recovery device for ballistic athletes, tuned by activation and stiffness in the obliques. More on tuning the obliques later. We recommend that athletes develop their "natural" belt.

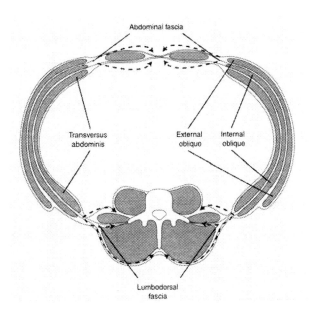

Figure 4.10 The abdominal fascia anteriorly, and the LDF posteriorly, are passive parts of the abdominal hoop. The lateral active musculature (transverse abdominis and internal oblique) serves to tension the hoop. Courtesy of S. McGill, Low Back Disorders, Human Kinetics, 2007.

Pain

Pain: Pain is often attributed to the back muscles. While the pain may be "felt" in the muscles, they act in sympathy as the pain is more often due to underlying pathology.

Predominant pain generating mechanisms in athletes: Given our work over the years, our opinion is that pain is due to overuse of the weak link – in this case, poor technique makes the back the weak link. For example, poor bending technique causes repeated bending of a disc, or region of discs. They become pain generators. True cases of painful muscles are almost always due to poor training technique and/or poor rest and recovery approaches. The approach is to remove the cause of the pain. This involves changing the mechanical load exposure of the painful tissues in every activity of life, including postural components as well as specific training efforts. To build the superior back, address the cause and optimize the treatment.

Sciatic symptoms: Sciatica can be caused by tension of the sciatic nerve, the lumbar nerve roots or within the cauda equina. It also can be caused by pinching at numerous locations along its length or by being irritated by rough surfaces such as arthritic bone or extruded disc material. The symptoms range from radiating pain to sensations in the leg or foot. Back pain may or may not be present. Tragically, cases of foot pain, ankle pain or leg pain caused by lumbar nerve compromise are often stretched for therapy. This just keeps the nerve sensitized and angry. We take two approaches: First, spine sparing motions are adopted to avoid end-range of motion and associated nerve tension, and reduce possible disc bulging. The second approach involves nerve flossing (see *Low Back Disorders* for more on nerve flossing).

Sacroiliac pain: Is it from the joint? Bogduk and colleagues (1996) proved that some low back pain is from the sacroiliac joint itself. However, we have noted the large extensor muscles that attach over the sacroiliac region and assessed the enormous loads resulting in a high risk of sustaining microfailure, resulting in pain at the attachment site (McGill, 1987). Such loads would lift a small car off the ground! Consider the tonnage that some athletes lift everyday in training - the potential for cumulative trauma is significant. This mechanical explanation may account for local tenderness on palpation associated with the many "SI" syndrome cases. The treatment approach is to remove the cause – reduce the loading on these muscle attachment sites with changes in technique and training approach. On the other hand, to assess true Sacro-iliac joint pain, compress the iliac crests while they perform a painful movement. This is done be placing a hand on each iliac crest and squeezing together to stabilize the SI joints while the athlete rises from a chair, walks, or squats etc. If this reduces pain then the temporary use of a sacral belt may be considered.

Staying within the "biomechanical envelope": Optimal health of the spine comes from an optimum of loading – not too much and not too little. For example, earlier it was shown that too much bed rest actually puts the spine into an over stressed state.

Ultimate training for the back results from exposure to the appropriate overload. An athlete cannot avoid injury mechanisms, but understanding the injury pathways facilitates training that minimizes the risk. Every single one is addressed with technique and program design. Consider the following:

- Reducing peak (and cumulative) spine compressive loads to reduce the risk of end-plate fracture.
- Reducing repeated spine motion to full flexion to lower the risk of disc herniation (reducing spine flexion in the morning helps alleviate symptoms).
- Reducing repeated full-range flexion to full-range extension to reduce the risk of pars (or neural arch) fracture.
- Keeping within tolerable levels, peak and cumulative shear forces to reduce the risk of facet and neural arch damage.
- Keeping within tolerable levels, slips and falls to reduce the risk of passive collagenous tissues such as ligaments.
- Keeping within tolerable levels, the length of time sitting when training and resting, particularly exposure to seated vibration, to reduce the risk of disc herniation or accelerated degeneration.
- Reducing cyclic twisting motions, when under compressive load, to reduce the risk of annulus layer delamination.

Biomechanical, Physiological and Motor Changes Following Injury

While the foundation for good clinical practice requires an understanding of the mechanism for injury, an understanding of the lingering consequences is also helpful. Unfortunately, too many athletes only become interested in their backs following injury.

Pain and central sensitization: An interesting point for athletes is that pain can be both a blessing and a curse. Working through pain (assuming muscular pain) is a training necessity, but pain from tissue damage is another story. It is well established that one does not get used to pain from tissue damage, rather the process of central sensitization ensures the person becomes even more sensitive to the pain. In other words, for this type of pain, the nervous system actually gets better at sensing pain. And pain inhibits normal motor patterns, which is disastrous for performance. The approach to break this type of pain cycle is to accommodate pain free motion - "winding down" the nervous system. This helps to justify the five stage approach detailed in the third section of this book.

Motor control changes

It is conclusive that patients reporting debilitating low back pain suffer simultaneous changes in their motor control systems. Recognizing these changes is important since they affect performance. Again, these are well documented in *Low Back Disorders*.

Among the wide variety of motor changes researchers have documented, many clinicians have paid particular attention to the transverse abdominis and multifidus muscles. Interestingly, others have found much larger disturbances in other important muscles that are involved in spine mechanics (eg Cholewicki et al, 2002). Further evidence shows changes include muscle fatigue rates, fibre type specific changes, together with muscle activation patterns in walking and a host of other activities. Our opinion is that there is stronger evidence for perturbed patterns in muscles other than transverse abdominis following pain that are more important for performance. They are discussed here.

The crossed-pelvis syndrome and gluteal amnesia: Dr. Vladamir Janda proposed the crossed-pelvis syndrome where those with a history of chronic low back troubles displayed characteristic patterns of what he referred to as "weak" and "tight" muscles. Specifically, he described the features of the crossed-pelvis syndrome as including a weak gluteal and abdominal wall complex with tight hamstrings and hip flexors, and developed a technique to "correct" this aberrant pattern. While I have difficulty in integrating the terms of "weak" and "tight" from a scientific point of view, Janda's general insights were generally true. From measuring groups of men with chronic back troubles during squatting types of tasks, it is clear they try and accomplish this basic motion/motor pattern of hip extension emphasizing the back extensors and the hamstrings – they appear to have forgotten how to use the gluteal complex. Noticeable restrictions in the hip flexors may or may not be present but without question the gluteals are not recruited to levels that are necessary to both spare the back and to foster better performance. I refer to this as *gluteal amnesia.*

It is common for athletes to arrive at our research clinic with chronic back troubles with a crossed pelvis overlay. Traditional strength approaches to rehabilitating their backs usually fail. This is because strength squat patterns were attempted on aberrant motor patterns – namely the gluteal complex was not able to contribute its share to hip extension, loading up the back as the erector spinae crushed the spine. Sparing the back during hip extensor training demands healthy integration of the gluteal muscles. Specific training to re-program gluteal integration is described and demonstrated in the third section of this book.

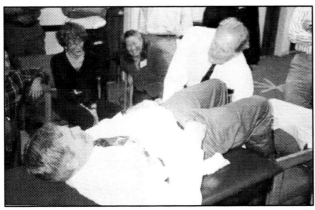

Figure 4.11 I worked in several clinical workshops with Dr Janda prior to his death. He taught me many clinical wisdoms which we were able to evaluate and quantify.

Other lingering deficits following back injury: In a recent study (McGill et al, 2003), we extensively tested 72 workers. Of those workers, 26 had a history of back troubles resulting in lost time, 24 had some back troubles not severe enough to ever lose worktime and the rest had never had any back complaints. All were asymptomatic and back to work at the time of testing. The litany of differences between groups is explained elsewhere but included several motor control deficits. This seminal study for us collectively justifies the training regimens described in section three of this book. It is critical to address basic motion and motor patterns first, before serious back training begins in earnest. This is the way to establish the foundation for ultimate performance, and to do it in a way that breaks chronicity in those with history of back troubles.

This chapter has briefly introduced some notions about function and dysfunction. In fact, effective training cannot occur without an understanding of how the spine works and how it becomes injured. The Russians for many years have understood the importance of education when training top athletes. Match your physical training efforts with equal effort toward knowledge gain.

References

Adams, M., and Dolan, P. (1995) Recent advances in lumbar spinal mechanics and their clinical significance. *Clin Biomech,* 10 (1): 3.

Axler, C., and McGill, S.M. (1997). Low back loads over a variety of abdominal exercises: Searching for the safest abdominal challenge. *Med.Sci.Sports.Ex.,* 29 (6): 804-811.

Bogduk, N., Derby, R., Aprill, C., Lous, S., and Schwartzer, R. (1996) Precision diagnosis in spinal pain. In: Campbell, J. (Ed.). *Pain 1996—An updated view* (pp. 313-323) Seattle: IASP Press.

Callaghan, J.P., Gunning, J.L., and McGill, S.M. (1998) Relationship between lumbar spine load and muscle activity during extensor exercises. *Physical Therapy,* 78 (1): 8-18.

Callaghan, J.P., and McGill, S.M. (2001) Low back joint loading and kinematics during standing and unsupported sitting. *Ergonomics,* 44 (4): 373-381.

Callaghan, J.P., Patla, A.E., and McGill, S.M. (1999) Low back three-dimensional joint forces, kinematics and kinetics during walking. *Clin. Biomech.,* 14: 203-216.

Cholewicki, J., McGill, S.M., and Norman, R.W. (1991) Lumbar spine loads during lifting extremely heavy weights. *Med. Sci. Sports Exerc.,* 23 (10): 1179-1186.

Cholewicki, J., Greene, H.S., Polzhofer, G.R., Galloway, M.T., Shah, R.A., Radebold, A., (2002) Neuromuscular function in athletes following recovery from a recent acute low back injury. J. Orthop. Sports Phys. Ther. 32(11):568-575.

Cripton, P., Berlemen, U., Visarino, H., Begeman, P.C., Nolte, L.P., and Prasad, P. (1995) Response of the lumbar spine due to shear loading. In: *Injury prevention through biomechanics* (p. 111). Detroit: Wayne State University.

Freeman, S., Karpowicz, A., Gray, J.,McGill, S., (2006), Quantifying muscle patterns during various forms of the push-up: Implications for spine loading and stability, Medicine and Science in Sports and Exercise, 38(3): 570-577.

Frost, D., Fenwick, C, McGill, S.M., (in press) Hip and back mechanics during sled drag and mini band exercises.

Gunning, J.L., Callaghan, J.P., and McGill, S.M. (2001) The role of prior loading history and spinal posture on the compressive tolerance and type of failure in the spine using a porcine trauma model. *Clin. Biomech.,* 16 (6): 471-480.

Juker, D., McGill, S.M., Kropf, P., and Steffen, T. (1998) Quantitative intramuscular myoelectric activity of lumbar portions of psoas and the abdominal wall during a wide variety of tasks. *Med. Sci. Sports Ex.,* 30 (2): 301-310.

Lett, K. and McGill, S.M. (2006) Pushing and pulling: Personal mechanics influence spine loads, ERGONOMICS. 49(9): 895-908.

McGill, S.M. (1987). A biomechanical perspective of sacro-iliac pain. *Clinical Biomechanics,* 2 (3): 145-151.

McGill, S.M. (1991). The kinetic potential of the lumbar trunk musculature about three orthogonal orthopaedic axes in extreme postures. *Spine,* 16 (7): 809-815.

McGill, S.M. (1997) Invited paper: Biomechanics of low back injury: Implications on current practice and the clinic. *J. Biomech.,* 30 (5): 465-475.

McGill, S.M., and Axler, C.T. (1996) Changes in spine height throughout 32 hours of bedrest: Implications for bedrest and space travel on the low back. *Arch. Phys.Med.Rehab.,* 38 (9): 925-927.

McGill, S.M., van Wijk, M., Axler, C.T., and Gletsu, M. (1996). Spinal shrinkage: Is it useful for evaluation of low back loads in the workplace. Ergonomics, 39(1): 92-102.

McGill, S.M., (2007) Low Back Disorders: Evidence based prevention and rehabilitation, Second Edition, Human Kinetics, Champaign, Illinois.

McGill, S.M., Grenier, S., Bluhm, M., Preuss, R., Brown, S., and Russell, C. (2003) Previous history of LBP with work loss is related to lingering effects in biomechanical physiological, personal, and psychosocial characteristics. Ergonomics, 46(7): 731-746.

Fenwick, C.M.J., Brown, S.H.M., McGill, S.M. (in press 2009) Comparison of different rowing exercises: Trunk muscle activation, and lumbar spine motion, load and stiffness. Journal of Strength and Conditioning Research.

McGill, S.M., Karpowicz, A., Fenwick, C. (in press 2009) Ballistic abdominal exercises: Muscle activation patterns during a punch, baseball throw, and a torso stiffening manoeuvre. J. <u>Strength and Cond. Research.</u>

McGill, S.M., Karpowicz, A., Fenwick, C. (in press 2009) Exercises for the torso performed in a standing posture: Motion and motor patterns. <u>J. Strength and Conditioning Res.</u>

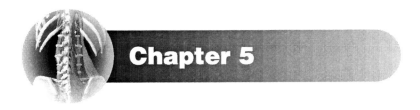

Chapter 5

Enhancing Lumbar Spine Stability

We have been studying and attempting to quantify spine stability for over 20 years. This process involves complex engineering analysis of biological systems – not conjecture about observations of the EMG records of a few muscles, or from readings from devices that people push on. Once again, a more detailed and referenced overview can be found in the book *Low Back Disorders*, together with a few of our original papers found at the end of this chapter. Here is a very brief synopsis relevant for back fitness: In our opinion, too many people confuse whole body stability with joint and spine stability to the point that they poorly train any sort of stability. No doubt you have heard about the great importance of muscles such as transverse abdominis and multifidus for stabilizing the back. No study that has measured stability has warranted that these muscles receive special attention. No doubt you have heard about some very specific exercises to train them. For the most part, many of the exercises are ill-founded to enhance stability. In fact, athletes must do so much more to maintain sufficient spine stability and minimize the risk of injury.

Findings about spine stability can be summarized as follows:

- All muscles are important. They are arranged to work and enhance the action of each other.
- Muscles that are farther away from the spine (have a larger moment arm) create more stability than an identical muscle acting closer to the spine.
- Longer muscles enhance stiffness over larger regions of the spine and their efficiency is enhanced by the activity of the shorter muscles.
- Shorter muscles create stiffness with less length change but this "stability efficiency" is compromised by these muscles typically being small, and closer to the spine.
- Muscles create both force and stiffness: Force may or may not be stabilizing.

Stiffness is always stabilizing.

- The symmetry of muscle stiffnesses and forces all around the spine is critical. No single muscle must exert too much force or too little – its activation level must be in "balance" with all the others.
- Endurance and motor control are needed to maintain stability; rarely is strength needed.
- Training a single muscle in many cases may actually compromise stability.
- The amount of muscle co-contraction is important at any instant in time, particularly in the moment antagonists.
- The geometry of the muscular guy wires is important - specifically, the width of the base of support together with their angle of pull. A "neutral" spine is required together with a broad abdominal base. DO NOT suck in or "hollow in" the abdominal wall. This causes the spine to buckle at lower loads.
- Activation of all three muscular layers of the abdominal wall together results in a "superstiffness".
- Activation of all three layers of the abdominal wall, called "abdominal bracing", also causes the lumbar extensors to activate, which buttresses those with painful shear instability.
- Stability of the spinal column is enhanced with the "guy wire" effect and compression imposed from muscle contraction. Muscles that run parallel to the compressive axis of the spine impart stabilizing compression.
- Muscles that have their fiber orientation parallel with the impending joint instability are important. For example, buttressing lumbar vertebra anterior shear instability is best buttressed with the lumbar fibers of longissimus and iliocostalis due to their line of action.
- A stabilization exercise is any activity that grooves motor patterns that ensure stability, and do so in a way that does not produce excessive loading of the spine.
- Instances of instability are more likely to occur during very high loading of the spine when a minor motor control error is all that is required to compromise the very small margin of safely, and during instances of very low loading since only a few muscles are assisting with stiffness enhancement.

A few crucial issues to enhance fitness and stability training

A Classic – viewing instability and injury: A number of years ago in a classic paper, we reported filming the spine of a powerlifter's spine buckling (Cholewicki and McGill, 1992). We used video fluoroscopy (which is real time dynamic x-ray video) to obtain a sagittal view of the lumbar spine while they lifted reasonably competitive loads. However, during the execution of a lift, one lifter reported acute discomfort and pain. Upon

examination of the video fluoroscopy records, one of the lumbar joints (specifically, the L2-L3 joint) reached the full flexion calibrated angle, while all other joints maintained their static position (2-3° away from full flexion). The spine buckled and caused injury (see Figures 5.1 to 5.3). This is the first observation we know of reported in the scientific

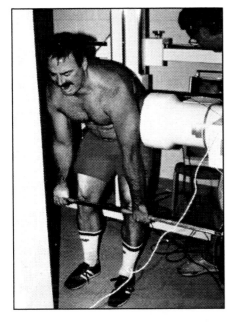

Figure 5.1 During our study of a group of competitive power lifters we filmed a buckling injury.

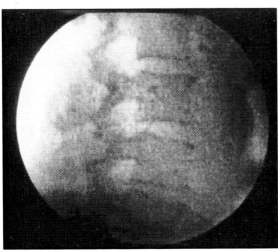

Figure 5.2 This fluoroscopy image of the power lifter's lumbar spine shows how individual lumbar joint motion can be quantified in vivo. Only one joint subtly rotated as the buckling incident occurred.

literature documenting proportionately more rotation occurring at a single lumbar joint; this unique occurrence appears to have been due to an inappropriate sequencing of muscle forces (or a temporary loss of motor control wisdom). This motivated the work of my colleague and former graduate student Jacek Cholewicki to investigate and continuously quantify the stability of the lumbar spine throughout a wide variety of loading tasks (Cholewicki and McGill, 1996).

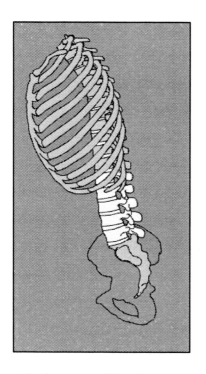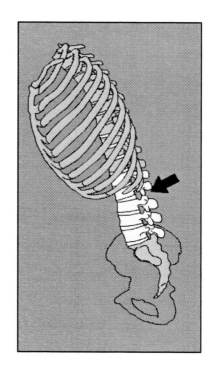

Figure 5.3 The power lifter flexed to begin the lift (left) and began to extend the spine during the lift. As the weight was raised a few inches from the floor, a single joint (L2-L3) flexed to the full flexion angle, and the spine buckled (right).

Illustrating the important conditions for stability: Typically, a lumbar spine from a cadaver will buckle under approximately 90 N (about 20 lb) of compressive load (first noted by Lucas and Bresler, 1961) – ie without any guy wires. This is all that a spine can withstand! Using a fishing rod as an analogy, the following demonstration of structural stability illustrates key issues. Suppose the fishing rod is placed upright and vertical, with the butt on the ground. If the rod were to have a small load placed on its tip, perhaps a pound or two, it would soon bend and buckle. Now suppose the same rod has guy wires attached at different levels along its length, and those wires are also attached to the ground in a circular pattern (see figure 5.4). Each guy wire is pulled to the same tension (this is critical). Now if the tip of the rod is loaded as before, the rod can sustain the compressive forces successfully. If you reduce the tension in just one of the wires, the rod will buckle at a reduced load. We could actually predict the node or locus of the buckle. It is the vital and difficult role of the motor control system to tune and arrange muscle forces (and stiffnesses) to ensure sufficient stability and produce the appropriate torque for posture control and motion. Just the right amount at the right time is needed to produce ultimate performance.

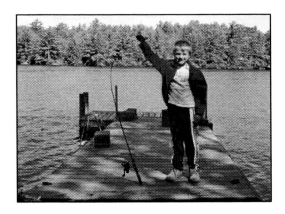 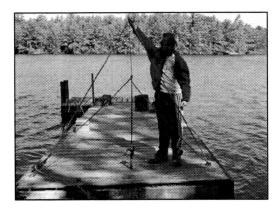

Figure 5.4 A fishing rod placed upright with the butt on the ground is a good model of the spine. When compressive load is applied downward to the tip, it will buckle quickly. Attaching guy wires at different levels and in different directions, and most importantly, pulling each guy wire to the same tension, will ensure stability even with massive compressive loads. Note that the guy wires need not have high tension forces but that the tensile forces must be of roughly equal magnitude. This is the role of the musculature in ensuring sufficient spine stability. Every guy wire, and every muscle plays a role.

Stability myths, facts and clinical implications

It is helpful to provide some data to establish a foundation for the critical issues. There is no such thing as a muscle that is the best stabilizer of the back (Kavcic et al, 2004b). The most important stabilizers continually change as the task changes (figure 5.5). In addition, different stabilizing exercises produce different amounts of spine stability (Kavcic et al, 2004a). This means that there is no ideal motor pattern to ensure stability in all tasks. Stability must be trained with a robust selection of challenges, loads, speeds, etc.

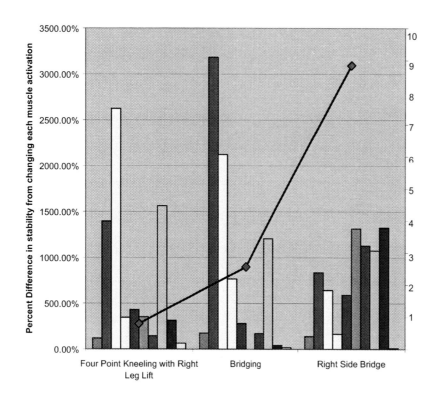
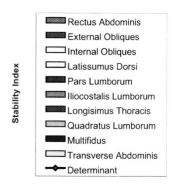

Figure 5.5 The contribution of some torso muscles to spine stability is shown in three exercises performed by a single person. The most important contributors continually change. In this individual, the four point kneeling and back bridge show that the obliques of the abdominal wall together with quadratus are most important. Changing the task increases the role of quadratus lumborum, latissumus dorsi, iliocostalis, longissimus and multifidus as seen in the side bridge exercise. Subtle shifts in posture and technique would change these relative contributions.

Ensuring sufficient stability usually needs only modest levels of muscle activation

Muscle contraction results in both force and stiffness. A muscle's stabilizing potential is dependent upon its stiffness and its tension. During conditions of static equilibrium, stiffness in a muscle is always stabilizing, however, its tension may act to either stabilize or destabilize. Consider the rectus abdominis, where too much force could actually buckle the spine into flexion (Brown and McGill, 2005). The force must be just right – not too much or too little. In the same way, too much stiffness when movement is needed is as counterproductive as insufficient stiffness that compromises the control needed to prevent unstable situations.

Quantitative stability analysis suggests that for most tasks of daily living, very modest levels of abdominal wall co-contraction during the exertion (activation of about 10% of MVC or quite often, even less) is sufficient. For example, standing upright with 30kg in each hand usually only requires less than 5% of MVC. Again, depending on the task, co-contraction with the extensors, including quadratus and latissimus dorsi, will ensure stability. However, if a joint has lost stiffness because of damage, more co-contraction is needed. Certainly, sufficient stability for world record lifts requires special stabilizing strategies. "Tuning" of abdominal contraction for specific events where storage and recovery of elastic energy is optimized along with motion requirements is discussed later.

The special case of transverse abdominis: Since so much clinical focus has been placed on transverse abdominis, a special note is required here. Incidentally, others had made single muscle groups such as the multifidus a single focus as well, which will be addressed here also.

All the evidence supporting clinical emphasis on TrA has been indirect until now. Dr Hodges' work emphasized raw data of timing events - any relevance to spine stability was only inferred. In the original studies, only some LBP patients had delayed TrA EMG onset – not all. He rightly claimed that this simply demonstrated some pathology in the transverse abdominis – and perhaps this would have functional consequence. He described in his work to train transverse that it was to correct the motor control deficits manifested in the onset delay, not to enhance spine stability. Others have interpreted his work out of context, claiming that transverse is a superior spine stabilizer and a source of many spine troubles. Further, recent work has shown that many muscles, other than transverse, exhibit activation delays during a rapid arm raise and that their patterns form sub-groups of back pain patients (eg, Silfies et al, 2009). A critical question is whether EMG onset delay is important for stabilization once electromechanical delay has been considered which lengthens the mechanical production of force. Given the relative magnitudes, we think the mechanical importance is minimal; 30ms delay is buried in the filtering of the muscle transfer function. In addition, Cholewicki et al, (2002) found that all torso muscles have perturbed onsets during sudden loading events in an athlete population. Further, there have been several clinical trials on the efficacy of "stability exercise" training (for example, the trials by O'Sullivan et al, 1997). These studies were fairly reported by the authors but too many in the clinical community have interpreted them to support TrA emphasis. In fact, they did not isolate TrA, multifidus or any other muscle. The exercises trialed produced muscle patterns that involved all abdominal muscles. Patients cannot just activate TrA or multifidus - the ability to isolate the TrA is extremely rare at a functional level of contraction. Typically, isolated TrA activation can only be achieved in at 1-2% of MVC after which internal oblique is recruited together with the rest of the abdominal wall (and only a few people can do this!). We have measured this, as have many others (including Richardson et al,

1992, Allison et al, 1998, Vezina and Hubley-Kozey, 2000). I also believe the clinical literature has been polluted with papers claiming to measure multifidus with surface EMG. This has been shown to be a myth. As Stokes et al (2003) has shown, one cannot obtain multifidus from surface EMG; instead they were measuring from predominantly longissimus. Interestingly our most recent work (Kavcic et al, 2004b) quantified the role of TrA and multifidus and every other muscle in the torso to contribute to stability. The most important muscle continually rotated amongst the many muscles so that no single muscle could be justified as a clinical focus – certainly TrA and multifidus did not prove superior in this role and many labs have now shown this (eg Wilke in Germany, Cholewicki at Yale, Granata at Virginia). On this subject then, I cannot understand why the clinical community has embraced this literature with the interpretation that specific TrA training is important. Rather, it is the exercises themselves that are important. O'Sullivan's group (O'Sullivan et al, 1997, 1998) reported fine work showing that specific exercise can change activation patterns in the abdominal and extensor muscles. It is the total pattern of all muscles that determines spine stability. Another feature of the exercise trials needing interpretation is that when performing specific exercises, other activities for the subjects are naturally restricted (some which might exacerbate an unstable spine). Removing the exacerbators would produce a positive outcome. Stretching the back is a specific example – simply removing the stretching which is exacerbating of the unstable spine brings relief. A study by Koumantakis and colleagues (2005) attempted to isolate the effects of intentional TrA and multifidus training. They compared two patient groups: One received an exercise program which included variants of our "big 3" exercises together with some ball exercises while the other group performed a similar program (but not exactly) which included abdominal "hollowing" and multifidus "swelling" exercises. Not doing the hollowing and swelling exercises was more effective in reducing short term disability. It is important to note that all patients were classified as having non-specific back pain with no obvious signs of instability. My own observation from working with clinicians and patients is that those who are focusing on just transverse are creating dysfunctional spines! These unfortunate patients become paralyzed by their own hyper-analysis of what their transverse is doing. They would be far better off to forget their transverse, the point being that the muscle patterns the exercises produce are the "bracing" patterns documented to enhance spine stability, reduce pain in patients, and enhance performance in athletes.

Abdominal bracing vs. hollowing: Hollowing is an attempt to simply activate transverse abdominis in isolation, while bracing is simply contracting all muscles in the abdominal wall without drawing in or pushing out – it does not imply enormous contraction levels. An interesting consequence of bracing is that the extensor musculature is also activated to form a girdle around the torso. Comparing the mechanical consequence of hollowing and bracing is helpful. The discussion of two mechanisms demonstrate the mechanical folly in this proposal. First, the supporting "guy wires" of the obliques and rectus abdominis are more effective when they have a wider base, that is, when the abdomen is not hollowed. Second, the obliques must be active to provide stiffness with crisscrossing struts, which measurably enhances stability.

The brace appears to invoke an additional phenomenon. The muscles have stiffness when activated. However, when the entire abdominal wall is activated the three layers bind together forming a composite such that the total stiffness is greater than the sum of the parts. Our recent work using rat abdominal wall muscles confirmed the force transmission between layers of the abdominal wall creating "superstiffness" and stability (Brown and McGill, 2009). Curiously, Huijing et al, (2007) measured force transmission from agonist to antagonist muscles in a rat preparation. Bracing of the abdominal wall activates the back muscles forming a stiffening girdle. In terms of stability there are no agonists or antagonists as all muscles contribute. Bracing appears to be a highly efficient strategy to enhance stability.

Finally, hollowing is weakening of the abdominal muscles as it can only be done when the abdominal muscles are almost inactive. But is also causes weakness in other tasks. A simple demonstration can be performed by anyone, proving the functionality of the brace. Sit on the corner of chair and perform an abdominal hollow. Burst up in a power squat style. Then release the hollow, contract the abdominal brace and repeat the power squat. The superior performance with the braced abdomen is graphic.

Breathing and stability: Many sprinters and lifters do not breathe. That is because they would compromise stability and either buckle, or lose performance. Analysis of the links between breathing and stability is revealing (see figure 5.6). With full inhalation the stability increases and reaches a maximum as the abdominal wall tightens to force air out of the lungs, decreasing as air leaves the lungs. Clinicians/coaches aware of this relationship can identify poor stabilizing motor patterns. Place the hands on the lateral abdomen of the athlete after they have performed enough work that their ventilation rate is elevated. Feeling taut and continuously firm muscles throughout the breathing cycles is a good indicator. In contrast, ON/OFF patterns of firmness and relaxation within each cycle is an indicator of poor stabilizing patterns. A nice exercise to correct this is shown in the third section of this book.

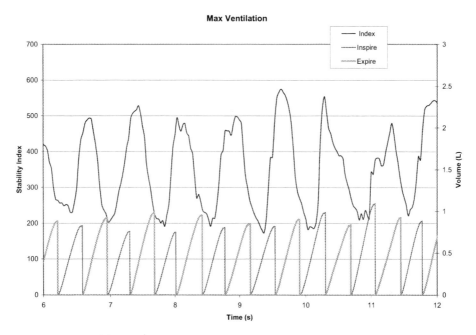

Figure 5.6 Normal breathing is characterized with the stability index rising as the lungs fill with air stiffening the torso. Maximum stability during the ventilation cycle actually occurs with the additional contraction of the obliques to assist in the expiration of air. In this example, the breathing challenge was increased by having the athlete breath through a large straw.

Summary: the lesson for athletes

Athletes training to ensure sufficient spine stability need the foundation of impeccable motor patterns (and the ability to maintain these patterns during all levels of exertion), impeccable motion patterns to control joint position and optimize stability and performance, and the muscle endurance to maintain the necessary muscle contraction patterns through the duration of the event. In addition, in many cases the best athletes must create stiffness extremely rapidly and then release the stiffness equally as quickly. Part III of this book will show you have to achieve these critical components.

References

Allison, G.T., Godfrey, P., Robinson, G., (1998) EMG signal amplitude assessment during abdominal bracing and hollowing, J. EMG and Kinesiol. 8:51-57.

Brown SH., and McGill SM., (2005) Muscle force-stiffness characteristics influence joint stability, Clin. Biomech. 20(9):917-922.

Brown,S., McGill, S.M. (in press, 2009) An ultrasound investigation into the morphology of the human abdominal wall uncovers complex deformation patterns during contraction. Eur. J. Appl. Physiol.

Brown, S., McGill, S.M. (2009) Transmission of muscularly generated force and stiffness between layers of the rat abdominal wall. SPINE, 34(2): E70-E75.

Cholewicki, J., and McGill, S.M. (1992). Lumbar posterior ligament involvement during extremely heavy lifts estimated from fluoroscopic measurements. J. Biomech. 25(1): 17-28.

Cholewicki, J., and McGill, S.M. (1996) Mechanical stability of the in vivo lumbar spine: Implications for injury and chronic low back pain. *Clin. Biomech.*, 11 (1): 1-15.

Cholewicki, J., Greene, H.S., Polzhofer, G.R., Galloway, M.T., Shah, R.A., Radebold, A., (2002) Neuromuscular function in athletes following recovery from a recent acute low back injury. J. Orthop. Sports Phys. Ther. 32(11):568-575.

Huijing, P.A., Langenberg, R.W., Meesters, J.J., Baan, G.C., (2007) Extramuscular myofascial force transmission also occurs between synergistic muscles and antagonistic muscles, J. Electromyography and Kines. 17:680-689.

Kavcic, N., Grenier, S., McGill, S., (2004a) Quantifying tissue loads and spine stability while performing commonly prescribed stabilization exercises, Spine, 29(20):2319-2329.

Kavcic, N.,Grenier, S., McGill, S.M., (2004b) Determining the stabilizing role of individual torso muscles during rehabilitation exercises, Spine, 29(11):1254-1265.

Koumantakis GA., Watson PJ., Oldham JA., (2005) Trunk muscle stabilization training plus general exercise versus general exercise only: Randomized controlled trial of patients with recurrent low back pain. Physical Therapy, 85(3):209-225.

Lucas, D., and Bresler, B. (1961) Stability of the ligamentous spine. In: Tech report No. 40, Biomechanics Laboratory, University of California, San Francisco.

O'Sullivan, P., Twomey, L.T., and Allison, G.T. (1997b) Evaluation of specific stabilization exercise in the treatment of chronic low back pain with radiologic diagnosis of spondylolysis or spondylolisthesis, Spine, 22(24):2959-2967.

O'Sullivan, P., Twomey, L.T., and Allison, G.T. (1998) Altered abdominal back recruitment in patients with chronic back pain following a specific exercise intervention. J. Orthop. Sports Phys. Ther. 27(2):114-124.

Richardson, C., Jull, G., Hodges, P., and Hides, J. (1999) Therapeutic exercise for spinal segmental stabilization in low back pain. Edinburgh, Scotland: Churchill-Livingston.

Silfies, S.P., Mehta, R., Smith, S.S., Karduna, A.R., (2009) Differences in feedforward trunk muscle activity in subgroups of patients with mechanical low back pain. Arch. Phys. Med Rehabil. 90:1159-1169.

Stokes, I.A.F., Henry, S.M., Single, R., (2003) Surface EMG electrodes do not accurately record from lumbar multifidus muscles, Clin. Biomech., 18(1):9-13.

Vezina, M.J., and Hubley-Kozey, C.L., (2000) Muscle activation in therapeutic exercises to improve trunk stability, Arch. Phys. Med. and Rehab. 81:1370-1379.

Part II   Individualizing Programs

Giving the same program to every athlete on a team or group will ensure mediocrity. To assist in developing the best individualized programs, this section provides information for evaluating each athlete, and their athletic task demands.

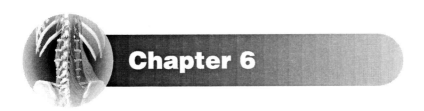

Chapter 6

Fundamental Principles of Movement and Causes of Movement Error

Working with some spectacular performance athletes, I am continually amazed that their "strength", when traditionally measured with conventional squat tests or bench press tests, is very modest. Yet their apparent strength-based performance is outstanding. Of course, their secret is to be able to coordinate their entire body to direct the forces into the ground, or into an opponent, by controlling their force sequence. They are able to "steer" their forces to have the optimal outcome. The purpose of this chapter is to assist in developing an algorithm to help you identify some critical basic patterns of movement for each athlete, which will become the basis of their training. In addition, the fundamental principles of human motion and movement errors are outlined to assist you in designing perfect exercise and training technique for any athlete/sport.

Section 1: Identifying the fundamental movement patterns

I am asked to consult with excellent athletes from all sorts of sports. But I am the first to admit that I have no pre-existing insight into the mechanics of the movements for each sport – so how do I know how to begin designing an optimal program for that athlete/sport? The first stage is to partition the required movements of the sport into the fundamental patterns that form the initial stages of training.

All movement can be broken down into six fundamental patterns which are:

- **squat/lift**
- **push/pull**
- **lunge**

- **gait**
- **twist**
- **maintaining balance**

Consider a baseball pitcher and the pitching motion. What do you see in terms of these fundamental patterns? Hopefully you see a lunge, a push, a twist, all within an upright balance environment. You have just identified critical movement components for the training program. In subsequent chapters you will learn the stages of building an athlete. Not all patterns can be trained during the initial phases of the training program. For example, in a twist intolerant athlete you would have to build twist tolerance before training twisting movement.

To illustrate how robust these fundamental patterns are in assisting the design of programs, I was asked to consult with a rock climber a few months ago. Having never rock climbed I asked to see them climb. Working through the checklist I saw in the movement the fundamental squat pattern, more specifically a one-legged squat close to the rock face. This formed a very unique balance environment for squats. The fundamental gait pattern was a crawl. Specifically the principle of dynamic correspondence was dominant – as one hip flexed the other extended. But the crawl also required the opposite arm (to the flexing hip) to reach out. Once again the six patterns greatly assisted in my being able to design a customized program of optimal functional training.

Once you have identified the fundamental movement patterns, you will discover many sub-patterns. The better consultants will be very creative in working within the sub-patterns, discovering and developing new customized exercises but always within the tolerance of the individual's back.

Section 2: Identifying movement errors and correcting their cause

Finding optimal movement and performance techniques

As I have stated before, having some expertise in spine function doesn't mean that I understand the best way to perform all performance tasks. Seeing all sorts of athletes for back problems and trying to prepare them for their sport requires several methods on my part to assist in understanding their specific requirements. In the previous section, I demonstrated how to identify the fundamental motion patterns; in this section I will discuss how to look for opportunities to improve their technique for better performance.

To help understand different sporting moves, and to help the athlete perform them better, we utilize the principles of mechanics that are universally applicable to all mechanical situations. For example, when training flat-out sprinting speed, the variable that often limits more speed is hip flexion power (not extension) – in other words bringing the recovery leg through the flexion range for the next heel strike. It is interesting that many keep training hip extension but predictably no further gains in top-end speed are realized. Assuming that optimal high speed hip flexion training was achieved, eventually the upper capabilities of muscular strength and contraction velocity will be reached. At this point, the only remaining variable to enhance the speed of the recovery phase of the swing leg is to reduce the resistance of the leg being flexed. This can be accomplished through the principle of "manipulation of the moment of inertia". This involves concentrating the mass of the leg and foot towards the centre of rotation – or in this case the hip. Most people understand how figure skaters spinning on the ice with their arms outstretched gain faster rotational speed when they bring their arms closer towards the spinning axis. To give the extreme example, running without much knee flexion in the recovery leg causes the leg to have a large moment of inertia requiring a large hip flexion torque to flex the leg – such a stiff-legged technique could not allow running. Fully flexing the knee during the recovery phase drops the moment of inertia, and a much smaller hip flexion torque can create much higher angular flexion speed. World class sprinters often look as though they are kicking themselves in the buttocks as they run – in fact they are skillfully minimizing the moment of inertia to overcome the dominant impediment to top end speed.

Many experts tell their athletes to "drive harder", for example – likely if the athlete could, they would. But thinking in mechanical terms, producing the force and directing it in the most beneficial direction provides specific guidance for technique improvement. Further, this approach helps to identify the causes of non-optimal performance, which can be corrected rather than simply being an exercise to identify the symptoms. Inappropriate force development as a cause can be corrected, but the symptom (eg ankle collapse) cannot be directly "corrected".

The first component in the approach is to identify the purpose of the task – for example to produce maximum horizontal speed, to maximize jump height, to encourage an opponent to move in a particular direction or to direct an object at a target etc. Since the body segments form a linkage with joints, and the muscles and ligaments produce torque at each joint, albeit with many anatomical constraints, "viewing" motion must be from several levels of "camera zoom". For example, optimization of movement can be conceived at both the level of the whole body, and the level of a particular area of the body. This mechanical linkage is subject to the Newtonian laws of motion such that general mechanisms can be listed and considered when determining optimal performance technique. The following list forms a checklist to find movement errors and potential technique improvements to enhance performance. The final three principles are intended to minimize the risk of injury during intense sporting effort.

1. Clearly identify and state the purpose of the task.
2. Consider the movement or task from a whole body perspective and from a segment-by-segment perspective. This requires careful observation of the whole body motion, the performance, and then areas of the body in isolation.
3. Apply the following principles for optimizing performance:

- Summation and continuity of joint forces and moments
- Production of linear impulse
- Direction of force application
- Principle of stability
- Summation of segment velocities
- Production of angular impulse (rotational motion)
- Conservation of momentum
- Manipulation of moment of inertia
- Elimination of energy leaks

- Principles for safety:
- Minimization of tissue stress
- Optimal joint positioning
- Minimization of fatigue

Principles for optimizing performance:

A description of each principle to optimize performance and correct movement error is provided here. Think of inefficient movement sources. For example, unnecessary muscular co-contraction, jerky movements, or holding a body segment against gravity when it is unnecessary. These are obvious and easy to correct. Correcting the errors rather than the symptoms will help you to incorporate perfect technique in the exercises that you design – the mark of the master consultant. The following list will help you become better at correcting more involved movement errors.

Summation and continuity of joint forces and moments

All sorts of examples could be used here but I have chosen the need to optimize terminal segment velocity and power. Boxers creating a hard punch need to develop force through the forearm and arm segments. If the shoulder force and moment is not matched by the elbow force and moment, both in terms of magnitude and in timing, the elbow will collapse as it is forced into eccentric contraction. The punch becomes non-optimal. But there is so much more to the story at the elite level. Elite boxers and martial artists understand the mechanics of the wrist and the compliance between the ulna and radius in the forearm during axial compressive blows. Stiffening the forearm is essential so that the forces developed higher in the linkage (in the "core" and torso) are not lost. This is sometimes optimized with wrist pronation just prior to the instant of impact to create more forearm longitudinal stiffness, assisting the final "snap" to have the greatest devastation, but even more is needed to optimize the impact impulse. Developing the necessary forces in the arms requires stiffening of the torso to transmit the forces to the floor, together with initial driving forces developed in the legs. Clearly, a chapter could be devoted to the analysis of developing the punch. But for this example, the reader appreciates the need to scale the magnitude of each joint force and moment together with timing them in a way that all joints are contributing exactly when needed. The boxer who doesn't utilize the abdominals cannot develop punching power as the leg driving forces cannot be transmitted through the sloppy torso. This example shows how the cause of the non-optimal movement task has been identified in a context that provides direct information to train the correction. The symptoms will resolve themselves.

For a back specific example, consider an athlete training the squat. The athlete has a history of chronic back troubles and exhibits the classic crossed pelvis syndrome noted by Dr. Janda. These individuals tend to not fully involve the gluteal muscles during hip extension but rather compensate by over utilization of the back extensors and hamstrings – creating poor performance and overload of the low back. The cause is inhibited gluts – correct the motor pattern in the gluts first and then resume training the squat.

Production of linear impulse

Think of a time-history of force in a rower pulling on the oar. The sum of the area under the plotted curve is the impulse – or the total sum of force. The first principle (previous paragraph) of optimally generating joint forces and timing them optimally results in a force on the oar. Slow development of force, together with a slow decline of force would result in a triangular waveform shape applied to the oar and the total impulse (area under the force curve) is low. In contrast, more rapid force development maintains the peak longer on the oar increasing the impulse. Some people may think this is better technique. However, generating too much force too early "pinches" the boat because the angle of the oar blade is directed away from the boat rather than in the direction of travel. Clearly, several specific technique considerations and how they affect force projection are necessary. In a jumping situation, the time to create force is limited and the rate of force development becomes the critical variable. Athletes who may be ultimately stronger than their competitors will lose if their competitors can generate forces faster (although their magnitude may be lower) since they were able to generate more impulse faster (see chapter 2).

Direction of force application

For every force, there is an equal and opposite reaction force. Forces applied to the ground will cause the body to move in a specific direction. If the identified objective of the task is to create maximal upward velocity (eg take-off for a volleyball spike) then all forces applied to the ground that have some horizontal component are wasted. Thus it is critical to identify whether a forward projection, or some other direction of force is needed. Static situations are fundamentally different than dynamic ones. Balance training during resistance exercises trains control of the projection of force to the ground. It ensures that the "line of drive" is directed through the base of support. If this is not accomplished, the amount of force is limited as the individual becomes unbalanced – performance suffers. However, in dynamic situations, the force is applied for several different objectives, perhaps to "corral" the center of mass and bring it back within a base of support – this happens with walking, running, and bike riding. In other situations, forces are directed to create rotational motion (see the principle of angular impulse below) which may be desirable or which may be unwanted and detrimental to performance. Finally, the direction of force application is a factor in developing technique to avoid injury (see principles for safety).

Principle of stability

An athlete who is not in balance and is having to expend effort to not fall over cannot exert optimal strength, speed etc. Whole body stability (not joint stability, which is addressed elsewhere in this book) is determined by the position of the body center of mass within the base of support. The "ready position" in racquet sports, martial arts, and in the football linebacker etc, are all examples of attempts to enhance stability. Specifically, the center of mass is lowered by flexing the knees and hips, and the base of support is broadened by spreading the feet. Much more force is required to move a person from this position, which is often a desirable objective. The person will fall over when the center of mass travels outside of the base of support. On the other hand, some tasks require a quick start. A sprinter in the blocks creates a base of support with the hands and feet on the ground. The fingers are placed on the starting line and the center of mass is positioned right up to the edge of the base of support (the fingers). In this way maximal horizontal projection forces on the feet can be developed. If the center of mass were positioned farther back, some projection would have to be misdirected vertically to pass behind the CofM and push horizontally. Thus, the concept of stability must be considered within the context of the desire to be immovable and the objective to move quickly. The soccer goal keeper must continually change his foot placement, and the distance between his feet, to react optimally for each challenge.

Summation of segment velocities (and storage and recovery of elastic energy)

The purpose of throwing, striking or kicking tasks is to obtain maximal velocity of the terminal segment at the instant of release or impact. The forward velocity of the hand at the time of release of a baseball or the velocity of the head of a golf club at impact determines the distance that the ball will travel. The speed of the terminal segment is produced by all of the contributing links in the chain that have been optimally sequenced. Rare is the example where maximal segment velocities occur at the same instant in time. For example, the baseball throw begins with the windup and the center of mass falling in front of the single legged base of support. The force to the ground is directed to drive the CofM forward and a lunge position unfolds. The resulting forward velocity of the pelvis, and all segments above the pelvis, is augmented with torso twisting, adding more forward velocity to the shoulder and all segments above. The hips lead the shoulders to store and quickly recover the elastic energy. Timing is critical. Subsequent arm rotation, forearm rotation, wrist rotation and finally finger rotation all contribute to optimizing the release velocity of the ball. Non-optimal rotation in any of the involved segments can reduce performance, but this does not always mean that torso rotation should be maximized. Developing maximal speed and power in terminal segments sometimes requires a stiffer torso to minimize energy losses between the pelvis and shoulders. The speed at which the elastic energy is stored and recovered in the torso is more important than the range of torso motion. Coaches often refer to the quick "snap" rather than the full range of motion which is slow. The discus throw, for example, begins with massive leg drive to begin maximal whole body rotation. The centrifugal forces on the discus developed in the outstretched arm are supremely important and require a relatively stiff link between the legs and shoulders with only a quick, but shortened, lead with the hips. Certainly there is an optimal tradeoff between torso stiffness and motion, and motion at other joints.

Production of angular impulse (rotational motion)

Rotational motion is created by segment muscular forces which can then be directed to the ground. Friction between the feet and ground allows projections of the force to create body rotation. Two important concepts enhance the improvement of generating rotational movement. The "eccentric thrust" requires the projected force to be transmitted along a line well away from the CofM. Consider the springboard diver who projects the foot force behind the center of mass to create forward angular motion. More rotation would require more force. Perhaps this rotation is unwanted and the movement correction would be to reduce the "eccentricity" or direct the thrust line closer to the CofM. Consider the hockey player lining up an opponent for a body check. An effective strategy is to contact the opponent in the body but project the force away from the opponents CofM to cause them to spin. The force that is delivered by the "hitting" player is directed through their own center of mass, having no "eccentric" component. Thus they remain in balance, are quickly underway for the next task and their opponent is crumpled on the ice – hence the effectiveness of the "hip check". Finally, an example from boxing shows why the knockout blow is often the uppercut or cross to the jaw. The brain is designed to absorb linear accelerations but more damage occurs under angular acceleration. During high angular acceleration the inertial brain tends to stay stationary in the skull while the skull rotates around it – damaging the connective tissues and concussing the brain. The "eccentric blow" directed to the jaw and not through the skull CofM causes this rotational acceleration.

Another variation for creating rotational motion is to apply the "hinge" moment principle. Here a hinge is created about which the body forces are directed. For example, a judo competitor thrusts his hip deep into the pelvic area of the opponent to create a low hinge so that hand forces applied to their upper body have a much greater distance to work through, creating a more devastating rotational throw. This provides clues for both offence and defense!

Conservation of momentum

The volleyball spiker projects the jumping forces to the floor vertically to maximize the height jumped, but while in the air they must generate maximum forward velocity of the striking hand. The rotational forces generated in the striking arm cause the body to react with rotation in the opposite rotational direction. Two problems emerge: if the rotation in the body is not corrected they cannot land on their feet (so they do not attempt maximum striking effort), or they cannot produce maximal striking effort because the rest of the body is not buttressed to support the reaction of shoulder contraction. Maximal striking effort is achieved by simultaneously flexing the knees during the windup and extending them during the strike. Torso motion and control augments this buttressing effect. Consider the ski jumper who has made an error in jumping force projection during takeoff and is slowly rotating so that if left unaddressed they will land on their face. Winding their arms causes rotational reaction forces in their body to de-rotate and correct the orientation of their body for landing. In this example, momentum is considered together with manipulating the whole body moment of inertia (the next principle).

Manipulation of moment of inertia

The sprinting example provided in the section introduction illustrates how technique is used to facilitate rotational motion with less muscular force. Returning to the ski jumper example in the previous paragraph, as the arms rotate over the head, the moment of inertia of the whole body is maximal and the rotational reaction is minimal. As the winding arms pass by the torso, the moment of inertia is much lower and the rotational reaction is larger. The net effect is to cause the body to rotate.

Springboard divers use the combination of the last two principles to control the amount of rotation while in the air (as they are unable to exert force externally). A tighter tuck position causes faster rotation if rotation already exists.

Elimination of energy leaks

Optimal transmission of forces developed in the arms and legs needs a stiff torso. Motion in the lumbar spine during sprinting would be an example of an energy leak. Leaks can also occur within a limb - for example, during explosive hip extension, if the foot were not flat to the floor it, being the weaker joint, it would be forced into eccentric contraction. More on this important principle in the third section of the book.

Principles for safety:

Optimal performance must not be achieved at the expense of safety or injury to the athlete. An entire chapter (see chapter 8) is devoted to explaining principles to protect the athlete from injury. Explanation of the safety principles as they are used to guide exercise design and optimize movement technique are explained here.

Minimization of tissue stress

Joint position determines the loads developed in the passive tissues – ligaments, joint capsule, and sometimes the bony constraints of the joint. Avoiding the end range of motion keeps these stresses to a safe level. For example, the squash player digging the ball out of a corner cannot use a full arm swing. Instead, one must use just the wrist which can "slam" into the bony and ligamentous stops at the end range of wrist motion which is problematic. A typical spine example could be in golfers who "slam" their spines into the passive tissues at the end range of lateral bend during ball contact. This causes troubles and symptoms for many a golfer.

Warm-up is also a consideration to minimize tissue stress. Consider the athlete who may stand for a period of time. The cartilage interface at the knee femur-tibia junction will slowly conform to the pressure, resulting in a small "dent". If forceful motion, particularly at a high speed, is suddenly performed, huge stresses develop at the edges of the "dent". This destroys cartilage. This is prevented with a warm-up consisting of gentle motion slowly progressing in vigour. The spine experiences a similar effect with the viscous discs which need to have gentle motion to reduce the internal friction to make subsequent motion less stressful. This principle is incorporated into the programs in the third section of this book.

Optimal joint positioning

While joint position determines the passive tissue forces and subsequent joint loading, position also determines muscle and ligament mechanics. For example, in the anatomy chapter, the influence of lordosis on the line of action of the lumbar longissimus was documented. When the lumbar spine is flexed, these muscles lose their ability to buttress imposed anterior shear forces on the spine. Furthermore, the interspinous ligaments become taut, exacerbating the anterior shear. In this way, lumbar position is an important determinant of risk and safety.

Joint position also influences the ability of muscles to generate force through the force-length relationship. Depending on the athlete, tighter hamstrings can enhance performance, but also may affect injury risk. While tighter hamstrings spare the cruciate ligaments of the knee, they may cause pelvic rotations loading the back. There is no set formula for perfection - each athlete must be considered as an individual.

Minimization of fatigue

Physiological fatigue causes poor technique, leading to poor performance and elevated injury risk. Efficiency of movement and of training sessions reduces fatigue. However, often the goal is to increase physiological fatigue to build tolerance to its effects. In this situation periodization of training is critical. However, periodization is sometimes ignored or misused. For example, I have experienced the coach who builds prolonged and deep fatigue into their team over a season due to unrelenting daily regimens. The team goes into a sustained slump, the coach works them even harder. My recommendation is usually to take three days off. The identification of the training objectives, and its placement into a long term plan, will result in optimal fatigue training.

Qualitative biomechanics to analyze the movement: putting the principles together

These principles will guide analysis of the task demands of any movement and also assist in matching the eventual demands with the most appropriate training exercises. Furthermore, optimization of any of the previous principles requires the consultant/coach to view the movements from a variety of vantage points. First the movement is viewed from a distant perspective where the principles are considered. Then various parts of the movement and various parts of the body become the focus. This is followed by consideration of the various planes of movement. Is there a dominant plane to apply the principles? Is the movement multi-planar? What are the most important joints or combination of joints? Linear muscle forces create angular motion of the body segments, but is the subsequent planar motion optimal? Answering these questions will assist in more insightful mechanically-based analysis to produce error free and optimal movement.

Final thoughts: control feedback and proprioception

Even with this systematic approach, the coach will soon realize that the whole movement is often more than the sum of the parts since the proprioceptive system is organized this way. This is the rationale to mimic the performance environment during specific phases of training. For example, the task of squatting, which is fundamental for rising from a seated posture to standing, requires full proprioceptive integration to be optimal. This cannot be achieved with a seated leg press machine where the legs will be extended with simple knee torque or with simple hip torque or with both. No control over body balance, or joint stability or synergistic torque control at several joints simultaneously is required. Mimic the environment of performance. For the most part, avoid machines that artificially stabilize, constrain motion to a joint, minimize the effect of gravity and which are so often performed in a sitting posture. They starve the athlete of proprioceptive feedback and training opportunity.

Section 3: Understanding the stages of motor skill development to better teach motor skills

Teaching motion/motor patterns, like any other skill, is a progressive process. Whether a pro athlete is re-grooving motor patterns or an adult is engaged in the rehabilitation process, we use a similar philosophical approach based on evidence from motor learning and skill acquisition in developing children. A foundation of basic movements must be developed long before any special skills are grooved. Consider the most basic skills for locomotion or simply moving from one place to another, then consider basic manipulation skills where objects are moved with the hands and feet. On top of these skills are the proprioceptive awareness and sensory awareness skills of vision, auditory and tactile awareness and processing which must be challenged to optimize reaction time, body position etc. Spatial and joint position awareness together with processing of vestibular information assists in ensuring balance so that subsequent optimal force can be developed and optimally directed. Returning astronauts are a poignant example of what happens when the constant challenge of training motor skills is neglected for a short period of time: They have difficulty walking and balancing. While there is much evidence about the best time to develop each of these skills in developing children, they still must be continually re-affirmed in adults.

With this background, I will list the textbook stages of motor skill development based on the experience of the individual:

Cognitive Stage:
- Individuals use environmental cues and past experience.
- Visual/verbal cues are more important than proprioceptive cues.
- Coaching is continually needed.

Motor Stage:
- Effective movement is obtained, which becomes consistent.
- Individuals are able to identify their own mistakes.
- Proprioception feedback is more important than visual feedback.

Automatic Stage:
- Movement "happens" on its own.
- Movement becomes independent of attention demands.

How to utilize knowledge of the stages to be the most effective coach:

Cognitive Stage:
- Use your hands to place clients into position.
- Have them use their own hands.
- Remember that you cannot activate what you cannot feel!
- Repeat until they can achieve optimal positioning on their own.

Motor Stage:
- Once the athlete can find their own optimal position then practice, practice, and practice more to groove the pattern.
- Have the athletes perform exercises and movements regularly at home.

While not specifically noted in these "mechanical" principles, the ability to quickly activate and de-activate muscle, to produce force quickly and then to relax, is paramount. This notion is inherent in these principles and will be specifically and practically addressed in subsequent chapters.

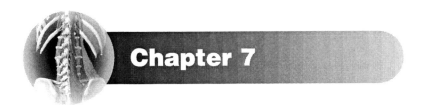

Chapter 7

Injury Prevention and Injury Proofing

Preparing the athlete

Athlete preparation for training and eventual competition can be made easier with systematic approaches. This book describes the steps for developing the physical athlete from grooving the motion/motor skills through to enhancing strength, power and agility. However, there is another component to the complete athlete – that is psychological preparation. I can claim no expertise in this area. My wife, Kathryn, is a sports psychology consultant and she has helped me appreciate the enormous potential that can go undeveloped in too many athletes. The reader of this book is encouraged to develop their expertise in this area to be come a more complete and effective consultant/coach/athlete.

Another critical component for optimal athlete preparation is the need to consider physical and psychological restoration. Training taxes the body systems which are only restored with rest. The "no pain, no gain" approach has a place in training but there is a line that, when crossed, weakens the athlete. Physiological systems can develop deep chronic fatigue, and tissues can accumulate cumulative trauma that go beyond the optimal levels for training adaptation. The point is that very rigorous training is necessary, but it must be within a periodized progression with peaks and tapers to coincide with competition. I have consulted for sporting teams driven into chronic fatigue states by coaches who are frustrated with a performance slump. This was compounded by the unavoidable rigours of league scheduled play. They would be far better performers and sustain fewer injuries with fewer competitions and, in many cases, less training during specific phases of the periodized plan. I have also seen more "mediocre" performing athletes that try to improve by "exhaustion" training approaches. Too many become injured. Compromising rest is foolhardy. The top athletes understand the importance of the periodized blend between training intensity and restoration to fully optimize the adaptations stimulated from training. There are several good books on periodization approaches. As in other aspects of achieving optimal training, there is a general approach but it must be modulated with individual athlete characteristcs.

Another component for athlete preparation is to receive appropriate nutrition and again I claim no expertise here. It is mentioned to assist in developing a checklist. The following section guides the discussion on injury prevention, or developing the health needed for optimal performance.

Reducing the risk in athletes - Guidelines

The injury mechanisms documented in chapters 3 and 4 form some of the foundation for the recommendations listed in this section. Athletes and teams from a variety of sporting activities—from world-class professionals to amateurs—have sought my advice as a low back injury consultant. In many cases, their bad backs were ending their careers, but as we have seen in preceding chapters, success in dealing with bad backs requires efforts to address both the cause of the troubles and the most appropriate rehabilitative and training therapy. In many cases, addressing the cause meant that athletes had to change their technique. Without exception, they had to change the way they trained. In a few cases this meant they had to live with small decrements in their performances, but these technique changes enabled them to remain competitive, and financially rewarded. An example would be a professional golfer who was unable to continue because of their back troubles. Shortening the backswing and mid-swing crunch reduced his drive distance but he remained competitive due to his great skill with accuracy. On the other hand, others have experienced great improvements in performance since their back troubles were greatly reduced once they changed their technique.

The examples contained in the following section illustrate how biomechanical principles can be applied effectively to virtually any sport. The following questions are often asked about how to minimize athletic back troubles. The answers should be used as a checklist to determine the most effective approach to reduce the irritants of a specific athlete's back troubles.

Should athletes avoid end range of spine motion during exertion?

Generally, the answer is yes—if the sporting objective allows for this strategy. In previous chapters, I documented the many complications that arise from taking the lumbar spine to the end range of motion in any activity. Athletic tasks often have the additional stressor caused by high rotational velocities in the spine, which often force the passive tissues to experience impulsive loading as they act to create the mechanical stop to motion. Following are examples in which technique change has improved some athletes' spines.

A baseball catcher was experiencing debilitating spine troubles when rising from the crouch and throwing the ball to catch runners stealing second base. Without technique change and symptom reduction, his career was finished. A combination of abdominal bracing and learning a spine kinematic motion profile that reduced the spine range of motion helped greatly (see figure 7.1). The athlete's throwing speed was compromised to a small degree, but he remained competitive.

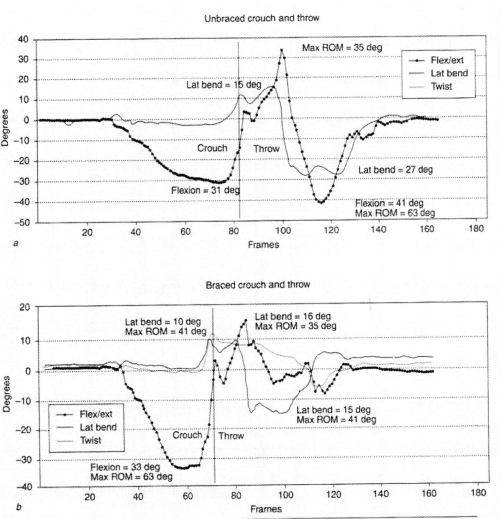

Figure 7.1 This baseball catcher's low back was troubled in particular by rising out of the crouch and throwing the ball to second base to deal with a runner stealing second base. Documentation of the lumbar kinematics revealed large excursions in flexion extension axis (a). In fact, the lumbar spine was extended to its full range of motion (35°) and flexed to 41°. Teaching abdominal bracing together with spine position and motion awareness reduced the range of lumbar motion to 16° in extension and 33° in flexion (b). As a result, the symptoms lessened. Reprinted with permission, S. McGill, Low Back Disorders, Human Kinetics, 2002.

Golfers typically take their spines through full ranges of motion in the lateral bend and axial twist axes. In an example from a professional golfer, the spine reached 100% of the lateral bend capability and 96% of the twisting capability. This spine brutality was performed with each swing of the golf club. He swung the club at least 300-400 times per day whether he played or practised! There was little hope for recovery without reducing this loading. The spine-sparing approach was to reduce the backswing and lateral crunch grooving abdominal bracing patterns that locked the rib cage to the pelvis on the follow-through. Spine range of motion was diminished (see figure 7.2) and this golfer lost a few yards from the ball distance during a maximum drive effort. But as professional golfers play a game of accurate ball placement, this reduction paled in comparison to the possibility of losing the capability to play at a high level of competition.

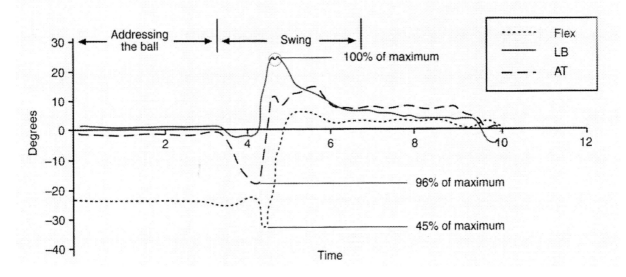

Figure 7.2 This professional golfer suffered chronic low back troubles. The lumbar kinematic analysis of the swing revealed that the spine was taken to 100% of the lateral bending capability and 96% of the twist capability with each shot. In fact the impact of the spine slamming into full bend is actually seen (inside circle). The only way to help this back was to remove the cause— that is, reduce this end range motion. Retraining the abdominals to brace and control, reducing the lateral bend at ball contact and to some extent, reducing the backswing lessened the symptoms.

The principle to avoid end range can be applied to training exercise. See the example of the rower in figure 7.3.

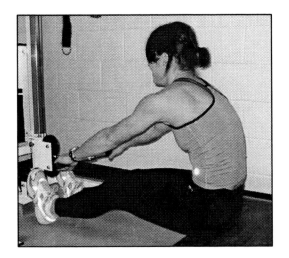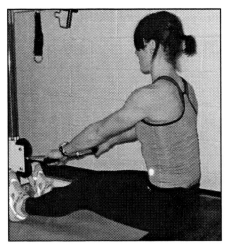

Figure 7.3 This principle is extended to training. For example, in the rowing exercise, the back is spared through technique selection. Allowing the spine to flex, considered to be poor technique (left panel), is risky. The back can be spared by maintaining a back posture that does not flex (right panel).

Minimize spine power – maximize hip power

Power is the product of force and velocity. If the spine is experiencing high angular velocity (actual spine bending) together with high bending torque, the risk of injury is high. This concept is an extension of the concept in the previous paragraph. If high velocity is required, it should be accompanied with lower torque. Moreover, the ability to manage high torque is enhanced with minimal spine bending velocity. The "power" in the protected athlete comes from the hips, not the back. Many studies have shown that the superior weightlifters (eg. Burdett, 1982) develop relatively higher hip power and lower back power than their poorer performing colleagues. Even in the much slower moving power lifters the ratio between higher hip and back torque characterize the better dead lifters (eg. Cholewicki et al., 1991) as do the squatters (eg McLaughlin et al., 1976).

How do you use technique to reduce the reaction moment?

The reaction moment about the low back results from the applied force vector and the perpendicular distance from the force to the lumbar spine (explained in chapter 2). A smaller reaction moment results in lower internal tissue loads necessary to support the moment. This spares the spine. Generally, however, in sporting activities, a reduced force is undesirable. The better option is to reduce the lever arm, or the perpendicular distance of the external force to the fulcrum in the low back. Martial artists take advantage of this technique, as do football linemen. Directing the external force vector through the lumbar spine minimizes the moment and the resulting compressive forces (see figure 7.4). The external force is still high for maximum performance, but the loads on the spine are minimized.

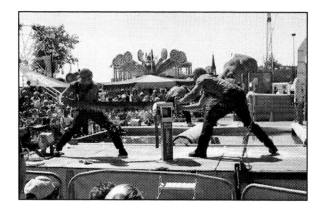

Figure 7.4 These lumberjack games athletes are directing the hand forces of sawing through the low back while locking their low backs in a neutral and abdominally braced posture. They are enhancing safety and performance.

Is there a problem with prolonged sitting on the bench?

Recall that prolonged flexion exacerbates discogenic back troubles, together with ligament-based syndromes. The position of most athletes when sitting on the bench results in prolonged full lumbar flexion (see figure 7.5). The spine postures adopted by some of the tall basketball players are tragically comical. Sporting tradition dictates this posture even though it is so detrimental to many troublesome back conditions. What can be done? Simply having athletes with back troubles not sit on the bench in this way reduces their symptoms. Some find relief from standing and pacing, while others find relief from sitting in chairs with an elevated seat pan that is angulated forward to minimize spine flexion. For years, physiologists have shown the muscular, vascular, and ventilatory changes from warming up. Warm-ups affect spine mechanics, too. A recent study documented the increased spine compliance in a cohort of varsity volleyball players (Green et al., 2002) following a warm-up. After sitting on the bench for 20 minutes, however, this compliance was lost. Twenty minutes is a typical sitting time for volleyball players (and for athletes in many other sports as well). The lasting effect of the warm-up is quite short lived if activity is interrupted with rest—particularly seated rest. Players should re-prepare their backs following a prolonged period of seated rest. Again, this includes sitting in higher chairs and standing and sometimes pacing prior to resuming play. One approach is to maintain the spine in a neutral posture while seated. A "lumbAir" inflatable support is helpful for some athletes (see figure 7.6).

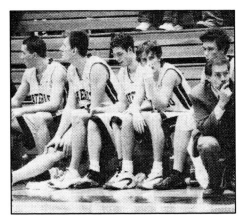

Figure 7.5 Sitting on the bench with a flexed lumbar spine is problematic for two reasons: this posture creates and/or exacerbates a posterior disc bulge, and it causes loss of the compliance obtained from warming up the back. Sitting in taller chairs with an angulated seat pan reduces lumbar flexion and the associated concerns.

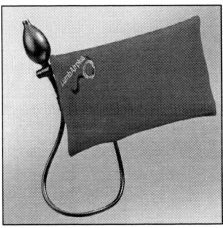

Figure 7.6 A wonderful device for supporting the low back while sitting is the "LumbAir" which is inflated to the appropriate level for each individual. Athletes will find less inflation is needed in the morning compared to more later in the day. Our recent study showed how disc stresses are reduced when sitting in an airline seat using this device (McGill and Fenwick, 2009)

Some athletes must sit flexed as demanded by their sport. Road cyclists have this challenge (see figure 7.7) for which there is no solution. Sitting upright would create too much wind resistance. The only solution would be to try some extended postures during breaks when not riding.

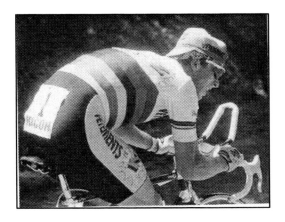

Figure 7.7 Prolonged training postures can be problematic for some backs. In this case, many road cyclists have back troubles due to the prolonged flexion posture. Frequent rests is one intervention strategy.

Should athletes train shortly after rising from bed?

The answer is no if a large amount of lumbar motion is required. Researchers have documented the increased annulus stresses after a bout of bed rest. In particular, full bending exercises are contraindicated. Yet many athletes and laypeople alike get up in the morning and perform spine stretches, sit-ups, and so on. This is the most dangerous time of the day to undertake such activities. It is standard athletic lore for rowers, for example, to rise very early and train on the water since the water is calm this time of day. Rowing requires large amounts of spine flexion during the catch phase. (We have had to train rowers with disc troubles to adopt a technique strategy that avoids full lumbar flexion.) Rowers pay dearly for their early-morning flat water; their backs would be much better served by training later in the day. Another option based on this reality is to rise earlier and arrange a progression to spine loading that produces progressive fluid loss in the disc to reduce the bending stresses.

Should athletes breathe during a particular phase in the exertion?

Many recommend that athletes exhale when raising a weight—or the opposite. We hear, for example, that when performing the bench press exercise one should exhale upon the exertion. What evidence is this based on? This pattern will not transfer to the athletic situation in a way that will ensure sufficient spine stability. As I emphasized in chapter 5 on stability, the grooving of transferable stabilizing motor patterns requires that lung ventilation become independent of exertion. The spine must be stabilized regardless of whether the individual is inhaling or exhaling. We recommend that the athlete train to breathe independently of the exertion. The rare exception may be for the one-time maximum effort that requires supreme spine stiffness for a brief period (for example, weightlifting). Hopefully, this would be a rare occurrence for most athletes in training.

Should the trunk musculature be co-contracted to stabilize the spine?

The answer is generally yes. Many athletic techniques require core stabilization to more effectively transmit forces throughout the body segment chain. Stiffening the torso is taught for many tasks. This approach also reduces the risk of low back injury. The optimal amount of stiffening depends on the task. Larger amounts of stiffness can be needed in the following situations:

- When the athlete might experience unexpected loading, as in contact sports;
- When combinations of simultaneous moments and applied forces develop, as in a basketball player setting a post; and
- After speed and acceleration of body segments are required, as in a golf swing or delivering a blow in martial arts.

I have also come to appreciate how many people interpret "stiffness". Stiffness is thought by many to mean no motion. However, a stiff torso (or any joint) can still enable motion, but the co-contraction about joints ensures that the joints remain stable.

Is specificity of practice regimens important for low backs?

Spine-sparing kinematic patterns and stabilizing motor patterns need to be practiced and grooved into movement repertoires. Since practice makes permanent, it is crucial that routines done in practice replicate as closely as possible the movements and skills demanded by the sport. You don't want the "permanent" you achieve to be incorrect! Ask, for example, will an exercise with free weights or an exercise machine that isolates a body part better replicate the conditions of the sporting task? Is strength really the primary requirement for a particular task? Is spine range of motion a requirement, or does the athletic task at hand require a stiff spine to transmit forces from the upper body through to the legs and the ground? Every athlete and coach must examine the requirements and objectives of their performance tasks. Time and again, I have seen training that included objectives not required by the athlete's particular event that greatly compromise spine health. For example, recently in England, Professor Yeadon simulated some gymnastics moves and then increased various components of fitness to see if performance was enhanced. For some tumbling and somersault tasks, increasing strength did not help; rather, takeoff speed was the component that enabled more rotations in the air. Unfortunately, the principles of bodybuilding have penetrated training for many athletes, leading some to train to look good rather than to focus on regimens directed solely at enhancing performance. The no pain, no gain approach is the misdirected nemesis of many a bad back. Remember, a strong spine in isolation may not necessarily be a stable spine. A stable spine, maintained with healthy and wise motor patterns and higher muscle endurance, protects against back troubles and generally enhances performance.

Can a variety of training movements help?

The issue here is to not do too much of one thing, meaning that variety in training will reduce the risk of overtraining one body mechanism until it fails. Of course this would be sport specific and may seem contradictory to the principle of grooving perfect motion patterns. Rowing is an example of a motion pattern that is repeatable and prolonged without much opportunity to spare the loaded joints with other motions. Depending on the individual, dry-land training can become more important in avoiding injury. In contrast, a basketball player has much more opportunity to train a variety of motion skills on the court while actually playing the sport.

Can imagery help protect low backs?

The steps in using imagery for developing back-sparing patterns for both performance and health are listed in chapter 10. While these are for spine position awareness and grooving motor patterns, they can be very helpful to athletes.

Can general fitness help?

Even though the literature does not always support general fitness as a protective feature, I explained in chapter one why I believe that this is an artefact. Developing the complete athlete requires the full complement of capabilities and components of fitness.

What coaches need to know

Many athletes' backs are ruined in training—not in competition. This sometimes results from the circumstances that are traditional to the sport, circumstance that must be changed. A good example comes from Australia where cricket bowlers typically develop pars fractures. After scientific research clarified the mechanism of injury, protective legislation was developed. Legislation now dictates the maximum number of bowls a cricket bowler can perform in a certain period.

Athletic preparation by its very nature requires overload, which is counter to training for health objectives. As such, it exposes athletes to more risk. When coaches add bodybuilding regimens to their athletes' programs, they can further increase the risk to their athletes. Coaches are well advised to define clearly the training outcome objectives and design a training program to attain them in a way that spares the back and other joints. The process of developing a stable core described in the third section of this book is designed to spare the spine. An encouraging study was reported by Durall and colleagues (2009), where using the "Big 3" stabilizing exercises described later in his book, a gymnastics squad avoided new back pain cases. A back-injured athlete has no chance for success.

Coaches who ask me to provide training programs for their athletes and teams are often amazed to find that I cannot do so without a penetrating analysis of the individual(s) and the task-specific objectives. Optimal preparation of an athlete is not achieved by following a cookbook recipe; every athlete and event or sport is different. Even the experts have to put forth the effort to continually improve their skill and practice to optimally prepare an athlete. There are no rules – only guidelines.

References

Burdett, R.G., (1982) Biomechanics of the snatch technique of highly skilled and skilled weightlifters, Research quarterly for exercise and sport, 53(3):193-197.

Cholewicki*, J., McGill, S.M., and Norman, R.W. (1991) Lumbar Spine loads during lifting extremely heavy weights. Med. Sci. Sports Exerc. 23(10): 1179-1186.

Durall, J., Udermann, B.E., Johansen, D.R., Gibson, B., Reineke, D.M., Reuteman, P., (2009), The effects of preseason trunk muscle training on low back pain occurrence in women collegiate gymnasts, J. Strength and Conditioning Res., 23(1):86-92.

Green*, J., Grenier, S., and McGill, S.M. (2002) Low back stiffness is altered with warmup and bench rest: Implications for athletes. Med. Sci. Sports Exerc. 34(7): 1076-1081.

McLaughlin, T.M., Lardner, T.J., Dillman, C.J., (1976) Kinetics of the parallel squat, Res. Quarterly, 49(2):175-189.

McGill, S.M. and Fenwick, C.M.J. (in press 2009) Using a pneumatic support to correct sitting posture in airline seats. Ergonomics.

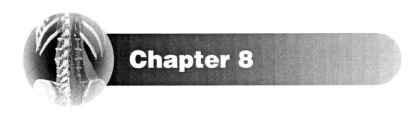

Chapter 8

Evaluating and Qualifying the Athlete/Client

In my consulting, I see the result of prescribed exercises that cause back troubles, or that are detrimental to performance in athletes/workers/patients. Where does one start in the process of finding the most appropriate and suitable exercise? While I have developed a general algorithm to assist in this decision process, I must admit that it is not an exact science. Generally we blend several perspectives, beginning with qualitative approaches and finishing with quantitative information. First we assess the patient's current exercise status within our own knowledge of spine tissue loads that result from various activities. Then we blend our knowledge of injury mechanisms to qualify an individual for a specific exercise progression. We then make an "educated" guess as to the best program and monitor patient progress to ensure a positive slope in the improvement in symptoms and function. In this way, we act as "medical detectives" where we try to view the person and then the exercises all within the context of their sporting and lifestyle environment. When I am teaching physicians, physical therapists or conditioning experts to "view" the client/patient, I suggest that they approach the task as if they are the student. What can they learn from the patient that will help them prescribe the optimal program? What do they see when they observe the client move, or sit, or stand? What do they hear when the client answers their questions? What do they feel when assessing co-contraction and muscle dominance in a particular test? In summary, form a working hypothesis and work to strengthen or weaken the hypothesis with each stage.

In many cases, pathology will be present particularly if there is a history of back pain. High expertise is usually needed to sort these disorders out. In *Low Back Disorders*, I have described many common pain and injury-induced syndromes that need assessment and a suitable corrective exercise. While many of you will be familiar with this material, others are urged to either become very proficient with this material or collaborate with experts who are. Given the scope of this book, which is focusing on back fitness and performance, I have listed only a few relevant tests. See *Low Back Disorders* for assessment of specific tests of:

1. Testing muscle endurance
2. Testing for aberrant gross lumbar motion
3. Testing for lumbar joint shear stability
4. Testing for aberrant motor patterns during challenged breathing
5. Determining suitability for ROM training and stretching
6. Distinguishing between lumbar and hip problems
7. Using many provocative tests to determine the cause of pain
8. Using functional screening tests of postural and movement variables

The qualitative approach described above provides an overall philosophy for assessment. The quantitative approach in *Low Back Disorders* is more systematic in obtaining helpful information from the individual who may have back symptoms. Both approaches are important. Sometimes an athlete may say something in the qualitative approach which, when given the context obtained from the quantitative approach, helps formulate the optimal exercise program. I have added a few more tests that are performance-specific at the end of this chapter.

The first consultant-athlete (with back symptoms) meeting:

A general algorithm is described in this section to help you maximize the information you can learn from the athlete/client in the first meeting that you have with them. The components are listed first to form a checklist and are described subsequently. Of course it should go without saying that if you are working with a patient/athlete that you should proceed with this approach only once you have ensured that your athlete has been screened for all red flag conditions (these include the medically serious sources of back pain such as tumours). In addition several of the tests suggested below should be conducted by clinicians that have the expertise to both perform them and to interpret the clinical results (for example the testing for dermatomes and myotomes). However they are listed here to form a list for those who should know about these tests, and for those who have the capability to perform them.

1. Identify the training objectives (specific health or performance objectives).
2. Consider athlete age and general condition.
3. Note sporting specific and lifestyle details.
4. Consider the injury history and mechanism of injury.
5. Have the athlete describe any perceived exacerbators of pain or symptoms.
6. Have the athlete describe the type of pain, its location, whether it is radiating, and specific dermatomes and myotomes.
7. Perform provocative tests.

1. Identify the training objectives (specific health or performance objectives)

The rehabilitation objective determines the acceptable risk-to-benefit ratio. A performance objective carries higher risk due to the need to create overload. Since the principles of bodybuilding and athletic training are so pervasive, you need to be sure that all patients understand the difference between athletic performance objectives and those of pain reduction and improved daily function. For example, if an athlete/client wants to prepare to waterski but has a chronic or repetitively acute back problem, they need to adjust their objectives to first minimize the back problem. Only then can they seriously train to waterski. Failure to pay the "back gods" causes trouble to linger with compromised performance.

2. Consider athlete age and general condition.

Age specific movement development features have been described earlier. Regarding back troubles, younger people tend to have more discogenic troubles (from the teens to the fifth decade), while arthritic spines tend to begin developing after 45 years, with ensuing stenotic conditions. Note how the client walks and sits. Have they noticeable deficits?

3. Note sporting specific and lifestyle details.

Generally, you should begin by documenting the athletes' daily routines: when and how they rise from and retire to bed, meal routines, exercise and recreational habits. Then direct specific focus toward areas of concern. For example, if the athlete reports sitting at a computer or watching TV for two hours in the evening, ask for details on the type of chair, range of postures used, and so on. After gathering information about the patient's daily routines, inquire about any other special demands. All of this information, when added to the clinical presentation, will help you evaluate common links. Discogenic troubles are linked with prolonged sitting (particularly prolonged driving) and repeated torso flexion. Arthritic conditions, facet troubles and the like are more linked with activities that involve large range of motion and higher loading. Former athletes such as soccer players also fall into this category, although long-distance runners do not since they do not, presumably, take the spine to the end range of motion.

4. Consider the injury history and mechanism of injury.

Attempts to recreate injury mechanisms are fruitful only when the real mechanisms are understood. These are detailed in *Low Back Disorders*. Once identified, the mechanisms can be linked with specific tissue damage (much of which is otherwise not diagnosable). Not only will this assist in designing the therapeutic exercise, it will also help in teaching patients to avoid loading scenarios that could exacerbate the damage and symptoms. Note that some of these will have acute onset, while others progress slowly. Slow onset may result in some patients being unable to identify the mechanism of injury. Nevertheless, a "culminating event" is usually involved. Careful questioning about events leading up to the culminating event will provide clues as to the mechanisms of injury.

5. Have the athlete describe the perceived exacerbators of pain and symptoms.

Prompt the athlete to describe the tasks, postures, and movements that exacerbate the pain. Examine these reported tasks from a biomechanical perspective to determine which tissues are loaded or irritated. These tissues should be spared in the exercise therapy/training, and the exacerbating movements minimized.

6. Have the athlete describe the type of pain, its location, whether it is radiating, and specific dermatomes and myotomes.

Description of the type of pain is sometimes helpful; athletes may describe their pain as deep and boring, scratchy, sizzling, at a point, generally over the back region, continually changing, and so on. You may need to help some people describe their pain by offering adjectives to choose from. Keep in mind that changing symptoms over the short time of an examination generally suggests more fibromyalgic syndromes, which can sometimes be resistive to exercise therapies. With radiating symptoms, the dermatomes and myotomes can assist in understanding the involved segmental levels and whether the pain originates from a specific nerve root. Direct pressure can indicate a unilateral disc bulge or end-plate fracture with a loss in disc height and root outlet foramen size.

7. Observe basic movements

Observe the hip and spine motion during sitting and standing and rising from sitting to standing. Look for spine "hinges" where excessive local motion occurs together with stiff regions of the spine. Paradoxically, the flexion intolerant patient typically sits in flexion. The extension intolerant patient often sits with the spine in extension. Others will demonstrate locked thoracic spines with large hinges occurring in the lumbar spine upon sitting, and by default often during squatting. But not always – some patients have good form during athletic squats but flop when simply sitting on a chair. Observe walking and running. Then watch warm-up A's and B's performed by track athletes. Has a spine hinge formed? These observations will guide you in determining the corrective exercise introduced in the next chapter.

8. Perform provocative tests

Once you suspect that specific tissues are damaged, you can load them to see if loading produces pain - provocative tests help identify motion and motor patterns and applied loads that cause pain. As noted earlier, certain expertise is required here. Many patients have more complex presentations, with several tissues involved. Nonetheless, the provocative procedure still indicates which postures, motions and loads should be avoided when designing the therapeutic exercise. Generally, athletes' descriptions of the activities they find exacerbating their pain will guide your decision as to which specific tissues to load and stress. For example, lumbar extension with a twist can provoke the facets, while the anterior shear test may be warranted for suspected instability (for the interested reader my first book "Low Back Disorders" described many of the pain provocation tests).

So what have we learned?

Performing the items listed in the previous checklist will reveal opportunities to prevent exacerbating scenarios, develop corrective exercise and progress exercise that is tolerable. Specifically, you will uncover whether an athlete does not tolerate sitting or flexion, for example. The corollary is that you will find motions and loads that are tolerable. The items that you learn about from each individual may form a consistent impression. If this happens your job is easier – develop the program to begin with tolerable exercise. However, if the impression of the athlete is not consistent it does not mean that they are malingerers or catastrophisers. It may mean that the source of their troubles is more complex, with more tissues involved.

The first meeting for those without back troubles

Rarely do I consult if back issues are not involved. However, for such instances, I focus on the current capabilities of the individual, and then on the necessary demands to be the best in what they do. Assessment of the mismatch between these two is used to guide the design of the training program. Sometimes this assessment results in the elimination of some current approaches that the athlete has been using. Sometimes the changes are subtle. Sometimes the recommendations are radical including elements of program design, such as time of day, number and frequency of sessions, changing of equipment, adding techniques for speed or direction of force generation, etc.

Some additional performance specific tests

Here are a few back performance-based tests that will aid in deciding what exercises are suitable for an individual, and rate of exercise progression.

Assess posture: Strong individuals stand with little tension reserving their capacity for work to be fully directed toward training. Poor posture saps capacity (see figure 8.1).

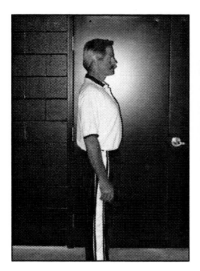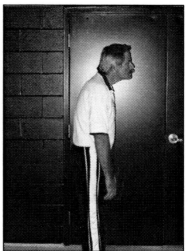

Figure 8.1 An upright and aligned posture (left) vs slouched shoulders and a "poked" chin (right).

Basic movement – The squat: I will use a squat example here to illustrate the point. Prior to allowing an athlete to train squatting with resistance, a simple test of their balance and range of motion could be accomplished by having them "potty squat" or snatch squat. Are they capable of achieving the hip-knee-ankle-torso confirmation necessary to spare their joints (see figures 8.2 and 8.3)? If not, what is the source of the problem – can it be addressed? Have they a troublesome ankle restriction? Is the athlete able to activate the gluteal muscles with powerful contraction or are they tending to overuse their hamstrings and back extensors? If so, they would be candidates for the specific training to address the crossed-pelvis syndrome described elsewhere. Observe facial expressions once you have studied and have become familiar with the athlete/client. Qualifying the athlete and staging their progression with specific exercise is the most important thing that the consultant can do. Interestingly, it is this aspect that many trainers fail to understand. They prescribe set exercises but never achieve more than a mediocre result.

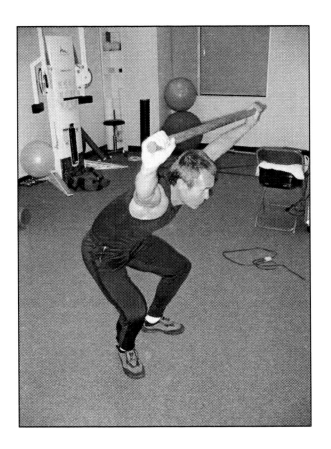

Figure 8.2 Qualifying the athlete to train the squat requires several considerations. World Champ Jerzy Gregorek models a snatch posture characteristic of those athletes who are simply unable to obtain the starting position needed to spare the back, and to groove motion/motor patterns needed for injury prevention and high performance. These deficits must be addressed prior to training the squat. For those interested in a world class lifting lesson from a world champ I recommend contacting Jerzy at www.thehappybody.com.

Basic movement – The squat – choosing optimal hip and foot width: The depth of the anterior labrum of the hip joint acetabulum is a major determinant of the ability to squat deeply. In order to find the optimal hip width (or amount of standing hip external rotation), have the athlete adopt a 4 point kneeling stance. From neutral, rock or drop the buttocks back to the heels (see figure 8.4). Mark the angle at which spine flexion first occurs. Then repeat with varying amounts of space between the knees. Look for the optimal knee width that allows the buttocks to get closest to the ankles without any spine motion. This is the hip angle that will produce the deepest, and ultimately the highest performance squat. It is much wider than most people think. Observe the world champs squatting.

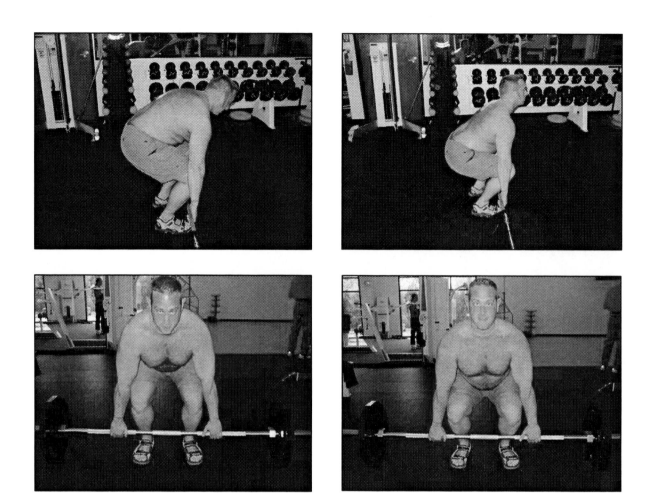

Figure 8.3 The postures achieved in the left panels suggest that the athlete would not be qualified to perform the dead lift with the bar at this height (modelled by lifter Vince Catteruccia). Ankle and hip mobility appear to be the culprit. Obtaining the necessary flexibility to achieve impeccable form qualifies the athlete to perform (shown in the right panels).

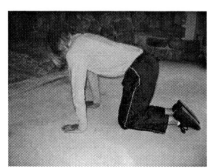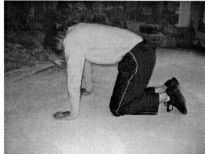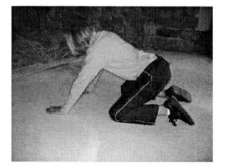

Figure 8.4 Begin on all fours with the spine in a neutral posture (left). Then rock the buttocks back to the heels noting the hip angle of the "back break" (middle). Now widen the knees and repeat searching for the deepest angle without a "back break" (right).

Looking for spine "hinges": Spine hinges occur at local segments which provide more motion than their counterparts. These are often a focal point for pain. Once identified, they can be braced and stiffened to reduce symptoms. Flexion hinges, for example, in a lifter are sometimes buttressed with additional latissimus dorsi activation (see figure 8.5 and 8.6). Twisting hinges are more difficult to address and often require focus on reduced gross range of twist motion and abdominal wall bracing (see figure 8.7).

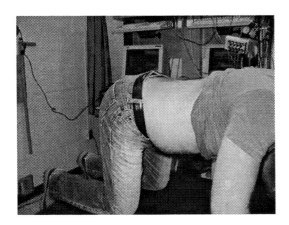 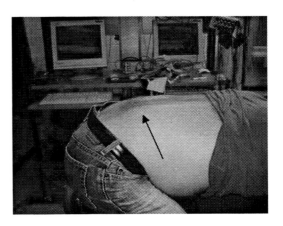

Figure 8.5 A flexion hinge (arrow) at L2-3 is the site of pain in this flexion intolerant former athlete. Here the patient starts on the hands and knees and rocks the buttocks back to the heels trying to maintain a neutral spine. General abdominal bracing removed his pain together with spine-pelvis position awareness training.

Poor control in torsional tasks: Other forms of aberrant motion may indicate poor lumbar control which is in contrast with the local spine instabilities shown above. For example, rotational disconnect of the rib cage and pelvis during this next test can indicate more work is required for enhancing lumbar control. Taking a push-up position, lift one hand and place it over to the other. Repeat to the other side. The pelvis and rib cage should remain level if torsional control is achieved (see figures 8.8 and 8.9). A similar indicator of control is achieved with one-legged hip extension.

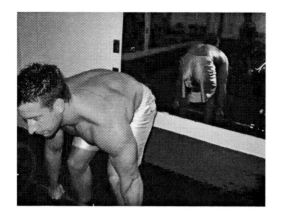
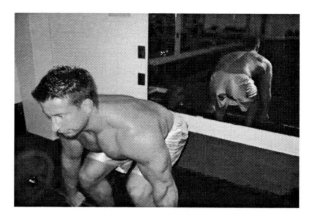

Figure 8.6 This high performance lifter has a thoracolumbar hinge (left panel) which is corrected with latissimus dorsi activation (better seen in the mirror image on the right panel).

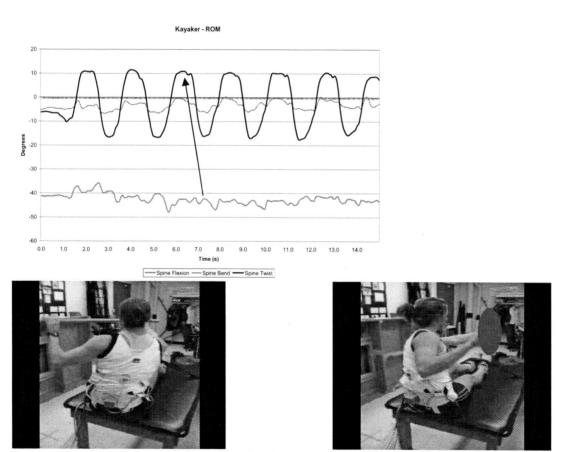

Figure 8.7 This athlete paddles a kayak. The twisting hinge is associated with both flexion intolerance and extension intolerance, and not surprisingly twisting pain. The excessive twist is shown in the top panel together with the collision of the tissues at full left twist (arrow). Here there was no option but to reduce the twisting range to allow the disc and facet irritation to resolve. A stiffer torso also helped to better store and recover elastic energy.

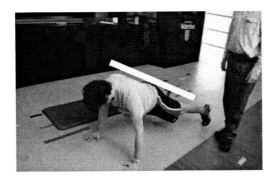 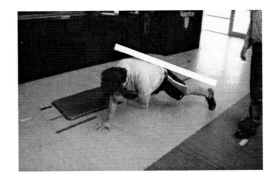

Figure 8.8 Starting in the pushup position one hand is lifted over to the other. The pelvis and ribcage should remain locked. An elevated pelvis on one side would indicate poor lumbar torsional control.

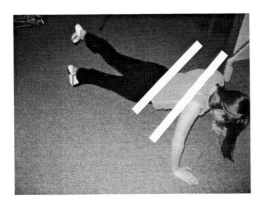

Figure 8.9 A locked pelvis to ribcage while raising one leg with hip extension also indicates lumbar torsional control. Hiking the pelvis indicates poor lumbar torsional control.

Stable patterns during challenged breathing: In the lab, we can test the ability for athletes to breathe heavily while not compromising spine stability. The best test for aberrant motor patterns during heavy breathing is rather sophisticated. Many individuals will not show pathology in tests performed at low levels of exertion. The pathology only shows at high work rates. Candidates for this type of test include high performance athletes and also occupational workers with high levels of fitness such as construction workers, warehouse employees, and so on. While the sophisticated lab test involves the breathing of CO_2 with torso muscle activity quantified with EMG (shown in *Low Back Disorders*), a test is described here that can be performed by an "aware" individual.

During this test the person ventilates heavily. The "expert" places the fingers on the abdominal obliques lateral to the navel and rectus. They feel the level of contraction in the abdominals. If the contraction level entrains to the breathing cycle then stability may be compromised. Constant abdominal contraction shows that the diaphragm is performing well and that torso stiffness and spinal stability are not compromised. To increase the challenge, weight can be added, or any other resistance to better represent this athletic ability. (see figure 8.10).

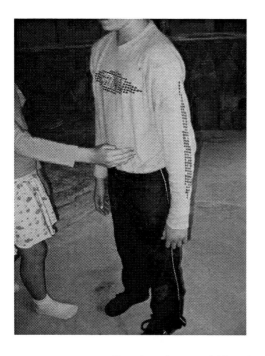

Figure 8.10 Challenged breathing test for high performance athletes. Athletes breathe heavily while their abdominal obliques are palpated. Constant contraction indicates an athletic ability to stiffen without compromise to stability. Various loads can be added.

Good spine stabilization patterns observed in the muscle EMG signal obtained during the challenged breathing test include constant muscle co-contraction ensuring spine stability. Of course too much contraction can occur. In the absence of our lab technology, detection of this requires expert judgement.

Endurance Testing: Protocols for testing torso muscle endurance are discussed in "*Low back Disorders*" together with normal/abnormal ratios. While absolute endurance is known to be protective for injury in the normal population, some coaches have observed that certain scores appear to be protective in athletes. For example, a few pro hockey coaches feel that the ability to maintain the side bridge posture for longer than 70 seconds is protective for the "sports hernia".

Specific Movement Screens: Several movement screens are available and there is no question that they reveal movement pathologies that are linked to future injury. We know that runners with asymmetric hips are the ones who develop back pain first – the same for road cyclists. However, movement screens do not reveal the muscle activation patterns that account for the movement disorder which sometimes causes the incorrect corrective exercise to be prescribed. Nor will these screens reveal the way a person will move in an athletic situation or even during a movement of daily living. Thus it is important to follow up every movement screen with a good observation of how a person moves during the tasks of daily living and during their sport/training performance.

Virtually any athletic task becomes a test: Use any task as a test for proper form, efficiency, joint sparing etc. Be aware of joint alignment, inefficient patterns of contraction, poor direction of force generation, to name a few. Refer back to chapter 6 for the list of determinants of optimal motion.

A philosophical approach for selecting specific tests, and designing the program

Once it has been decided that the training will be designed either for performance or more for general health or for rehabilitation, then the question becomes, "How will the training program be designed?" Several approaches may be considered depending on the age/development of the individual, the sport/activity, together with their current deficits. Movement and performance skills develop with age. General movement (eg balance, running etc.) may be a better objective in younger athletes. Specific objectives are better left for more developed individuals (lifting technique, developing the back for throwing potential etc). Another approach is to perform a battery of tests to identify specific deficits which become the subsequent focus for training prior to challenging specific sport demands. The final approach borrows from the industrial worker process of defining job demands, defining worker capabilities and matching the two – or in this case, focusing on related weaknesses that impede performance in the athlete. Usually a blend of these approaches is required.

Step 1: What are the demands of the sport/activity?

These may be basic demands (running, quick stops and starts, directional change) or they may be specific demands (buttressing torsional movements with core strength to transmit arm forces to the legs during a discus throw). More detail on assessing the sporting demands were addressed earlier. Nonetheless this cataloguing of demands reveals the essential elements for training. For example, a wrestler would spend some time in a ready position, execute a specific number of explosive contractions, transition heights from high to low, work on the knees etc all within a round. This cataloguing reveals some of the elements for designing the training program.

Step 2: What are the capabilities of the athlete – together with current deficits?

Basic capabilities/deficits could include balance, stability, endurance, strength, and agility. Specific capabilities could include throwing accuracy, golf ball distance etc. Some of the spine-specific tests were listed previously in this chapter.

Step 3: Design the program

Develop the program considering age, development deficits, the rhythm of the playing season and the need to protect previous injury etc. Overlay the results of the spine specific tests described here. Make the program practical, personal, and planned. Specific strategies for program design are discussed later.

A final note on qualifying the athlete for specific training exercises and optimal program design

The risk of performing any exercise depends on the current ability of the athlete. The algorithms described previously in this chapter will help uncover some of the current capabilities and deficits of the athlete. The intention is to match them to the demands of the exercise. However, there is no magical formula to guide this process – the best consultants use science together with their own experience to know when, and how much, an athlete should attempt. Other chapters provide information on progressive training.

In summary, here is a rather random list of items that, if considered in the proper context, will lead to better results:

1.   When testing a team at the beginning of the season, an endurance run is often a component (eg how far did they run in 12 minutes, or what was their time for a mile). Remember that the last place finishers may well be the most explosive athletes. They need different training, and different opportunities to showcase their talents. They will have the best performance in a standing long jump for example.
2.   Train shorter periods when recovering from injury. Train shorter but more intensely for performance training. Consider honing the quality of a training session – before adding quantity.
3.   Optimal training volume, whether for rehab or performance varies widely among individuals. Giving the same program to all members of a team indicates that other expertise is required.
4.   A keen eye is needed to observe technique deterioration within a training session. This is usually an indication to stop. Capacity changes from day to day and so should the program.

Note: I am in the process of finishing a new book, and a DVD, cataloguing and quantifying provocative tests and functional screens for the back. Stay tuned to www.backfitpro.com for updated information.

References

McGill, S.M., Low Back Disorders – Evidence Based Prevention and Rehabilitation, Second Edition, Human Kinetics Publishers, Champaign, Illinois, 2007.

Part III
Building the Ultimate performer: Putting it all together

The scientific analysis conducted and documented in this book provides guidelines for selecting, grading and progressing exercise. A systematic approach for building the ultimate back is provided here, together with several case studies to provide examples of what has proven successful with many athletes.

Chapter 9

Developing the Program

The components of the 5 stage program presented in this book have been quantified to enhance the various components of performance. Different stages have been proven effective with experimental study groups. The overall program has helped many individuals when all else failed. We know that many traditional approaches used with other areas of the body simply do not work with the back.

Choice of the starting challenge for any stage in the program is difficult, as is the determination of the progression. High performance athletes can be as delicate as patients in that there is little margin for error. The dose of exercise is critical, in terms of both magnitude and the fundamental components that include the motion/motor patterns utilized with the dose. The dose determines whether tissue is stimulated to adapt or overloaded to break down. The approach in this book is designed to tip the scale towards successful performance enhancement with minimal risk of injury. Too much athletic potential is wasted due to inappropriate training.

A summary of the components of the program is introduced here. Optimal training programs require thoughtful consideration of every component. Each component must be designed and justified to meet an objective. Identification of the objectives is a critical first step – is the objective for pain reduction and rehabilitation of problems or is it for performance? Health objectives demand a focus on motion/motor patterns, stability and endurance resulting in low tissue loads, and a low risk environment. Performance requires more overload with an elevated risk naturally occurring. The trick is to stay within the "lowest risk possible". Exercise designed to focus on minimal spine load while establishing the three initial stages of spine function, is discussed first. Stages four and five are reserved for higher level performance. It is stressed that taking shortcuts in the foundation stages will compromise success at training true strength and power. While we begin by focusing on the objectives in the first stage, training progresses to add additional components in parallel.

The trained athlete continues training to maintain all components.

Stage 1: Groove motion patterns, motor patterns and corrective exercise
- identify perturbed patterns and develop appropriate corrective exercise
- build basic movement patterns through to complex activity specific patterns
- build basic balance challenges through to complex/specific balance environments

Stage 2: Build whole body and joint stability
- build stability while sparing the joints
- ensure sufficient stability commensurate for the demands of the task

Stage 3: Increase endurance
- develop basic endurance training to build the foundation for eventual strength
- incorporate activity specific endurance (duration, intensity)

Stage 4: Build strength
- spare the joints while maximizing neuromuscular compartment challenge

Stage 5: Develop speed, power and agility
- develop ultimate performance with the foundation laid in stages 1-4
- focus on optimizing elastic energy storage/recovery
- employ the techniques of superstiffness

Overlay for all stages:
- the position of performance
- the balance environment

Within each stage and as the athlete progresses, there are several progressions. Typically, the stage will begin with an element of basic conditioning and basic skill development which is then progressed through advanced forms of conditioning and advanced specific skill development.

Some preliminary matters

Before presenting the exercises, I will review some of the basic ideas discussed in the text thus far, and establish how they may be put into practice.

Some notes for the chronic back

While my first book, *Low Back Disorders*, described various rehabilitation progressions together with several techniques to ensure maximal rehabilitation success, a few of the techniques are applicable to the performance trained athletic back. For example, specific endurance deficits may be addressed with quantitative and defined objectives. In addition, there are several other variables and tasks that assist in the process of building the superior back – they are listed here.

The return of function and reduction of pain is a slow process. Athletes still have "bad" days although these should become fewer and less intense as they progress. But having "good" and "bad" days is educational. By studying daily activity, the athlete learns what activities cause trouble, and which ones result in a higher work capacity the following day.

Keeping a journal of daily activities

Many athletes keep a training log that may also include nutritional components. I also advocate documenting daily back pain, or other musculoskeletal concerns. This information is essential in identifying the link with mechanical scenarios that exacerbate the troubles. Two critical components should be recorded in a daily journal: how the back feels and a log of the training regimen together with all other tasks and activities that were performed. When the athlete encounters repeated setbacks, he/she should try to identify a common task or activity that preceded the trouble. Likewise, even when progress is slow, the athlete/patient will be encouraged to see some progress nonetheless. Without referring to the journal, the athlete sometimes does not realize there is improvement.

Ensure continual improvement

Performance needs constant improvement within the confines of the peak-and-taper program design. Those with a history of back troubles may, on occasion, regress and experience symptoms. If this occurs, we usually drop back a stage to the "foundation" and work at that level until the symptoms resolve. Then review what caused the symptoms to return and "tweak" the program design. Those simply experiencing a performance plateau need to alter their training program and/or their execution technique.

How long should each stage be?

There is no single answer for all backs. Some will progress quickly, while others will require great patience. Progressing from one stage to the next is not a serial process as an athlete may be training in a few stages in parallel. Nonetheless, these decisions are the job of the clinician and coach—to determine the initial challenge, to gauge progress and enhance the challenge accordingly and to keep the patient motivated, even during periods of no apparent progress. The great clinicians blend keen clinical skills and experience with scientifically founded guidelines and knowledge.

Training with labile surfaces underneath the athlete

Gym balls, for example, have become quite popular. Certainly, these labile surfaces challenge the motor system to meet the dynamic tasks of daily living or specific athletic activities. But might this type of training be of concern for some patients? Our recent quantification of elevated spine loads and muscle co-activation when performing a curl-up on labile surfaces (Vera-Garcia et al., 2000) suggests that the rehabilitation program (or those concerned about spine compression) should begin on stable surfaces. In this case, we assessed the simple curl-up for the effect of a labile surface on muscle activation patterns (see figure 9.1). Simply moving from a stable surface to a labile surface caused much more co-contraction, which in some cases virtually doubled the spine load (see figure 9.2). The practice of placing patients/athletes on labile surfaces early in the rehabilitative program can delay improvement by causing exacerbating spine loads. We therefore suggest beginning exercises on a stable surface and establishing a positive slope to improvement. Introduce labile surfaces judiciously only once the patient/athlete has achieved spine stability and sufficiently restored load-bearing capacity, and can tolerate additional compression. This same principle can be extended to sitting. Sitting on a gym ball greatly elevates spine load through increased muscle co-activation. For this reason, non-patients should avoid prolonged sitting on gym balls, and patients should use them only once they have achieved spine stability and increased load-bearing capacity. There is a time and a place for labile surfaces. The progression shown later in this chapter demonstrates how they can be effectively used to train functional stability.

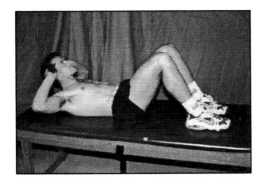
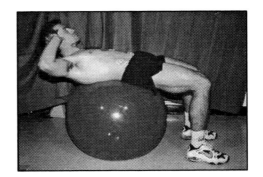
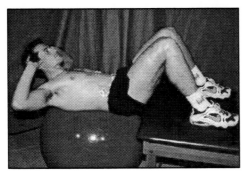
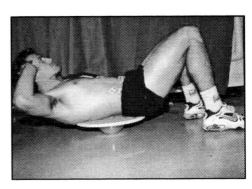

Figure 9.1 The simple curl-up assessed for the effect of a labile surface on muscle activation patterns. Simply moving from a stable surface (upper left) to a labile surface causes much more co-contraction, which, in some cases, virtually doubles the spine load. Reprinted with permission from Physical Therapy, Vera-Garcia, F.J., Grenier, S.G., and McGill, S.M. 80(6): 564-569, 2000.

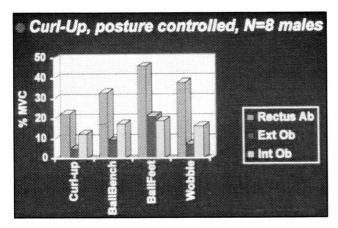

Figure 9.2 A curl-up with the torso over a ball and the feet on the floor (seen in figure 9.1) virtually doubles the abdominal muscle activation and correspondingly, the spine load.

Training harder and longer is not always better

Some of the greatest athletes would appear to undertrain. Others criticize their work ethic in training. Yet when I study their training regimens, they often emphasize motion and motor patterning and skill practice. Many of the athletes that I am asked to see work too hard at the wrong things. They brutalize their body with ill-chosen exercises, believing that doing them even harder will result in higher performance. The point here is that often this approach will result in injury, or in not achieving the performance that is possible. Squeezing a few more reps out of an exercise set is rarely productive for performance. It is simply stupid to destroy the body. Always consider skill development, perfection of motion and motor patterns, and avoidance of technique-compromising fatigue.

Some final thoughts on reps, sets and sessions

Recall the discussion of capacity and tolerance from chapter 1. A painful back that is exacerbated by walking 20 meters will not benefit from training 3 times per week. Rather train 5 times per day in short brief sessions that never exceed the capacity or tolerance of the individual. As tolerance and capacity increases, reduce the number of sessions, and increase the workload within a session. I will often start an athlete on 2 or 3 brief training sessions per day until they can tolerate more work. Further for these people, I will eliminate a warmup simply because that would use too much of the compromised capacity.

Stages of athlete progression

Hopefully those with back concerns will have familiarized themselves with the preliminary process of finding and removing activities that exacerbate low back troubles (in my book *Low Back Disorders*). This is a crucial part of the exercise design process. Provocative testing should also be performed at that time. Once this has been done, the training can proceed with the 5 stages described in the next chapters.

References

Vera-Garcia, F.J., Grenier, S.G., and McGill, S.M. (2000) Abdominal response during curl-ups on both stable and labile surfaces. Phys. Ther. 80(6): 564-569.

Chapter 10

Stage 1: Groove Motion/Motor Patterns and Corrective Exercise

It is assumed that assessment of basic motions (sitting, standing, walking, perhaps running and lifting) has been completed and faults documented. Are parts of the spine unstable? Are parts of the spine too stiff and stable resulting in an unnecessary crushing down of the spine with over-activation? During provocative testing and the testing of some functional screens - what failed? Not that the failed tests themselves should be trained but rather will give insight into the causative faults. The appropriate corrections must be understood and repeated until they become automatic behaviour (described in chapter 6). Success is enhanced by removing the faults first, before optimal performance can be trained.

How many times have we heard the discussion about what is the perfect arm curl? Should one stand against the wall, flex the elbow with the upper arm braced? Think about the mechanics – the motion is restricted to the elbow and the supinated forearm helps to isolate biceps, minimizing the contributions from brachioradialis. This follows the isolation principle from body building – not functional training for performance. Think of one activity where this is an essential component for success. Assume that you are training a football lineman and that you are following the process outlined in this book. Firing out of the squat stance position and ripping with the forearm was identified as an essential motion (from the analysis you conducted following the principles in chapter 6). The fist-forearm is in a neutral position – neither pronated nor supinated. The motion requires elbow flexion with simultaneous shoulder flexion in an environment of balance and dynamic thrust to the ground. For this lineman, training "the perfect curl" would involve a lunge with simultaneous elbow and shoulder flexion. This trains the fully integrated elbow and shoulder flexion complex without weakening the potential by muscle isolating postures. Using a dumbbell with a hammer grip will optimize brachioradialis integration, while stepping into the lunge with simultaneous elbow and shoulder flexion completes the functional motion/motor pattern (see figure 10.1). This is a graphic example of a popular "body building" training approach versus functional performance training. But now let's focus on back integration.

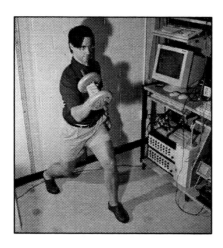

Figure 10.1 For a football lineman, stepping into a lunge with simultaneous elbow and shoulder flexion forms a functional training exercise to train "ripping" power. The hand is in a hammer grip to maximize elbow power and the upright lunge demands proprioceptive integration in the position of play.

A note on the training environment

The environment of the clinic/gym/training room is important to ensure optimal progress. It is popular among many to consider the process of ingraining motion/motor patterns as a subcortical process. That implies that muscles are facilitated by other patterns. While this may be important for some approaches, we insist on mental focus from the athlete. Mental imaging techniques, together with direct mechanical contact applied by a clinician and by the athletes palpating and "feeling themselves" is employed to assist with the activation process. This requires great mental focus and concentration by the athlete. The environment needs to be quiet, no background music, and no distracting stimuli.

Awareness of spine position and muscle contraction

Some people are very "body aware" and are able to adopt a neutral spine or a flexed spine on command. Others, even some high performance athletes, can be frustratingly unaware. I recall working with a motor bike trials event athlete who was unable to exert maximal control of the bike through the knees and hips because of poor positioning and control of the torso and legs. Developing the spine positional awareness greatly enhanced his bike/body control but in his case, it took a lot of effort to develop.

- **Finding the "neutral spine"** employs the concept of elastic equilibrium (minimal elastic tissue stress). The posture, or curvature, of the lumbar spine when standing is close to elastic equilibrium. This posture may be modified by those with pain who find relief with slightly more lumbar flexion, or extension. This modified position becomes their neutral spine.

Lumbar spine proprioceptive training

Given our research on the importance of spine position awareness to spare the spine and our experience in teaching positioning, we became interested in proprioceptive training for the back. The fact that very little evidence was available to validate the use of proprioceptive rehabilitation for the lumbar spine motivated our recent work on spine proprioception (Preuss and McGill, 2006). The purpose of this work was to quantify the effects of a six-week training program designed to improve lumbar spine position sense and sitting balance. Twelve subjects with a previous history of LBP were evenly split into a training group and a control group. Subjects in the control group received no intervention, while the subjects in the training group received a 20-minute rehabilitation session three times per week emphasizing spine stabilization exercises with a neutral spine. Lumbar spine repositioning error in four-point kneeling and sitting balance for the training group showed significant improvement over the study. This small but initial study demonstrated that proprioception and position awareness in the lumbar spine can improve through active proprioception exercises.

Corrective standing approaches

Upright standing should produce minimal contraction in the low back extensors. Those who are "chin pokers" or who have a slouched standing posture waste precious capacity by wearing out these muscles with chronic low level contraction. Some of the great strongmen and east European trained weightlifters believe that this chronic contraction compromises their efforts to build more "white", or fast twitch, muscles fibres. Here is a simple test to determine the contraction level. In a standing posture, palpate the lumbar extensors with one hand. If they are active, and hard, extend about the hips to shut these muscles off. Then adjust head posture and shoulder posture, together with the hip angle, to stand in a way to cause relaxation in these muscles (see figure 10.2).

Here is another technique to assist those who have difficulties positioning their shoulders and chest. When standing, make a fist with the thumbs out. Then rotate the thumbs, steering them around with maximal external rotation at the shoulders (see figure 10.3). This naturally lifts the chest, while positioning the thorax into a posture of strength. Now relax the arms. Re-check that the low back extensors are relaxed.

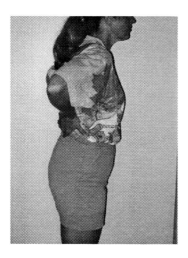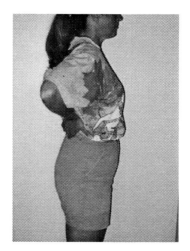

Figure 10.2 Learn to find the relaxed posture that shuts the lumbar extensors "off" with manual palpation. Slouched shoulders and "poked chin" cause chronic extensor contraction (left). Retraction of the chin and shoulders are two helpful strategies together with extension of the hip. Once the upper body center of mass is over the supporting lumbar spine, the extensors will relax (right).

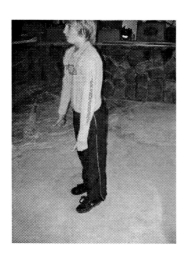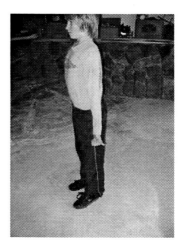

Figure 10.3 Steering the thumbs around with shoulder external rotation lifts the rib cage and retracts the shoulders.

Corrective walking approaches

Similar posture cues are used for establishing athletic walking gait (see figure 10.4). Typical patterns that characterize pain, or simply poor athletic performance, include a slouched posture, small steps, arms not swinging or swinging with low amplitude about the elbow and feet externally rotated.

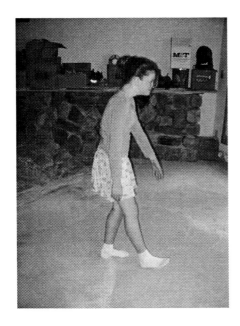 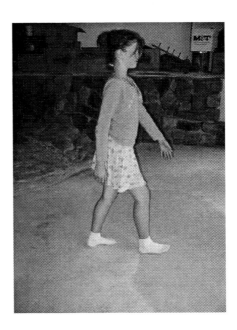

Figure 10.4 Poor walking posture wastes capacity (left). Correct posture builds capacity for training (right).

A convincing demonstration of the influence of posture on strength

A few years ago I met Pavel Tsatsouline, who is very clever in optimizing strength via technique. He uses the following technique to demonstrate the influence of posture on the ability to summon strength (see figure 10.5). With a partner, shake their hand and then squeeze it as hard as you can. Now fine tune your posture in the following manner. Take a wide foot stance and "grip the ground" with the heels and toes. Then, using the hip musculature, isometrically abduct and externally rotate to try and "spread the floor". Activate the gluteal muscles by squeezing an imaginary nut between the buttocks. Stiffen the abdomen with an abdominal brace. Lift the rib cage. Stiffen and depress the shoulder girdle with latissimus dorsi contraction. Make a fist with the non-shaking hand and squeeze. Now repeat the handshake. The strength gain should be impressive. This will convince you that posture modulates the ability to generate strength. Remember all of these steps and apply them to a bench press effort, or squat, for impressive gains. Or try it on a stuck jam jar lid and impress yourself.

The technique results in a neutral spine, a stiffened "core" and whole body stiffness, together with a redirection of neuronal overflow from the non-shaking hand over to the shaking hand.

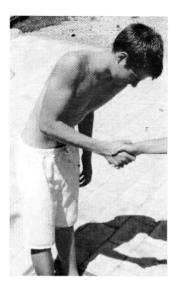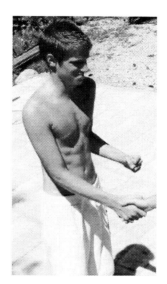

Figure 10.5 Maximum effort hand squeeze with a typical, but weakening, posture (left). Stiffening the feet, legs, hips, torso, shoulders etc enhances the strength (right).

Distinguishing hip flexion from lumbar flexion: teaching the motion pattern

Once static postures are easily attained, motion patterns are developed. The initial objective of this critical component of stage 1 is to continue the progression with the person consciously separating hip rotation from lumbar motion when flexing the torso. For the more difficult cases, we typically begin by demonstrating on ourselves lumbar flexion versus rotation about the hips. Other techniques that we have found particularly helpful are as follows:

▪ Have your patient place one hand on the tummy while placing the other over the lumbar surface. This way they can feel whether the spine is locked and motion is occurring about the hips (see figure 10.6).

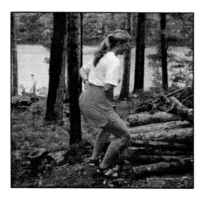

Figure 10.6 For people who are not "body aware" and are unable to adopt a neutral or a flexed spine on command, we suggest rehearsing the spine-neutral position and hip (not lumbar) flexion while doing squat motions before exertion.

- When all of these attempts fail, we resort to the final technique: having the athlete perform the "midnight movement" (rolling the pelvis). This is lumbar motion (no figure here)! Interestingly, some patients who found sex painful never associated pelvis tilting with lumbar flexion. Pointing this out to them often facilitates their making the next leap in spine position awareness.

Once you begin to see that any, or several, of the techniques just listed are helping these "difficult" patients/athletes, you may test to see if the concept of the neutral spine is becoming ingrained. One such task is to take a stick and ask the patient to knock down an imaginary spider web overhead in the corner of the room. If she loses the lumbar neutral posture, point it out to her so she can correct it.

Some people have a very difficult time remembering the protective neutral spine pattern. We tell these types of athletes to begin each training session or when performing an exertion in daily living:

1. Stop before performing an exertion,
2. Place the hands on the tummy and lumbar region,
3. Practise a few knee bends with the motion about the hips and not the lumbar spine, and
4. Then perform the lift (see figure 10.6).

This practice is effective for many people.

Perfecting the "hip hinge"

The motion in the previous section is called the "hip hinge". Some have more difficulty in perfecting the hinge than others. Here are two more movement cues to assist these people.

The first approach is to eliminate other joints in the body by having the person kneel, then drop their buttocks back to their heels (See figure 10.7). This isolates the hips and causes a 45-degree path of motion for the hips to drift posteriorly. This will also set up subsequent squat technique training.

Another technique has the person starting in a standing posture. Have them adopt the "shortstop" posture from baseball (see figure 10.8). The hands are placed on the thighs just above the knees. Upper body weight is rested through the arms on the hands. The pelvis drifts posteriorly and any lumbar flexion is corrected to a neutral posture. Then have the person "hip hinge" into an upright standing posture. Once again, this is another nice motion pattern exercise for the squat.

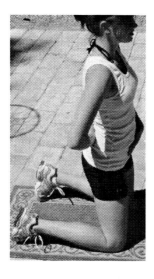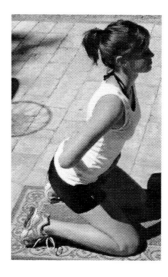

Figure 10.7 An isolation technique for grooving the hip hinge. All motion is constrained to the hips because of the kneeling posture.

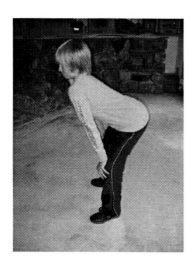

Figure 10.8 Moving from the "shortstop" posture to upright can also assist in grooving the standing hip hinge. Slid the hands down the front of the thighs to rest just above the patellas. The hips drift posteriorly. Slide the hands up the thighs only hinging at he hips.

A note on spine stability, spine motion and control

Clinicians who attend the initial clinical course that I am asked to teach indicate that they misinterpret my textbook writings. They sometimes comment that they did not realize that the spine is allowed to move and yet still maintain stability. The answer, once again, is that it depends on the person. Sometimes getting the intransigent bad back to turn the corner for symptom control requires restricted spine motion. As progress is made, and control is well established, spine movement may very well begin. I think the point of confusion lies in the paradigm shift to have a book like this emphasize stability first without motion, and if successful, pain-free motion will return. Yet other people present with their spine locked into a posture, fearful of any spine motion whatsoever, and they suffer from chronic crushing loads and muscle fatigue cramps. This class of person does not need more stability. Still others will have regional instability (usually lumbar) with regional stiffness (usually thoracic). They need different considerations yet again. The message here is to choose the appropriate clinical tool. The following are approaches to establish motion and motor patterns that assist for pain control and prepare for the loading that occurs with the eventual serious training for performance.

Locking the ribcage onto the pelvis

For many athletes, learning to lock the ribcage on the pelvis is essential for injury prevention and for performance – of course it is not for all. We have developed and used the following progression to salvage athletic careers from several sports. We use the wall roll to establish the locking pattern. The motion pattern is accompanied by the abdominal brace motor pattern (see figure 10.9). The progression continues with a floor roll and scramble. Discipline is directed towards maintaining a neutral spine with no spine motion at all in the entire motion of rolling, the scramble up, and perhaps the eventual bursting into a sprint or hopping pattern (see figure 10.10 and 10.11 for an exercise to reinforce the pattern). This way the foundation for developing optimal hip drive becomes pre-programmed. Another terrific exercise for transitioning into performance is the Turkish Getup (see figure 10.12), where the spine posture is controlled and the overhead weight is steered as the body learns more movement strategies that maintain torso stiffness while driving with other extremities.

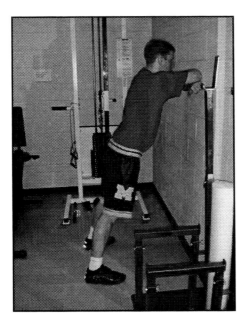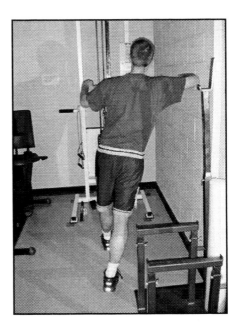

Figure 10.9 The wall roll begins with the athlete in the "plank" with both elbows planted on the wall. Focus is in spine/hip posture to find the "sweet spot" with minimal pain. The abdominals are braced and the ribcage is "locked" on the pelvis. The athlete pivots on the balls of the feet pulling one elbow off the wall. No spine motion is permitted.

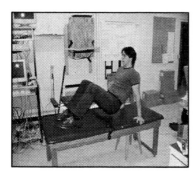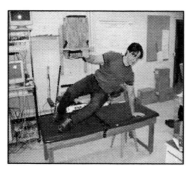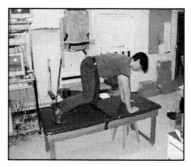

Figure 10.10 The floor roll begins with the athlete in contact with the floor with the hands and feet. The ribcage is locked to the pelvis with an abdominal brace. The athlete pivots and rolls completely about 360 degrees. No spine motion is permitted.

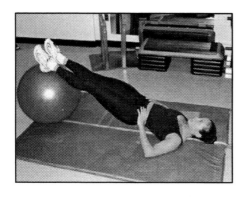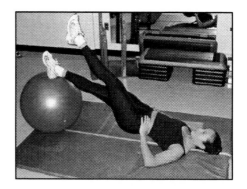
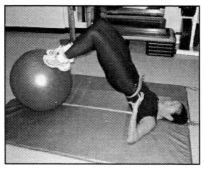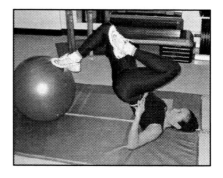

Figure 10.11 Advanced ball exercises can groove the "locked" back. No spine motion is permitted.

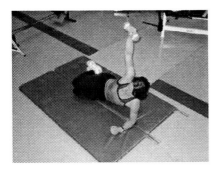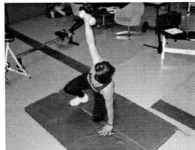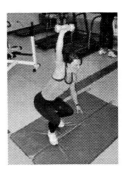

Figure 10.12 In the Turkish Getup, a neutral and braced spine teaches movement strategies to steer and drive the overhead weight.

Mental imagery

Mental imagery is useful for both spine position and muscle activation awareness, and is critical for ultimate performance. Imagery is more than simply visualizing the motion. It incorporates replicating the kinesthetic sensations associated with an action. The following is a general protocol that we have adapted from the imagery literature for use with spine training.

Steps of mental imagery:

1. Focus on feeling the surface under the feet/buttocks, etc. Whatever body part is touching a surface, be aware of the sensation. Be aware of the magnitude of the force. Is the force compressive, or are shearing components detectable? Should there be shearing or frictional components – or is it technique error? Correct kinesthetic sensations are critical.

2. Practice simple motions such as tightening and then relaxing specific muscles in different areas of the body. Then graduate to performing the abdominal brace.

3. Palpate, and have the athlete self-palpate, the muscle involved while he is attempting to tighten and relax it. Sometimes a full-body mirror is helpful. The focus for the athlete is on the specific muscle(s) involved.

4. Perform motions slowly, chunking them into segments and sequences, then image the total motion. For example, beginning with a simple task such as a forward reach, image the neutral spine, activate the extensors and the bracing abdominals and finally initiate the motion about the hips.

5. Practice the imagery independent of physical action. Of course, the athlete will have already been successful in learning spine position awareness, proper muscle control, and desirable motion patterns.

Other imagery exercises to develop motion/motor awareness

The imagery process can be enhanced with some simple techniques. We have athletes draw the movement on a piece of paper. Then we ask them to draw specific joint patterns of motion and other motion variables such as the center of mass, the base of support, and any others such as a hand-held bar trajectory. This is sometimes revealing and assists in documenting whether the athlete has the proper mechanics in their mind to image correctly.

In summary, a critical feature of imagery is to understand and "see" the entire motion and event. Imagery is about seeing and feeling each component needed for eventual success. Failure to image and control each component can be disastrous. Jerzy Gregorek, holder of several world records in Olympic lifting, related to me a wonderful story of imagery and outcome. The clean and jerk is a two-stage lift. In his final lift for the championship, the weight was cleaned and the bar was resting across the upper pecs as he prepared for the jerk. At that point he knew that he had won the championship. He "smiled internally" - not an external smile that any observer would detect, but a smile in his brain. He lost the lift and the championship that year. His imagery and mental control lost the moment and leapt forward to victory, allowing victory to escape. As a side note, several high performance people have suggested that "smiling" inhibits muscle activation. There is some evidence to suggest that this is true. It may well turn out that ultimate muscle contraction requires a "game face"!

Important abdominal patterns

Maintaining a mild contraction of the abdominal wall can help ensure sufficient spine stability and in some demanding tasks is essential, however this is the beginning of an enormous controversy. Many believe that intentionally activating the transverse abdominis and focussing training effort on this muscle with a "hollowing" procedure is helpful for bad backs and athletes alike. Hollowing involves intentionally sucking in the abdominal wall towards the spine. In fact, training transverse abdominis in this way compromises stability and creates spine dysfunction!

Abdominal hollowing is dysfunctional: abdominal brace instead

"Hollowing", while intended to activate the transverse abdominis, has been documented to actually decrease stability in some situations. In contrast, the abdominal brace has been proven to enhance stability (Kavcic and McGill, 2004). When the bracing contraction is performed correctly, no geometric change occurs in the abdominal wall. In other words, rather than "hollowing in" the abdominal wall, the athlete simply activates all the abdominal muscles to make them stiff. We call this contraction abdominal bracing.

Teaching abdominal bracing

We begin by having the athlete/patient standing palpating their active low back extensors while the lumbar torso is slightly flexed, extending slowly until moment equilibrium is reached and the extensors shut off. This is the position of rest for the spine and is often reported as a posture of least symptoms in many. This position can also be reached sooner in the extension motion by retracting the shoulders, holding the arms back and pushing the chest out (see figure 10.13). At this point, the athlete performs the abdominal brace and they feel the extensors re-activate, proving the general bracing girdle that is produced with the abdominal brace technique.

This is another critical difference between the hollow and the brace. The brace produces a true muscular girdle around the spine with both the abdominals and the extensors being active to buttress against buckling and shear instability. In a most recent study we have found that there is a missing component to spine stability when we quantify the role of all the abdominal muscles. We suspect that activating the entire wall (rectus, the obliques, and transverse) creates a binding of the three layers to produce an augmented stiffness and stability – similar to the glue between layers of wood in plywood. Again, this super-stiffness is only achieved with the brace.

Some individuals have difficulty in understanding the conscious abdominal contraction that constitutes the brace. For these people we do the following. Generally, to demonstrate abdominal bracing to the athlete, we stiffen one of our own joints, such as an elbow, by simultaneously activating the flexors and extensors. The athlete then palpates the joint both before and after we stiffen it. Then we ask the individual to attempt to stiffen her own joint through simultaneous activation of flexors and extensors. Once she can successfully stiffen various peripheral joints, we demonstrate (again on ourselves, with athlete palpation) the same technique in the torso, achieving abdominal bracing. Finally, we again ask her to replicate the technique in her own torso. Occasionally, we use a portable EMG monitor so the athlete can learn through biofeedback what 5%, 10%, or 80% of maximum contraction feels like (see figure 10.14). We use similar devices to teach patients how to maintain the contraction while on a wobble board and in functional situations such as when picking up a child, getting on and off the toilet, and getting in and out of cars. For athletes, we choose appropriate and familiar training tasks.

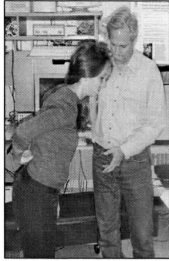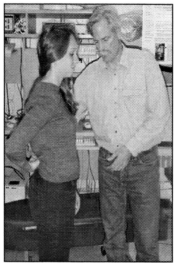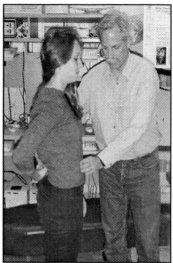

Figure 10.13 Teaching the abdominal brace. Feel the extensors contracted, then extend to an upright posture to the point where they shut off. Without moving, contract the abdominals and feel the extensors contract once again. This is a brace.

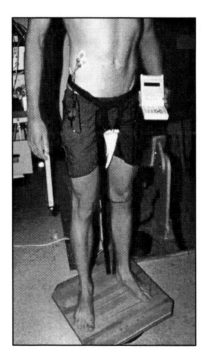

Figure 10.14 EMG biofeedback devices are an economical way to provide feedback to the patient regarding the level of abdominal activation during any type of functional task, from standing on a wobble board to lifting on a platform.

A note on "fascial raking"

Some low level patients are poor at activating the abdominal wall. This type of person can be assisted in contraction with a direct stimulus called "fascial raking". Yet other high performance athletes can use the technique to obtain more complete contraction of the abdominal wall to enhance the production of superstiffness for performance.

We have learned many things from our work with intramuscular electrodes that have to be implanted in the abdominal wall to monitor deep muscle activity. A valuable discovery involved the muscle activation facilitation mechanism. For example, as the canula (large bore needle) penetrates the skin in the abdominal region and touches the fascia of the oblique muscles, it creates a characteristic pain. The pain can be reproduced by taking a long fingernail, digging it into the oblique muscle and "raked". This produces a pain that can be referred to as "scratchy". Typically it causes the individual to respond by contracting the muscle wall.

To encourage complete activation of the abdominal wall, have the individual lie on their back. Prepare by having them place their hands under the lumbar region to prevent the spine from flattening to the floor (this results in spine flexion and an increase in the risk of injury – don't allow it to happen). Instruct them to contract the abdominal wall. Facilitate this by taking your hand with a wide grip, placing the thumb lateral to the rectus abdominis and the fingertips lateral to the other rectus – you are gripping into the oblique muscles (see Figure 10.15). Do not grip the rectus abdominis. Now instruct them to initiate a slight flexion motion with the locus of rotation in the middle of the sternum (not in the lumbar spine). The head, neck and shoulders hardly move. Now "rake" the abdominals, asking the individual to "fight with your abdominal wall", and "contract". Irritate the obliques by squeezing your thumb towards your fingertips, raking the fascia. Encourage good effort while you are stimulating the abdominal wall.

For the performance, athlete this procedure trains the abdominal wall for short range stiffness enhancement, forming the foundation for eventual plyometric training of the abdominal wall. Even accomplished athletes will report instant performance enhancement on tasks such as pull-ups with simultaneous fascial raking.

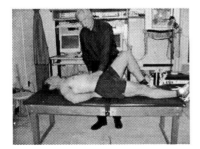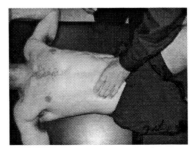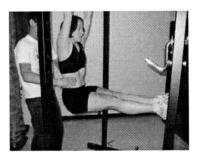

Figure 10.15 With the individual voluntarily contracting their abdominal wall, facilitate more complete contraction by "raking" the fascia over the obliques. Make sure that your fingers are lateral to the rectus abdominis. Try this while in a hanging kip (right panel) and feel the more robust contraction and better performance.

Building squat patterns

A good back needs healthy gluteal muscle function, while performance demands balanced hip power about each axis. This section describes some hip motor patterns that inhibit performance and compromise back health, together with documenting several training progressions to address them.

The crossed-pelvis syndrome was described in chapter 4, where the gluteal complex appears to be inhibited during squatting patterns and is very common in those with a history of back troubles (together with some others as well). Interestingly, we still do not know if the crossed-pelvis syndrome exists prior to back troubles or is a consequence of having them. Nonetheless, the syndrome is noticeable in both athletes and normals referred to our research clinic. This results in two concerns: First, those with aberrant gluteal patterns cannot spare their backs during squatting patterns since they use the hamstrings and erector spinae to drive the extension motion. Subsequently, the erector spinae loads up the lumbar spine. In this way, healthy gluteal patterns are needed to spare the back. Second, it is impossible to re-build optimal squat performance, either for strength or hip extensor power, without well integrated hip extensor patterns. In fact the reason why many athletes fail to properly rehabilitate is because of the emphasis on strengthening philosophies without addressing the aberrant gluteal patterns first. This failure by many strength coaches is one of the reasons for athletes to be sent to our research clinic. A strength and power athlete will continue to be compromised with chronic back troubles until these motor patterns are addressed.

Retraining the gluteals cannot be performed with traditional squat exercises that utilize a barbell on the back. Performing a traditional squat requires little hip abduction. Consequently there is little gluteus medius activation and the gluteus maximus activation is delayed during the squat until lower squat angles are reached (155 lbs was the bar load) (see figure 10.16). It's a quadriceps exercise. In contrast to the traditional squat, a one-legged squat activates the gluteus medius immediately to assist in the frontal plane hip drive necessary for leaping, running etc, together with sooner integration of gluteus maximus during the squat descent motion (see figure 10.17). Muscle activation levels at the bottom of the "squat" are compared in an experimentally naïve athlete performing a one leg "step up", back squat with a bar, and a single leg squat (see figure 10.18) A sample progression for retraining the gluteals is now provided.

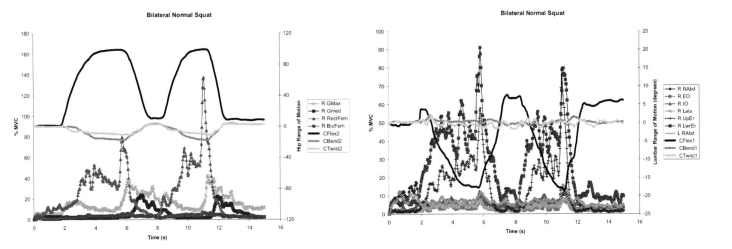

Figure 10.16 The traditional squat exercise with a barbell on the shoulders produces non-functional activation patterns of hip extension and spine stabilization for many athletes. Gluteus medius activation is too low, as is gluteus maximus activation until quite deep in the squat position. These types of squats are dominated by the quadriceps and can be good quad exercises, but fail the performance athlete.

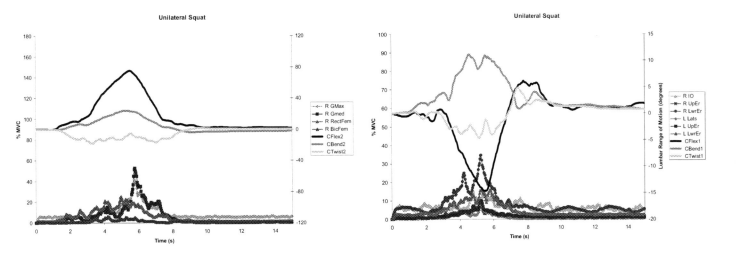

Figure 10.17 In contrast to the traditional squat, a one-legged squat activates the gluteus medius immediately to assist in the frontal plane hip drive necessary for leaping, running etc, together with sooner integration of gluteus maximus higher in the squat motion.

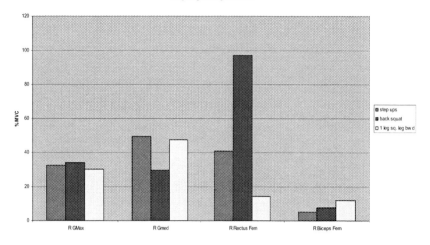

Figure 10.18 Traditional squats are superior for challenging the quadriceps. Single-legged squats, even with no additional weight, are superior for training the gluteus medius.

Re-training the gluteal complex

1. Learning to activate gluteus medius

The first stage involves isolating gluteus medius. Once again, the athlete needs to "feel" the muscle and perceive its activation. Lay on the side. Place the thumb on the ASIS and reach with the fingers posteriorly – the tips will be over the gluteus medius (see figure 10.19). With the hips and knees flexed, spread the knees apart with the feet remaining together acting as a hinge. Feel with the fingers the Glut Med activate. This manoeuvre is to simply activate the Glut Med and should not be considered a strengthening exercise. There is no need to offer resistance at this stage (resistance is imposed later during strength training); true isolation of the Glut Med is not possible and other muscles are active. In this posture, the external hip rotators are recruited. Extending the hips to a neutral posture and repeating the movement tends to activate the Glut Med with a greater integration with the Tensor Fascia Latae. An optional exercise that can be added to the progression is the lateral leg raise with the athlete maintaining finger contact with the Glut Med. This will add to the challenge and begin "strength" training (see figure 10.20). Finally, a weight bag can be added to the ankle for strength training. This progression will enable the athlete to develop skill in conscious and unconscious Glut Med activation during all activities. Those who do perform traditional barbell squats will now find that conscious external hip rotation and abduction will achieve higher Glut Med activation – and improved performance.

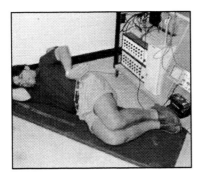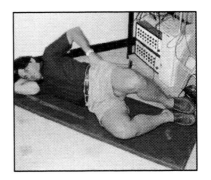

Figure 10.19 Anchoring the thumb on the ASIS and reaching around with the finger tips should position them to land on gluteus medius. Opening the knees like a clam shell will allow the athlete to feel the glut medius activation.

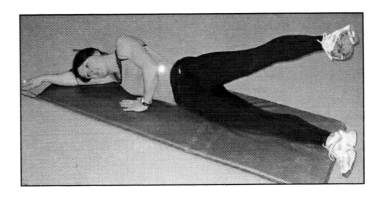

Figure 10.20 Lateral leg raises with isometric external rotation effort prepare the athlete for eventual "strength training". The abdominals are braced.

2. Learning to activate gluteus maximus

Lying on the back with the knees flexed and the feet on the floor, the athlete places the fingers on Glut Max to feel its activity. Image a coin placed in the gluteal fold which must not be dropped. Activate glut max by "squeezing" the buttocks, not by creating hip extension. Focus on the pelvis at this stage to ensure that no pelvic tilting occurs. The lumbar spine remains in neutral posture (see figure 10.21). Then, once the activation has been mastered, begin bridging the torso off the floor. The clinician/coach at this stage feels the hamstrings. Those who are hamstring dominant and gluteal deficient will immediately activate the hamstrings just prior to motion occurring. This pattern is very dominant in those who have the aberrant crossed-pelvic syndrome, but is also seen in some sport-specific athletes such as cyclists. Power athletes must override this hamstring pattern. The athlete must repeatedly try to begin the bridging action without hamstring activity (or at least only mild activity).

To override the hamstring dominant tendency in some athletes requires coaching and cueing from the coach/clinician. For these challenging cases we place our foot against the athlete's toes, instructing them to continue with the preparatory gluteal activation and stimulating the quads by very mildly attempting to extend the knees. Buttressing their feet with the clinician's foot assists this (see figure 10.22). A gentle stroke on the quads to assist their imaging and perception also facilitates this pattern. Then repeat the attempt to bridge with gluteal dominance. Now maintain the pattern and try a one legged bridge (see figure 10.23). This skill must be perfected prior to more challenging hip extensor strength and power training. Once mastered, squat performance will improve.

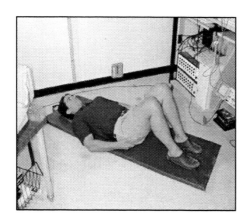 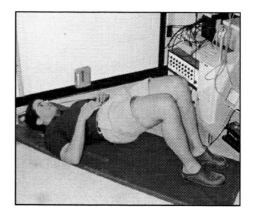

Figure 10.21 Imaging squeezing the gluteal cheeks prior to performing the back bridge will assist in grooving gluteal dominant hip extension patterns. Then perform the bridge with focus on the gluteals throughout the full range.

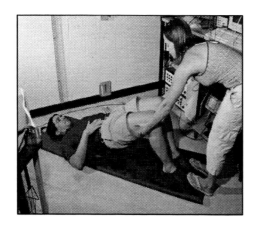

Figure 10.22 Some hamstring dominant athletes will need more assistance to learn to activate the gluteals. This is accomplished with mild quadriceps activation by pushing their toes into the coach's foot, creating knee extensor torque. Mild hip external rotation effort may also help. Focus on glutual activation to dampen hamstring activity.

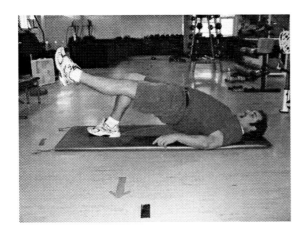

Figure 10.23 A one-legged bridge is now attempted while maintaining the gluteal dominance to create hip extension torque.

3.   Beginning basic squat patterns

After ensuring proper hip hinge mechanics, we would begin a basic squat progression with a "potty squat" (see figure 10.24). Sitting on the corner of a chair or a stool, the athlete positions the feet under the body to squat rise off the chair without using any momentum shifts. The lumbar spine is neutral and braced and this begins to groove a good two-legged squat position. Then progressing to a standing position, the arms are held out laterally and moved in front of the body as the athlete squats (see figure 10.25). Of course, emphasis is placed on maintaining a neutral lumbar spine and abdominal bracing. The "Goblet squat" from Dan John also has proved very effective in adding depth to the squat. The athlete can shift side to side while maintaining perfect spine posture working the hip joints.

Progressing to a single-legged squat involves the same arm motion to assist balance. As the single legged squat is performed, the free leg is held in front as if the athlete were reaching with the toes to a distant object in front of them on the floor. The free leg is held behind and the knee is touched to the floor, or the toe is reached with an outstretched leg to a distant object behind. Finally, the free leg is reached out to a distant object placed laterally during the squat. Variations include working the free leg to different positions "around the clock" (see figure 10.26, while muscle activation levels are shown in figure 10.27). This challenges the full hip extensor, flexor, and abduction torque generators together with keen motor control. Full integration with the pelvis and lumbar spine is achieved with emphasis on the appropriate motor and motion patterns. Specific focus is directed towards maintaining a neutral lumbar spine. Focus on hip motion and developing the extensor drive through the hips with a stiff torso.

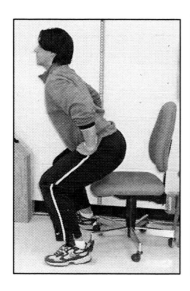
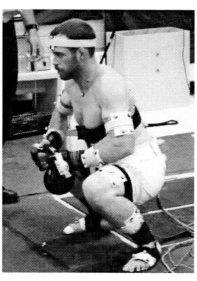

Figure 10.24 The potty squat (far left). Feet are placed so that no momentum is needed to rise from the seat. The goblet squat (left) while holding a kettlebell adds depth with balance and form. The weight is shifted between the feet working into a deeper squat.

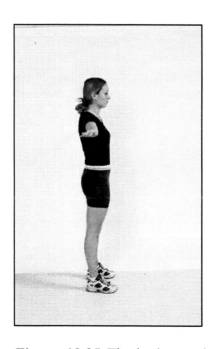
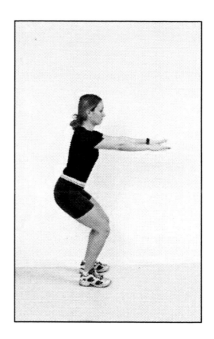

Figure 10.25 The basic two-legged squat emphasizing abdominal bracing and hip motion. The hips move along a trajectory that is about 45 degrees from the horizontal (back and down). Note that the knees hardly move yet they are flexing to allow the hips to translate back.

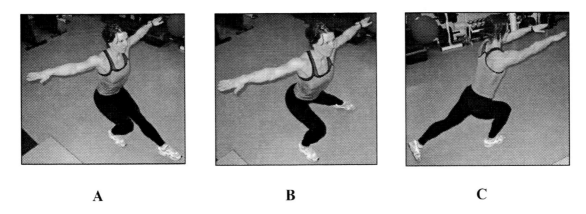

A   B   C

Figure 10.26 Single-legged squat progressions with the leg to the front (a), side (b) and behind (c). The abdominals are braced, the lumbar spine neutral and the mental focus of the athlete is on hip extension torque. Notice that the hips are drifted posteriorly during the descent to place more emphasis on the gluteals for hip extension, unloading both the knees and the back.

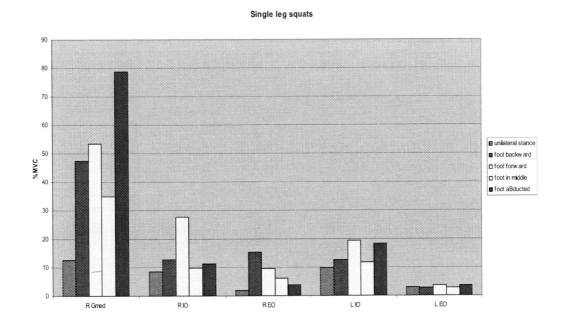

Figure 10.27 Muscle activation levels for standing and the 3 styles of one-legged squat shown in figure 10.26.

The progression may continue with the use of devices to add lability to the task or resistance challenge. Simply standing on a piece of "2x4" wood block increases the balance requirement and adds the challenge to integrate the motor control from the ankle up through all joints, including the torso. The "2x4" can be placed in line with the foot or across the foot to enhance the ankle plantar flexor challenge (see figure 10.28). Wobble boards may be used in various planes to achieve the same effect.

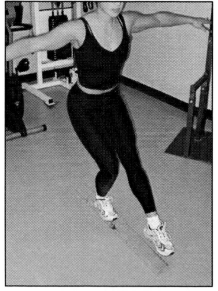 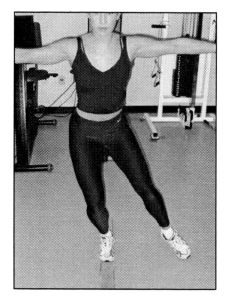

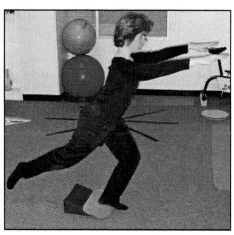 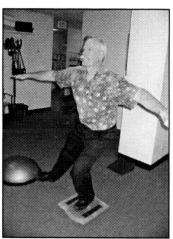

Figure 10.28 Adding lability to the squat with a piece of 2x4 wood block (top) facilitates more leg activation that progresses up the linkage. Note the emphasis to drift the hips posteriorly to focus on gluteal integration. More lability can be added to teach "steering" of the force (bottom).

One-legged squat progressions progress to the "bowler's squat" (see case study in chapter 14). Here, rotational balance and power is trained via integration of the swing leg generating torsional inertia. This is progressed so that the repetitions are performed at great speed. This can be very helpful for those training running change of direction, for example (see figure 10.29 where the progression helped an injured dancer achieve the arabesque).

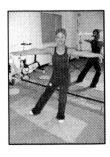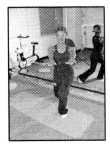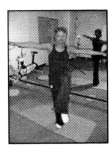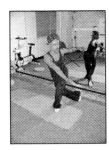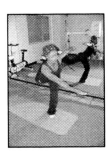

Figure 10.29 Progression of one-legged squats, to the bowler's squat, culminating in the arabesque.

Finally, the one-legged squat patterns can become as functional as possible by integrating arm reaches to the floor, adding weights (with dumbbells and cables) to the hands. Complex motions involving squatting with arm motions overhead can train all sorts of sporting manoeuvres (see figure 10.30).

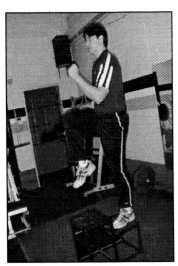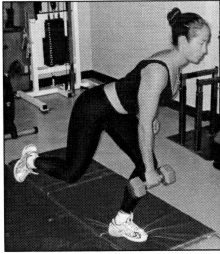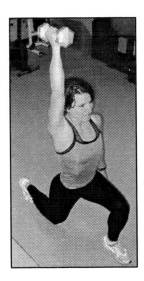

Figure 10.30 Some complex squat progressions including step-ups, one-legged weight pulls and lunge squats.

Star exercises

One method growing in popularity involves what is known as the star exercises. These are designed to promote range of motion and ability to move quickly, efficiently and safely in all directions and are very appropriate for athletes such as racket sport players. A plus sign (+) and an "X" are drawn on the floor with a common intersection. Participants stand on the intersection (see figure 10.31) and practice movement patterns that have been identified as essential by moving into each star quadrant. This is ideal for pre-training patterns that prepare for the grooving of skilled patterns such as a tennis serve, for example. Co-contraction of the abdominals is emphasized together with lumbar motion within the patient's safe zone.

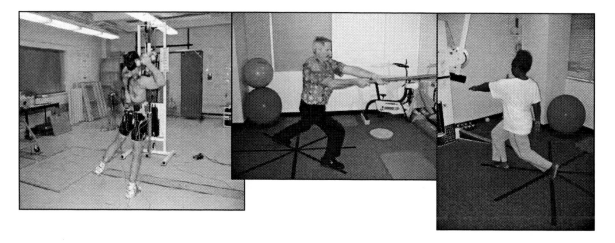

Figure 10.31 Star exercises facilitate basic squat and lunge patterns into all quadrants.

Active flexibility and stretching for back performance

The science of stretching has been covered previously in this book. While it is appropriate for some athletes, it should not be blindly considered appropriate for all. To summarize:

1.   Stretching immediately prior to exercise does not prevent injury. This is not to suggest that it has no role in training, only that one should question its emphasis during a warm-up.

2.   Stretching and bending the spine soon after rising from bed results in enormous strain in the annulus of the disc and reduces the load tolerance of the disc.

3. Stretching appears to increase the tolerance of the athlete to increased range of motion but not the actual stiffness. This means the athlete feels less pain with the same force applied about a joint but the joint does not necessarily gain more motion.

4. The neuromuscular responses to stretching together with performance indicators from a variety of athletes support replacing static stretching with "active flexibility", particularly for the back.

Active flexibility for the back

We have searched for the most spine-conserving method of moving, or mobilizing, the back. The cat-camel motion, while on all fours, proved to result in the lowest of spine loads and is often the best starting point (see figure 10.32). Emphasis must be made here that the cat-camel is intended as a motion exercise, NOT a stretch. The objective is to enhance active flexibility, specifically controlled motion. We have measured the viscosity in the spine/torso, which is the friction or resistance to motion, and have found that only 6-10 cycles of motion are required to reduce the friction. More cycles do not reduce the viscous friction further. Optimal technique involves several key points: Have the hands directly beneath the shoulders and the knees directly beneath the hips. The entire spine is engaged in synchronous motion with the cervical, thoracic and lumbar sections moving in flexion and extension. Proper form requires hip motion to enable proper lumbar function. "Sticking the butt out" when in extension is an image that works with many athletes. Before initiating motion lightly brace the abdominal wall. Cues may be provided by the coach/clinician by brushing the abdominal wall throughout the motion cycle to ensure that the brace is not lost. The emphasis is on motion rather than "pushing" at the end ranges of flexion and extension. If pain is present use it to guide the suitable range of motion – never move into a painful zone. Some athletes may wish to incorporate lateral bending motion while in this position as well.

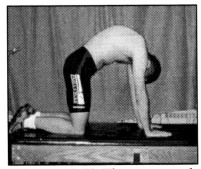 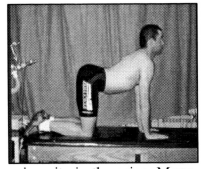

Figure 10.32 The cat-camel motion reduces viscosity in the spine. Many key points regarding this motion are listed in the text.

Progressions of "active flexibility" are highly sport and athlete specific. A butterfly swimmer is a rare athlete in that spinal motion increases power and efficiency. For them, utilize the gym balls to train spine motion with stabilizing control and endurance. However, for most other athletes, active flexibility requires whole body motions in "playing position" which is usually an upright position on the feet. For example, the "potty squat" was introduced previously in this chapter. Performing the potty squat with a bar on the shoulders requires active flexibility in the hips and ankles but without constant reminding from a coach, some athletes slip into poor form. It is still easy to cheat once the buttocks have risen from the stool if discipline is lost. Another active flexibility technique that is helpful for many athletes is the "snatch squat". It is very difficult to cheat while performing the snatch squat and it achieves the objectives of active flexibility. Namely, the extremities are challenged with motion, the back is locked into a strong and safe position and strength is required throughout the motion, as is joint and whole body stability.

The snatch movement is demonstrated by Jerzy Gregorek, a holder of several world records and superstar performance coach currently based in Los Angeles. Taking a light wooden dowel in the hands, the hands are raised overhead, over the ball of the foot (see figure 10.33). Hands are positioned close together on the bar and the knees are close together. See how far the athlete can descend with the bar kept over the shoulder and the mid-foot. This is an excellent qualifying test to see if an athlete is ready to begin lifting training. It is also an excellent exercise for revealing body locations that need enhancement. For example, a thoracic spine that is not extending properly will restrict the ability to place the hands over the shoulders. Likewise, compromised shoulder motion will cause the same movement symptom, but the snatch squat helps to locate the hitch in the active flexibility chain. A lack of leg drive and strength is also revealed in this exercise. A very flexible person may have perfect form on the descent but may not be able to rise. Adding some weight on a bar often is used to reveal a mismatch between available flexibility and strength. Those who have perfect form but are unable to rise are revealed.

Moving to other forms of the snatch squat, the hands are placed much wider on the bar. The athlete can groove the descending and ascending pattern. Progressing to the snatch squat, the bar is held directly over the shoulders while the perfect squat is grooved (see figure 10.34). Jerzy demonstrates some common technique errors that greatly increase the risk of back injury, usually involving a loss of the spine position, locked and braced (see figure 10.35). Lifting with a loaded bar, even with only a light weight is a good test of technique (see figure 10.36). Without a locked back and hands over the shoulders, the lift is impossible. Don't worry if the athlete cannot do the snatch – it is a very special and difficult lift.

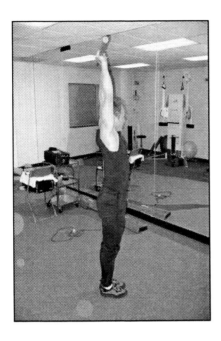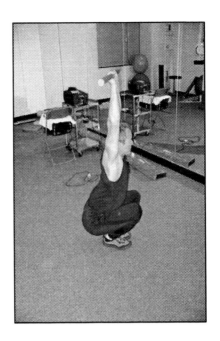

Figure 10.33 A good test of active flexibility for a lifter is to perform a modified snatch squat with the arms and knees together. Problem areas are easily located.

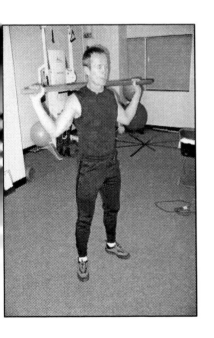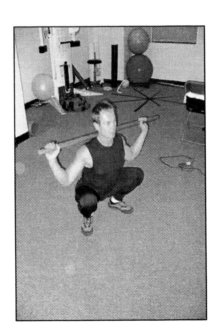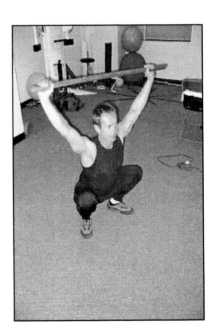

Figure 10.34 Grooving perfect snatch squat technique with the bar directly over the shoulders, elbow and mid foot.

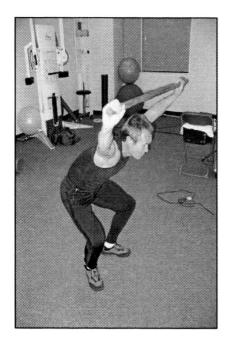 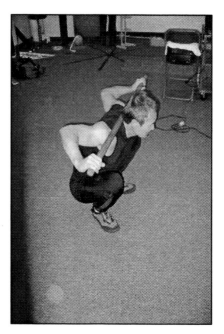

Figure 10.35 Common snatch squat errors usually include a loss of the locked neutral and braced spine (left) and poor bar trajectory, which may be caused by insufficient active flexibility at the shoulders (right), the thoracic spine in extension, the hips in flexion and the ankles in dorsi flexion.

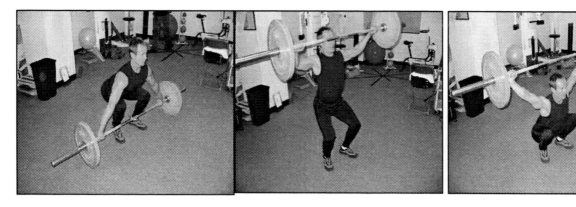

Figure 10.36 The snatch lift with weight is unique in that it is almost impossible without good uppe᷈ back and shoulder form. The lower back posture is critical.

An excellent active flexibility exercise from the squat family is the wall squat. Here, the athlete faces the wall and is only a short distance away from it. A hip-hinging squat is performed and the upper body is shifted from side to side challenging active flexibility from many different angles (see figure 10.37). Other athletes benefit from training the lunge squat to enhance active flexibility. The bar is maintained over the shoulders and an upright, braced spine (see figure 10.37).

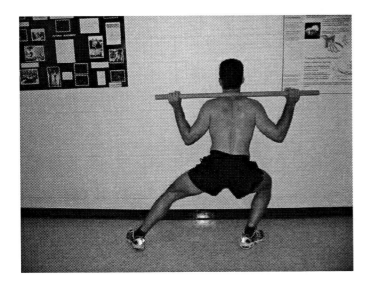

Figure 10.37 "Wall squats" are an excellent "active flexibility" hip exercise to enhance mobility and performance in many sporting tasks requiring hip drive and controlled torso stiffness. Shift the upper body from side-to-side. Try and cover as large an area as possible with the nose to the wall.

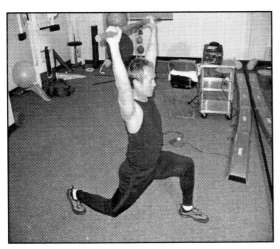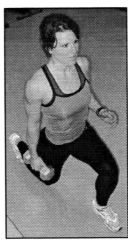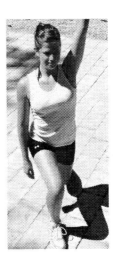

Figure 10.38 The lunge squat can be a wonderful active flexibility exercise given the combination of challenges: range of motion, strength, endurance and whole body balance. Focus is directed towards a neutral spine position and a muscular brace. The walking lunge adds dynamic mobility – emphasis is on pushing the arm straight up through the torso region.

Many squat and overhead reach tasks are compromised because of poor thoracic spine mobility. Squatters carry the bar too high loosing leverage for this reason. Here is a nice thoracic mobilizer that enhances lifting performance by assisting better bar carriage, and other upright tasks (see figure 10.39).

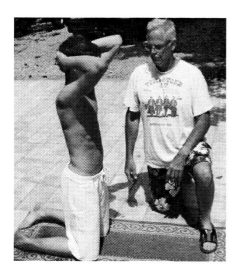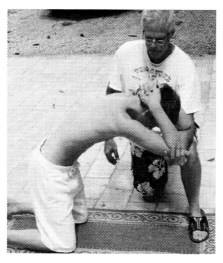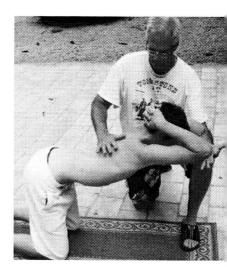

Figure 10.39 Thoracic mobility enhancement begins with the hands clasped behind the head. The elbows are planted on the assistant's thigh. Gentle pressure is applied through the elbow to the thigh for about 8 seconds and released. Then the assistant "draws out" the elbows causing gentle thoracic extension. The hand on the back cues this motion. This is repeated several times.

Controlled mobility in the extremities is essential for active flexibility. Some technique errors have lead to bad backs in athletes or hindered their recovery from episodes of back injury. To prevent this from occurring, some guidelines are provided here to spare the back and lessen the risk of back troubles. I must emphasize the importance of technique: Too many good athletes continue to compromise their backs with silly notions about spine stretching. This is unfortunate, particularly when the solution is so easy with technique change.

Sparing the back while stretching the hips and knees

A general guideline for sparing the back is to maintain an upright torso posture while performing hip and knee static mobility work. Preservation of a neutral spine protects its passive tissues while forcing more mobility in the target joints. An upright torso minimizes the reaction torques, the associated muscle contraction, and spine load. Abdominal bracing is sometimes required for pain control. An example of this principle is provided using the lunge (see figure 10.40). Some clinicians recommend keeping the back leg straight, which causes patients to flex the torso forward. This is poor form for sparing the back. Figure 10.41 shows correct postures for stretching the quadriceps and the hip adductors.

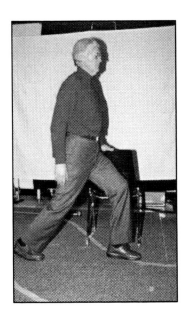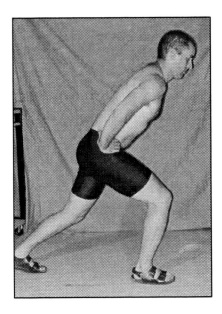

Figure 10.40 During early stages of active flexibility training the spine is spared, performing the lunge by maintaining an upright torso and a neutral spine curvature. This is good form (left panel). Some load their backs (right panel) by flexing the spine rather than the knee of the leg behind them, which is poor form.

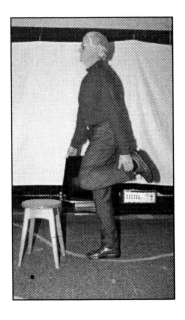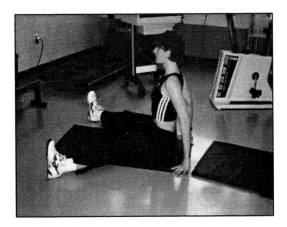

Figure 10.41 During stretching at joints other than the back, the spine is spared by maintaining the upright torso and neutral spine curve. This beginner is demonstrating that when stretching the quads, holding a chair for balance is a good way to ensure a straight back (left panel). The athlete shown (right panel) has sufficient hip flexion mobility to ensure an upright torso and a neutral spine during hip adductor work. Individuals who are unable to maintain this spine posture should forgo this exercise until they can achieve the required hip flexion mobility.

Once again Jerzy Gregorek demonstrates perfect form for hip flexion mobility which protects the back and enhances the hip mobilizing objective, together with demonstrating poor form. I am disheartened to see the poor form that is often accepted by clinicians and coaches alike in their athletes while stretching – be vigilant and create better athletes (see figures 10.42 to 10.46).

A terrific active flexibility exercise for the gluteal muscles – and one that takes the gluteus maximus through its range of motion under load with control is the "hip airplane" (see figure 10.46). This exercise has all of the components including balance and the need to steer strength through the supporting leg. It is a compulsory warm-up exercise for all lifters, runners, golfers, etc.

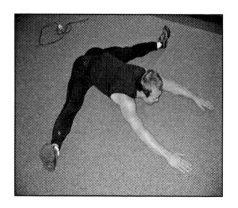
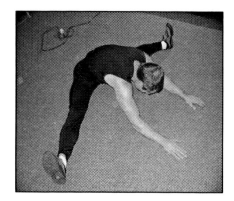

Figure 10.42 Enhancing active flexibility in hip flexion is performed with the torso braced and locked, directing more stretch to the hip (left panel). Poor form results with the misguided objective of flexing the spine and reaching the nose to the floor (right panel).

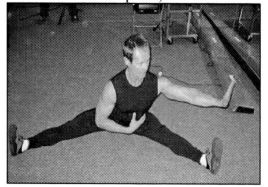
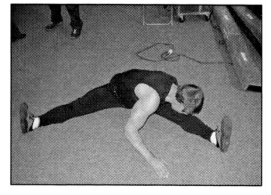

Figure 10.43 Variations to enhance hip mobility follow the same principles. Correct form on the left, poor form on the right.

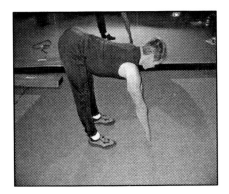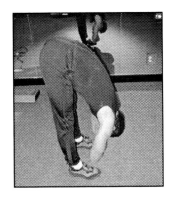

Figure 10.44 When standing, similar principles apply. The back locked in neutral position is correct and directs more mobility to the hips (left panel). Flexing the spine reduces the effectiveness of active hip flexibility for performance (right panel).

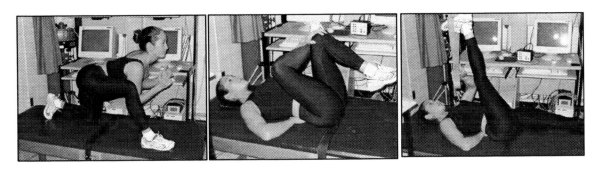

Figure 10.45 A sprinter demonstrates spine sparing but wisely chosen specific stretches. The back is buttressed in neutral with a hand placed in the lumbar region.

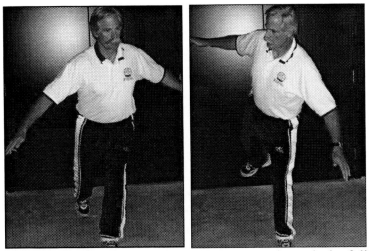

Figure 10.46 The hip airplane takes the gluteus maximus through the full range of motion, under load, in a balance challenge needing perfect steering of strength. The rib cage is locked on the pelvis with a brace, and the pelvis is flexed on the supporting hip. Then the hip is rotated in full internal rotation followed by external rotation where the opposite hip is directed up.

Spasms in the psoas, which produce a shortening and hip extension restriction, are common in those with back troubles (McGill et al, 2003). These people usually benefit from hip flexion "active flexibility" as will many athletes. Here the importance of the anatomy learned in chapter 3 is essential. For example, lunges are a good exercise for challenging strength, endurance, balance and mobility in the lower extremities. In this case, the objective is on hip flexion stretching in the extended hip. Many people talk about "iliopsoas" but there is no such thing to the elite athlete/coach/clinician. Iliacus crossing the hip is stretched in the traditional lunge. But psoas crosses the hip and all lumbar joints. It can only be isolated and stretched with a lunge that includes spine lateral bending with some twist and extension (see figure 10.47). A graphic illustration can be created by self-palpating the psoas tendon, which travels through the iliopectineal notch just medial to the rectus femoris tendon and under the inguinal ligament. Feel the soft psoas tendon with the traditional lunge and the subsequent tensioning as the spine is moved laterally, then slightly twisted and extended.

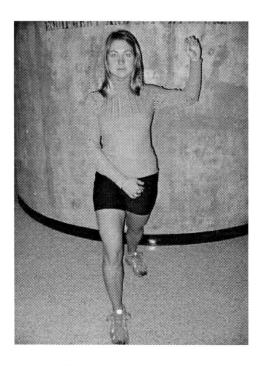 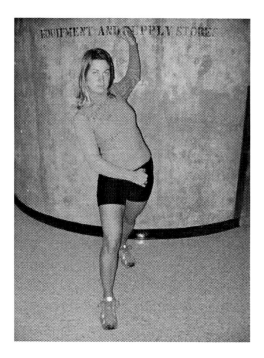

Figure 10.47 The psoas stretch is different from a typical "hip flexor" stretch which requires not only hip extension, but also torso lateral bending and slight twisting to isolate its tension from iliacus. "Feel" the psoas tendon tension just medial to the rectus femoris with the fingers.

The approaches introduced here form the essential first stage towards ultimate performance. Continually review and integrate these approaches as the progression continues through the next stages.

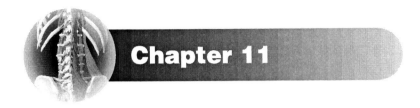

Chapter 11

Stage 2: Building Whole Body & Spine Stability

This section will address the building of whole body stability and balance first, followed by specific protocols for spine stability.

Whole body balance

As has been emphasized throughout this book, the optimal deployment of joint strength requires that the body be balanced to facilitate proper direction of force. Thus, balance is an essential pre-condition for performance. As well, we distinguish between static balance and dynamic balance. Achieving the ability to balance only requires a low volume of work, but it is best to perform daily as part of the workout routine. Several people have developed balance progressions from which many examples are shown here throughout (see figure 11.1). The following list consists of items to consider when developing balance progressions (from Gary Gray, 2002) and can form a checklist:

1. Bilateral stance
2. Unilateral stance
3. Arms and legs as counterbalance
4. No arms
5. Eyes closed
6. Varied surface
7. Apparatus (labile or reduced base of support)
8. Dynamic movement
9. Increase range of motion
10. Increase speed
11. Add reaction
12. Add external kinesthetic stimulus

Balance training examples that progress from less demanding to more demanding for the back

Leaning Tower
- Stand and begin swaying without moving the feet. First in the anterior/posterior direction, and then in the medial/lateral direction.

Hurdle Walk
- Step over object and then pause in one-legged balance and repeat for the next step.

Red Light/Green Light
- An excellent group exercise; athletes are provided with some instruction, either delivered verbally or by hand signal, to move. Upon the red light command, they stop dead and hold their balance. The cycle repeats itself with each red light-green light command.

Rhythmic Balance Exercises
- Use music to govern rate of movement and balance activity.

Wobble Board
- Practice throwing, catching, chopping, and sweeping movements while balancing – first on a 2x4 block of wood and then graduating to a wobble board. This was popularized by Dr Vladamir Janda in Prague.

90 Degree Jumps
- Jump and turn 90 deg and land, then jump back to the starting position. Close the eyes and repeat.

Scramble Up
- Start prone then scramble up (quickly) into a standing posture or a running gait. Then repeat with eyes closed. Note that for many athletes in rehabilitation training this demands excellent spine position awareness control. Each athlete would need to be qualified to partake in this training exercise to not risk exacerbating a back that could not tolerate rapid, but small, spine motions.

Perturbations on Wobble Board, add a Japanese Stick
- Begin standing on a wobble board. The athlete is then perturbed manually and must recover their balance. They may be prodded in different directions and at different levels of the body. The wobble board may by perturbed as well. Other stages to the progression may involve closing the eyes or standing on one leg.

Perturbations on a Swiss ball

- Take a balance position on a Swiss ball - perhaps sitting, kneeling for a motocross rider or lying for a swimmer. The athlete is perturbed or the ball is perturbed. Elastic bands may be attached to the hands or feet to create various effects on the athlete.

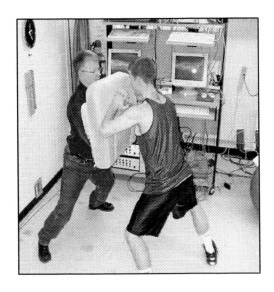 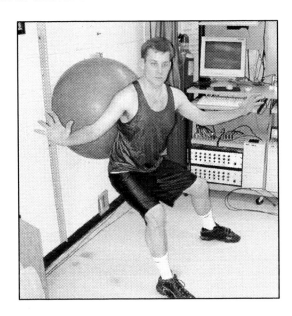

Figure 11.1 Balance tasks are only limited by a coach's imagination. Match them to the demands of the sport and use spine sparing principles. This example is "posting" training for a basketball player. Here the abdominals are braced, with fast and strategic footwork. Imprecise force application will result in rolling off the ball, making this exercise a good trainer.

Specific exercises to develop whole body balance

Soft Hands

Direct contact between client and patient/athlete can make a workout fun but when done to groove stabilizing patterns under controlled motion, it can be highly productive. The objective is to have the client motion patterns directed by the clinician/coach. In this way, the amount of mobility challenge can be controlled. This is a controlled way to begin training "active flexibility".

The client/athlete faces the coach holding his hand up, his palm touching the palm of the athlete's outstretched hand. The touch does not transmit force but simply stays in contact. Throughout the entire process, abdominal muscle control/bracing is performed together with conscious attention directed towards the position of the spine and torso. The coach then begins to make circular motions with their hand and the client follows, maintaining the lightest of touch. Squares and triangular patterns together with push-pull motions begin to develop the awareness needed for subsequent levels (see figure 11.2). Awareness will develop and the perception of touch will become enhanced. At this stage, the athlete will be able to progress to more complex motion patterns. Foot steps can be introduced with dance steps complete with pirouettes. The client can be lowered to their knees, onto their backs and into rolls on the floor, all the time both parties are conscious of spine position and muscular patterning with the coach offering cues when appropriate. The role of the coach is critical and to be a great coach requires the highest levels of observational skill. The coach may take the athlete into regions brinking on falling over, or into a pain zone. Progressions include closing the eyes and standing on one leg without falling. These challenges teach the athlete how to control postural deviations to maintain balance and minimize pain. The coach will observe problematic balance zones and troublesome motion patterns. The coach will then take the athlete in and out of these zones to groove successful patterns.

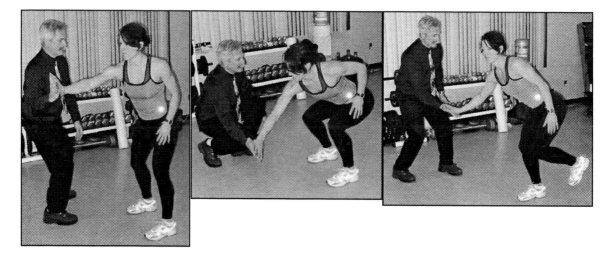

Figure 11.2 With soft hands, the "master" guides the athlete into positions to challenge the back. Progression may include single leg stance and closed eyes.

Higher levels of challenge may then be offered by having the client stand on one leg and move through motion patterns. Standing on a labile surface such as a wobble board offers additional challenges, as does the coupling of challenged breathing. In fact, any challenge that may eventually be experienced by the athlete can be incorporated into the soft hands training exercise. Some may even graduate to soft hands while blindfolded on a wobble board, etc.

Japanese Stick

The Japanese stick is a tool that helps many aspects of balance and general conditioning. It is similar to the soft hands technique in that it is also another wonderful way to build relationships between the trainer and the athlete. However, the Japanese stick exercise can be used to add much more vigor to the challenge and build strength in this demanding balance environment.

The athlete takes a grip on the stick and the coach usually takes a wider grip outside that of the athletes' hands. The progression begins with the coach trying to pull the athlete off balance – victory is achieved when the opponent is forced to take a step. Special focus is directed to the low back at all times to ensure that it remains in a strong position, or a neutral position for those with troubles (see figure 11.3). Again the progression may involve eyes closed, one-legged stance, labile surfaces etc. Remember when engaged in a "challenge", always ensure that the athlete/warrior wins!

R

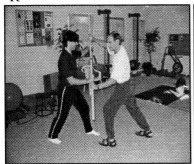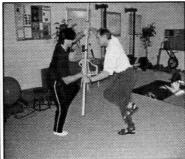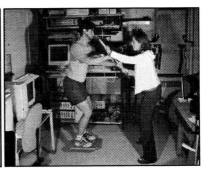

Figure 11.3 Japanese stick progressions from two leg support, to one leg support and a labile surface.

Exercises for training the stabilizing muscles

Recall from chapter 5 that all muscles are spine stabilizers. The way in which they contract together and stiffen will determine the amount of stability in the spine. So what are the wisest ways to challenge and train the stabilizers? This question will be answered in the following sections.

Training the stabilizers of the lumbar spine: The "Big Three"

Our work quantifying many different exercises for spine load and the resultant stability has allowed the selection of better exercises. This analysis has also revealed which exercises create redundant training features so that an "efficient minimum" of exercises can be suggested. Finally, the precise technique for each exercise has been assessed and comment will be provided. As has been stated before, it's not a matter of "doing" the exercise, It's a matter of executing the exercise with precision and skill.

We have been able to select three basic forms of exercises (known as the "Big 3") that ensure stabilizing patterns are being developed and minimal spine loading is maintained. For example, exercise forms such as sit-ups, or leg raises do not meet our criteria – they are poorly designed exercises unless hip flexion training is an objective. However, one cannot engage the hip flexors without creating very high spine compression, eliminating these types of challenges in the early stages of stabilization. Other forms of abdominal exercise have been recommended by others but deserve attention here. One example is the "press-heels" sit-up, which has been hypothesized to activate hamstrings and neurally inhibit psoas, was actually confirmed to increase psoas activation! (See figure 11.4) (Original data can be found in Juker et al.,1998; some clinicians and coaches who intentionally wish to train psoas will find this data informative.)

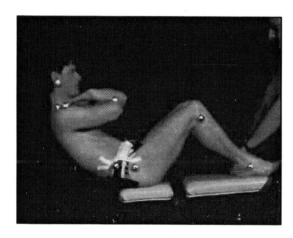

Figure 11.4 The press-heels sit-up, where the athlete attempts to activate hamstrings by pulling the feet towards the buttocks, does not neurally inhibit psoas as has been claimed.

In their basic form, the "Big 3" are comprised of:

1. The Curl-up
2. The Side Bridge
3. The Birddog

The following will assist in choosing the most appropriate form of the exercise.

The Curl-up

The curl-up is not really a curl-up at all, as little motion occurs when performed correctly. It is an outstanding exercise to begin training the abdominal spring used by many athletes, as it challenges the entire abdominal wall. Curl-ups performed with poor technique, however, can be counterproductive, either failing to activate the rectus abdominis sufficiently or unnecessarily overstressing the spine (see figure 11.5). Curl-ups with a twisting motion are expensive in terms of lumbar compression due to the additional oblique challenge. Higher oblique activation with lower spine load is accomplished with the side bridge, which is therefore preferred over twisting curl-ups for training the obliques. This will be presented in the next section. The highest level curl-up will be presented later.

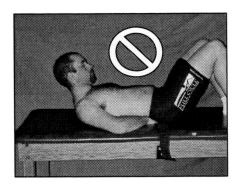 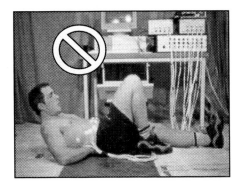

Figure 11.5 Poor form is to flex the cervical spine, loading the neck and not the rectus (left panel). Correct technique focuses the rotation in the thoracic spine. Another common type of poor form is to elevate the head and shoulders a large distance off the floor (right panel). This athlete is elevating far too much, which is closer to replicating the much higher stresses of the sit-up. The intention is to activate rectus and not to produce spine motion.

Beginning the Curl-Up

The curl-up technique is critical to spare the spine (McGill and Karpowicz, 2009). The basic starting posture is supine with the hands supporting the lumbar region. Do not flatten the back to the floor, which takes the spine out of elastic equilibrium and raises the stresses in the passive tissues. While elastic equilibrium is desired in the lumbar region, the hands can be adjusted to minimize pain if needed. One leg is bent with the knee flexed to 90° while the other leg remains relaxed on the floor (see figure 11.6). This adds further torque to the pelvis to prevent the lumbar spine from flattening to the floor. The focus of the rotation is in the thoracic spine; many tend to flex the cervical spine, which is poor technique. Rather, picture the head and neck as a rigid block on the thoracic spine. Individuals who report neck discomfort may try the isometric exercises for the neck that follow. In addition, particularly for patients experiencing neck discomfort, the tongue should be placed on the roof of the mouth behind the front teeth, and pushed upwards to activate the digastric muscles, which help promote stabilizing neck muscle patterns. Leave the elbows on the floor while elevating the head and shoulders a short distance off the floor. The tendency for many is to rise up too far. The rotation is focused in the mid-thoracic, or mid-sternum, region. The head/neck is locked onto the rib cage. No cervical motion should occur—either chin poking or chin tucking. The intention is to activate rectus and not to produce spine motion.

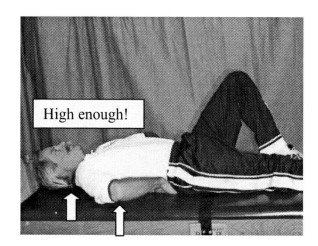

High enough!

Figure 11.6 Curl-up with proper form. In advanced forms the abdominals are pre-braced so that the athlete increases the challenge. The elbows are raised off the floor. Rising higher with the head and shoulders is not necessary – the challenge is increased with purposeful abdominal wall contraction and added deep breathing.

A trick to alleviate neck symptoms

Some people experience neck discomfort during the curl-up. It appears that many use a motor pattern where sternocleidomastoid contributes more of the flexor torque because the digastrics under the chin are not contributing. To solve this, just touch the teeth together and push the tongue to the roof of the mouth with vigorous effort. This activates the digastrics and helps to support the neck, often alleviating the discomfort (Skaggs et al, in press). In others, the neck is simply deconditioned.

Isometric exercises for the neck

Those who experience neck symptoms with curl-ups may also benefit from isometric neck exercises. In all of these exercises, the head/neck does not move, and the tongue is placed on the roof of the mouth behind the front teeth: (a) the hand is placed on the forehead, which resists neck flexion effort; (b) the hand is placed on the side of the head to resist cervical side flexion effort, and then repeated on the other side; (c) the hand is placed on the back of the head to resist cervical extension effort (see figure 11.7). Some find buttressing the chin and isometrically pushing the "chin down" into the fist more comfortable (see figure 11.8). The challenge should be created by performing an appropriate number or repetitions. The duration of hold should remain about 8-10 seconds in length.

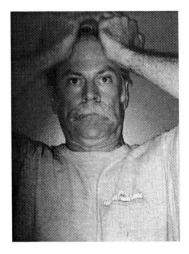 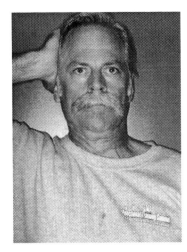 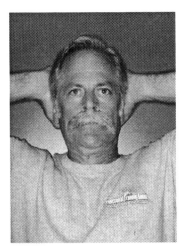

Figure 11.7 Neck isometrics

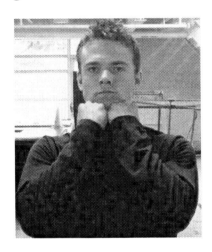

Figure 11.8 The fist is held while the chin is isometrically pushed down into the fist.

Curl-up progressions

To increase the challenge of the curl-up, the following techniques are employed: Since many beginners pry the shoulders up from the floor, we remove this advantage by having them raise the elbows just barely off the floor. In this way, more load is shifted to the rectus. Do not raise the head/neck any higher than in the beginner's form of the curl-up.

Even the most serious athletes can increase the challenge of the curl-up to ultimate training levels. First a pre-brace is performed by the entire abdominal wall. It is simply maximally activated – neither sucked in nor blown out. The secret is to curl (slightly) against the abdominal brace in such a way that the large resistance is provided by the activated abdominals – not by rising any higher from the floor. I have had some of the heavy pro athletes unable to master this curl-up. Some will perform a variation of an advanced curl-up where the hands are placed beside the head (never behind the head) as long as lumbar posture is controlled and no pressure is applied to the head by the hands.

Note: The head and neck must move as a unit, maintaining their rigid-block position on the thoracic spine, but it is emphasized again that the resistance comes from curling against the heavy abdominal pre-brace. This makes the exercise as challenging as the athlete wishes.

Fascial raking may also be employed for these high performing athletes (introduced in the previous chapter) to facilitate deeper contraction. Rake the obliques prior to, and during, the exertion. This may be done in the curl posture or in the hanging kip. In this way, the curl-up can be taken to the highest level possible. The athlete self-creates the matched resistance.

Finally, more challenge is created by having the athlete breathe deeply while performing the curl-up. The abdominal brace is maintained. This not only adds to the challenge but assists in training the breathing patterns that will be needed later.

More on the abdominal progression

Dynamic limb motion can be added once the curl-up has progressed to a high level. The "dead bug" involves first pre-bracing the abdominal wall with a neutral spine and the opposite arm and leg flexed at the shoulder and hip to mimic the motion of a bug on its back. Motor programming for control can be enhanced with the hands and feet scribing geometric motion patterns (circles, squares etc) (see figure 11.9).

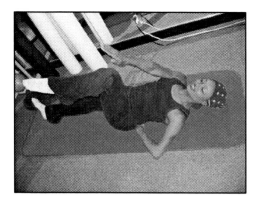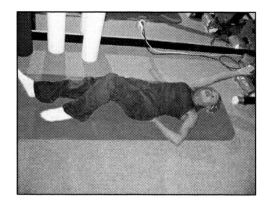

Figure 11.9 Dead bug: beginners can buttress their lumbar spines by placing the hand underneath. No spine motion occurs.

The side bridge

The side bridge is a wonderfully designed exercise. Spine loads are minimized as one side of the torso musculature has much lower activation. Stabilising patterns are ensured as long as the bridge posture is maintained. The many facilitation techniques enable all of the neuromuscular compartments of the obliques to be challenged. All three layers of the abdominal wall are activated, together with rectus, to optimise performance. Important stabilizers such as the quadratus lumborum are also trained. The abdominal spring is "tuned" with the torso in a neutral posture.

Many special patient cases deserve consideration, but are out of the scope of this book. Nonetheless, there are some special situations involving even high performance athletes which remind us that one can only work with the restriction presented. One example was a football player whose shoulders were so painful he could not tolerate the shoulder load. Some elderly women also fall into this patient group given a loss of shoulder strength and ability to handle body weight. This situation called for a modified side bridge on a 45° bench with the feet anchored, which spares the shoulders. The torso can either be elevated from the pad (figure 11.10), or bridged with the shoulder.

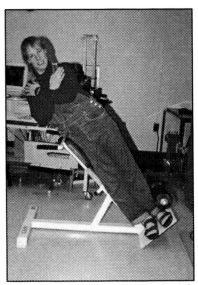 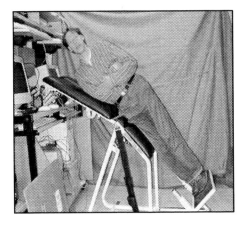

Figure 11.10 Remedial side bridges to spare the shoulder. They are not preferred for those with good shoulders since the important latissimus dorsi is not in the motor scheme.

The form of the side bridge must be matched to the individual. Here is a progression – choose the most appropriate entry form. The lowest lateral torso torque is obtained by bridging from the knees. In the beginning position, the athlete is on his side, supported by his elbow and hip (figure 11.11). The knees are bent to 90°. The free hand is opened maximally and capped over the deltoid on the opposite shoulder. Then pulling the hand down with the arm across the chest will help stabilize the shoulder. The torso is straightened until the body is supported on the elbow and the knee, with some input from the lower leg. Note that there is no lateral bending of the torso during the movement into the posture – it is accomplished with a hip hinge. This is spine sparing. The progression continues by placing the upper arm along the side of the torso—effectively placing more load on the bridge (see figure 11.12).

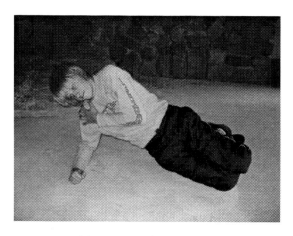

Figure 11.11 The hand caps the deltoid and the elbow is drawn tightly down the chest to help buttress the shoulder in this shoulder conserving form of the side bridge.

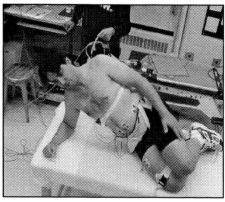
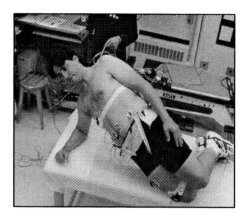

Figure 11.12 Using the "hip hinge" to achieve the Side Bridge. The hips may remain slightly flexed, or the challenge is increased with full hip extension.

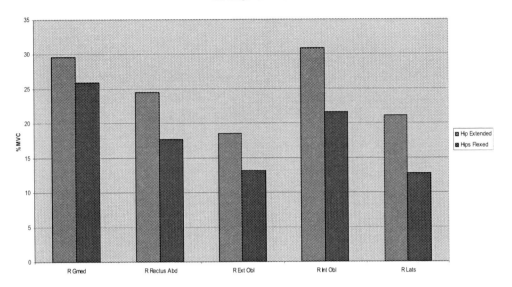

Figure 11.13 Pushing the hips forward in the beginner's side bridge (as in the previous figure) elevates all muscle activation levels.

The progression continues with straight legs so that the bridge uses the elbow and feet for support (Figure 11.14). When supported in this way, the lumbar compression is a modest 2500 N (about 500 lbs), but the quadratus closest to the floor appears to be active up to 50% of MVC. This is a preferred exercise for the obliques since they are active to similar levels.

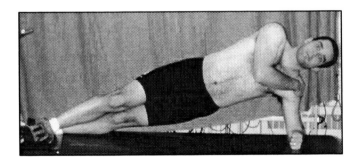

Figure 11.14 Side bridge with straight legs. Note that the "top" foot is placed on the floor in front of the bottom foot.

Placing the upper leg/foot in front of the lower leg/foot will enable longitudinal "rolling" of the torso. This is an important component of the progression as it is very effective for challenging both anterior and posterior neuromuscular compartments of the wall (see Figure 11.15).

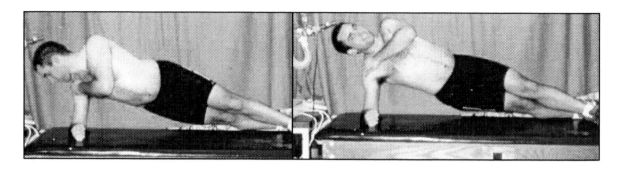

Figure 11.15 Capturing different neuromuscular compartments in the obliques by rolling about the shoulder.

An advanced form of the progression is designed to enhance the motor challenge of the side bridge. This is known as the "Roll". Transfer support from one elbow to the other while abdominally bracing (Figure 11.16) rather than repeatedly hiking the hips off the floor into the bridge position. Ensure that the rib cage is braced to the pelvis and that this rigidity is maintained through the full roll from one side to the other. Focus on the technique – not allowing the pelvis to move before the rib cage requires supreme strength, control and stability. Higher levels of activation would be reached with the feet on a labile surface (Vera-Garcia et al., 2000).

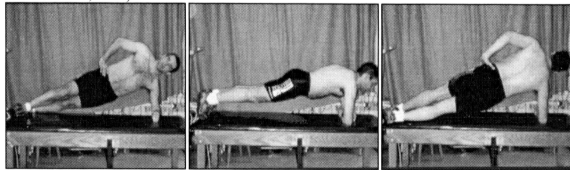

Figure 11.16 Rolling from one side into the plank, and then to the other side. Lock the rib cage to the pelvis. Be disciplined so that the pelvis does not lead the rib cage – this almost doubles the difficulty of the exercise and should be insisted upon. Generally hold each position for no less than 10 seconds with a few deep breaths.

Training spine stability during high physiological work rates

Consider the warehouse worker, firefighter, or football player who must work at a high physiological rate, resulting in deep and elevated lung ventilation. The inability to maintain constant co-contraction in the abdominal wall would compromise stability. For example, when the muscles tend to relax during deep inhalation spine stability is compromised, particularly when heavy external loads that demand a stable spine are required. These individuals must develop stabilizing motor patterns that will transfer to all activities.

For those athletes who require stability while breathing heavily, we train them by first increasing their ventilation rate by riding a stationary bike. They then drop into the highest level of side bridge. This ensures motor patterning of the diaphragm separately from the abdominal wall. If the athlete were to relax the abdominal wall he would fall out of the brace. In this way, dominating diaphragm patterns are grooved while spine stability is ensured with the constantly co-contracting abdominal wall. Our experience has suggested that tall athletes are prone to losing the ability to breathe heavily and maintain spine stability – such as 7 foot tall basketballers. This is a critical exercise for this type of athlete.

Birddog progressions

Training the back extensors is a challenge if the goal is to minimize spine load. For example, the "superman" is a commonly prescribed spine extensor muscle exercise that involves lying prone while extending the arms and legs (see figure 11.17). This results in over 6000 N (about 1300 lbs) of compression to a hyperextended spine, loading the facet joints and crushing the interspinous ligament. This is not a cleverly designed exercise for anyone. Further, recall that the mechanism for disc herniation is reproduced by back machines taking the lumbar spine from full flexion and through the range of motion under load from muscle contraction.

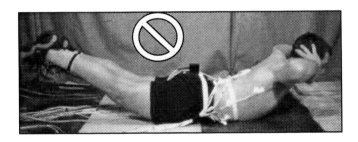

Figure 11.17 The "superman" is a commonly prescribed spine extensor muscle exercise that results in over 6000 N (about 1300 lbs) of compression to a hyperextended spine. It is a poorly designed exercise.

In contrast, our research has shown that the birddog is a much wiser exercise as it spares the spine of high compressive loads and ensures stable patterns of muscle activity. It challenges both lumbar and thoracic portions of the longissimus, iliocostalis, and multifidii with minimal spine loading. For example, a lower form of the birddog involves extending and raising just one leg that results in acceptable spine loading (< 2500 N) and activates one side of the lumbar extensors to approximately 18% of MVC. The birddog is achieved with the athlete raising the opposite arm and leg simultaneously, not raising either the arm or the leg past horizontal. The objective is to be able to hold the limbs parallel to the floor for about six to eight seconds. Good form includes a neutral spine and abdominal bracing. This full birddog increases the unilateral extensor muscle challenge (approximately 27% MVC in one side of the lumbar extensors and 45% MVC in the other side of the thoracic extensors), but also increases lumbar compression to well over 3000 N (Callaghan et al., 1998) (see figure 11.18). This exercise can be enhanced with abdominal bracing and by visualizing activating each level of the local extensors. Both latissimus activity during this exercise together with abdominal co-contraction make it a measurable superior stabilization exercise. Remember to emphasize abdominal bracing and a neutral spine throughout all versions of this exercise. Once again, technique for challenging the extensors should be guided by the athletes' status and goals. This is an individual clinical decision.

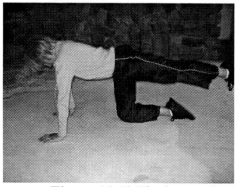 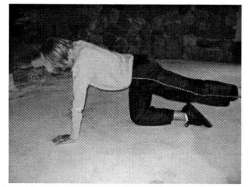

Figure 11.18 The lowest form of the birddog is to extend one leg (left). In the next level, the opposite arm and leg is raised (right).

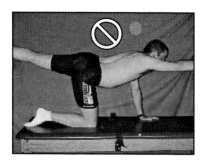

Figure 11.19 Poor form for the birddog includes "hip hiking" or any other configuration that causes deviation (twist, flexion, or lateral bending) to the spine. Also, all motion should take place at the hip and shoulder joints. There should be no motion in the spine.

Advanced motor patterns with the Birddog

The motor control challenge can be enhanced further in this exercise: instead of placing the hand and knee on the ground after each repetition, the athlete should sweep the hand and knee along the floor so that no weight is borne by either. Then they extend the active limbs back out into the birddog position (figure 11.20). This is called "sweep the floor".

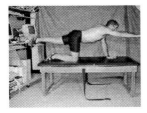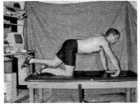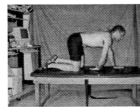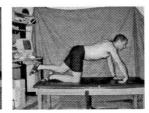

Figure 11.20 Birddog "sweep the floor"

Upper back contraction can be enhanced with the following technique: Help to facilitate co-contraction throughout the raised arm musculature by clenching the fist. Laterally draw the fist away from the midline and concentrate on extension in this new arm plane (see figure 11.21). The upper extensors, rhomboids, latissumus dorsi and lower trapezius will be greatly enhanced.

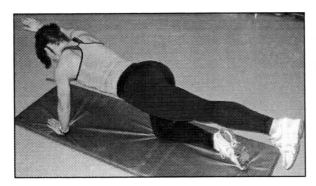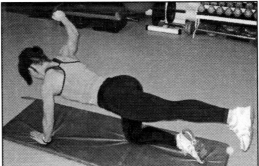

Figure 11.21 Activation of the upper extensors (right panel) can be facilitated by clenching the fist and drawing the arm into abduction. Then focus on extension and activating the upper extensors (conventional in left panel).

Building the stabilization program

Several pro teams and many individual high-performance athletes begin their team workouts with a stabilization routine. Some have claimed that it serves a neural reactivation function although I know of no data that confirms this. It does help to groove stable motor patterns that will remain for exercises that follow in the session. The following is an example of a popular sequence – choose the most suitable for your purposes.

   a. Begin with the flexion/extension cycles, also called the cat/camel motion, to reduce spine viscosity. Note that the cat/camel is intended as a motion exercise, not a stretch, so the emphasis is on motion rather than "pushing" at the end ranges of flexion and extension. We have found that five or six cycles is often sufficient to reduce most viscous stresses. For those individuals with sciatica, increased symptoms may occur during the flexion phase. If pain is present use it to guide the suitable range of motion.

b. Slow lunges, with an upright and braced torso, satisfy the objectives of sparing the spine while achieving hip and knee endurance and mobility. A one-legged squat matrix may be added.

c. These motions are followed by anterior abdominal exercises, namely appropriate curl-ups.

d. Lateral musculature exercises follow, namely the side bridge for quadratus lumborum and the muscles of the abdominal wall for optimal stability.

e. The extensor program begins with the birddog.

Safe progressions of back exercises

The curl-ups, side bridges and birddogs pictured can be made more challenging and yet reasonably safe for those who have mastered the earlier progressions. Use provocative testing to determine the starting level and the rate of progression (McGill, 2008). I have described more advanced progressions in the following chapter that involve plyometrics, however here is another concept that suits the birddog.

Once again, ensure that no motion occurs in the spine – only about the hip and shoulder. The birddog transforms into a more dynamic exercise by moving the foot and hand in geometrical motions. Drawing circles and squares is a favorite starting progression. As the foot and leg are abducted away from the midline, the arm follows – also moving from the midline. The foot and hand are dropped together, adducted towards the midline, and finally raised to complete the foot-hand square. The final arm-leg raising motion progresses to a ballistic contraction where the arm and leg "explode" up. Impeccable form is required, meaning no spine motion. Teach the hip extensors to explode with stiffening torso contractions (ie. no motion). This is a precursor to ultimate jumping and leaping drills, running with directional change, etc. The progression may continue to use small wrist and ankle weights (see figure 11.22).

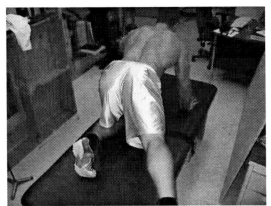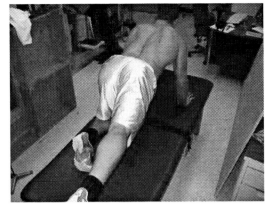

Figure 11.22 The hand and foot follow matching motion patterns – for example, a "square" shaped pattern. The progression continues to an "explosive" contraction as the arm and leg are raised where the motion is constrained to the shoulder and hip. This is a wonderful transitional exercise for back plyometric training.

References

Callaghan, J.P., Gunning, J.L., and McGill, S.M. (1998) Relationship between lumbar spine load and muscle activity during extensor exercises. *Physical Therapy*, 78 (1): 8-18.

Juker, D., McGill, S.M., Kropf, P., and Steffen, T. (1998) Quantitative intramuscular myoelectric activity of lumbar portions of psoas and the abdominal wall during a wide variety of tasks. *Med Sci Sports Exerc*, 30 (2): 301-310.

McGill, S.M., Karpowicz, A. (2009) Exercises for spine stabilization: Motion/Motor patterns, stability progressions and clinical technique. Arch. Phys. Med. and Rehab., 90: 118-126.

McGill, S.M. (2008) Therapeutic exercise for the painful lumbar spine: Where does one begin, Orthop. Div.Review CPA, pp. 12-18, March/April 2008.

Skaggs, C.D., Gray, J., McGill, S.M. The effect of forceful masticatory muscle activation on jaw and neck mechanics.

Vera-Garcia, F.J., Grenier, S.G., and McGill, S.M. (2000) Abdominal response during curl-ups on both stable and labile surfaces. Phys. Ther. 80(6): 564-569.

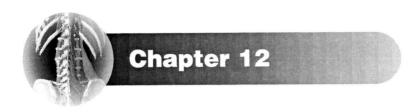

Chapter 12

Stage 3: Endurance

Endurance is a pillar for training virtually every athlete with very few exceptions. There is a progression to building endurance and it starts by doing so without becoming tired! Typically, endurance is built first with repeated sets, and for some athletes, the progression continues with longer holds.

Early endurance progressions usually begin with the isometric holds performed in the curl-ups, bridges, and birddog exercises. They should be held no longer than seven or eight seconds. The duration is based on recent evidence from near infrared spectroscopy indicating rapid loss of available oxygen in torso muscles contracting at these levels. Short relaxation of the muscle restores oxygen (McGill et al., 2000). The endurance objectives are achieved by building up repetitions of the exertions rather than increasing the duration of each hold.

Motivated by evidence for the superiority of extensor endurance over strength as a benchmark for good back health (McGill et al, 2003), we have documented normal ratios of endurance times for the torso flexors relative to the extensors and lateral musculature (see *Low Back Disorders* and also McGill et al 1999, McGill et al, 2009). Use these values to identify endurance deficits—both absolute values and for one muscle group relative to another—and to establish reasonable endurance goals for your athletes.

The reverse pyramid for endurance training

This approach to designing endurance sets is founded in the Russian tradition of maintaining excellent technique and form. The idea is to train endurance without becoming tired. For example, if one were to design sets for the side-bridge exercise using 5 repetitions then the workout would look like this. Five repetitions on the right side would be followed by 5 on the left. Rest. Then 4 on the right and 4 on the left. Rest. Finally 3 on the right and then 3 on the left. Finished. Good technique is facilitated as the repetitions are reduced with each fatiguing set. This is generally used to build the endurance base since the objective of maintaining sufficient O2 levels is met so that the failure is not oxygen starvation. As the progression continues, more reps are added to each cell rather than increasing the duration of the holding time (about 8-10 seconds). Once proficiency is enhanced with the Russian pyramid and technique is never compromised by fatigue, holding times for each rep may be extended if desired.

The Russian Reverse Pyramid for Rep/Set design.		
Right side	Left side	
5 reps	5 reps	Rest
4 reps	4 reps	Rest
3 reps	3 reps	

Training for endurance events

As athletes progress, some will need to train constant and prolonged contraction in the torso. An example of such an athlete would be a long distance swimmer. There are no specific guidelines here beyond seeking the optimal challenge for the back. Traditional endurance overload principles will be utilized within the sport specific endurance demands. These types of athletes will obviously train with much longer durations for a repetition (see figure 12.1), up to several minutes, or even hours in some cases.

Certain strength athletes have different endurance requirements. The chapter on stability highlighted the importance of maintaining torso muscle co-activation to ensure sufficient stability. Under large loads and when breathing heavily, the muscle patterns demand both strength and endurance capabilities. Consider the athlete who must step onto one leg under load – the power lifter for example, when unracking a heavy bar, or a competitor in a "strongman" competition. Many examples are observed in the occupational world among fishermen, construction workers and farmers. The compressive load down the spine must traverse the horizontal pelvis and progress down the femur. Even though the spine remains upright it is subjected to enormous compressive, bending, twisting and shearing loads. An excellent training exercise could be the one-armed dumbbell carry (sometimes referred to as the suitcase carry). The torso is braced and the athlete carries a substantial dumbbell load in one hand. Focus is on maintaining perfect torso bracing with no spine movement while breathing and supporting the load with each step (see figure 12.2).

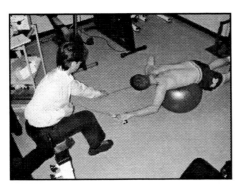

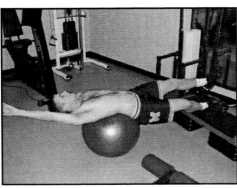

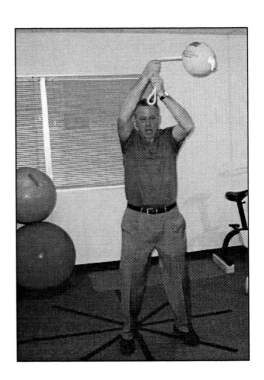

Figure 12.1 Endurance training for some swimmers, for example, may progress to holding these postures for substantial lengths of time. Turbo ball training (right panel) with a focus on the torso co-contraction greatly enhances neuro-muscular endurance. It is a tremendous endurance exercise.

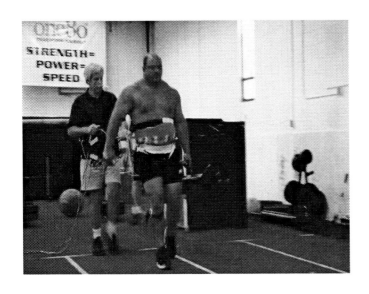

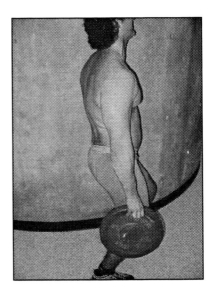

Figure 12.2 Endurance for some strength athletes require torso-bracing patterns while

under asymmetric loads. The one-handed weight carry can be an excellent trainer. This is one of the best activators of the quadratus lumborum which is an essential spine "carrying" muscle. Remember to accentuate the hand grip which will facilitate activation in the rotator cuff in the shoulder.

Breathing mechanics

Endurance events that require simultaneous strength, demand optimal breathing mechanics. Strongmen competitors are examples of those who must sustain spine stiffness while generating joint motion – but they must breathe efficiently. Training is begun with "crocodile breathing". Here the prone athlete stiffens the torso and pushes the abdomen into the floor, raising the body, with each breath (see figure 12.3).

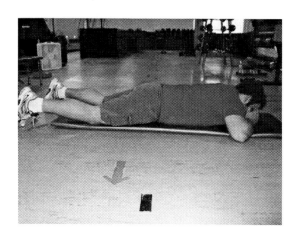

Figure 12.3 "Crocodile breathing" is trained by pushing the abdomen into the floor.

References

McGill, S.M., Childs, A., and Liebenson, C. (1999) Endurance times for stabilization exercises: Clinical targets for testing and training from a normal database. Arch. Phys. Med. Rehab. 80: 941-944.

McGill, S.M., (2007) Low Back Disorders: Evidence based prevention and rehabilitation, Second Edition, Human Kinetics Publishers, Champaign, Illinois.

McGill, S.M., Hughson, R. and Parks, K. (2000) Lumbar erector spinae oxygenation during prolonged contractions: Implications for prolonged work. Ergonomics, 43: 486-493.

McGill, S.M., Grenier, S., Bluhm, M., Preuss, R., Brown, S., and Russell, C. (2003) Previous history of LBP with work loss is related to lingering effects in biomechanical physiological, personal, and psychosocial characteristics. Ergonomics, 46(7): 731-746.

McGill, S.M., Belore, M., Crosby, I., Russell, C. (accepted March 2009) Comparison of two methods to quantify torso flexion endurance. Occup. Ergonmics.

Chapter 13

Stage 4: Developing Ultimate Strength

Ultimate performance is achieved when all components (biomechanical, physiological and motor control systems together with the technical and mental "skill" variables) are optimally functioning and peaking together. Three of the foundation variables were addressed in the previous chapter; strength, speed, power and agility complete the physical athlete and are addressed here. As has been clearly pointed out before, no athlete can exert strength if their joints or body position are unstable or the projection of the external force is misdirected. Nor can the back/torso make its critical contributions to the process if it has poor positioning, posture and muscle coordination – the foundation presented in the previous chapter to address this is a mandatory prerequisite. A healthy back requires excellent mechanics in the hips, pelvis and knees below it, and neck and shoulders above it. For this reason, special exercises that integrate these regions are also included here. "Surround the dragon" is a concept that can extend to all joints and body parts in the quest for the ultimate back.

World class athletes are for the most part, in my experience, mutants. Or, at least they are at the extreme end of the biological spectrum when compared with the population. Studying their dynamic form reveals techniques that, in many cases, are beyond contemporary sports and performance science. Scientific validation often lags behind athletic and training practice. Our use of the scientific method provides insight into enhancing performance and reducing the risk of injury, but not all of the techniques in this chapter of the book have been rigorously assessed. Nor can they be – individual behaviour is a function of the load and effort. In many cases, we have only performed limited investigations to obtain impressions and some of these are contained here. My suspicion is that most of these impressions will withstand more complete scientific scrutiny.

Stage 4: Strength training considerations

Training ultimate strength without injury is a difficult challenge. When searching for ways to obtain maximum myoelectric activity from the back extensor muscles, we discovered that isometric back extensor exercises do not recruit the full pool of motor units. With some extensor motion, many more motor units fire. For example, maximal effort deadlifts only appear to activate a very limited number of the motor units possible with isometric contraction. There appears to be a "fusebox" in the system that, if overcome, could enhance performance. But the fusebox performs a safety function and subduing this inhibition is at the peril of the athlete. Many superior athletes such as Bill Kazmaier, the "World's Strongest Man" for several years, have trained to activate the maximum number of motor units. Kazmaier, for example, used mental imagery together with clever exercise technique to accomplish this. He trained his ability to image the entire muscle and motor unit pool and potentiate the muscles. He worked to perceive optimal recruitment and complete contraction. With his mind controlling the preparation, goosebumps developed on his skin as he rallied the ability and determination to accomplish the task. A portion of his resistance training was directed towards enhancing the ability to activate every available motor unit. These techniques are described below. Other athletes who need supreme speed-strength developed regimens that incorporate elements to train slow strength, fast strength, concentric strength, eccentric strength, multi-articular complex strength, reciprocal inhibition strength, and "playing position" strength. The motor units recruited are very different within a muscle for each of these tasks. Machines, no matter how well designed or promoted, can never provide the rich environment to create the training challenges needed. Even athletes who perform slow-strength activities make substantial gains in strength with speed-strength training. Most NFL linemen will tell you that if you are squatting slowly then you have too heavy a load. Vasily Alexiev, the great Russian super heavyweight, limited the lifting of competitive loads in practice. Rather, he practiced lifts at great speed and with impeccable form. Ultimately, all athletes training for optimal strength will have to speed-strength train.

Qualifying the athlete

The clinical decisions involved in staging an athlete through the progression is an art that can be assisted with scientific data (some guidance was provided in chapter 8). Those who are looking for a set recipe, however, will fail. Of course, each individual must prepare by developing general fitness and balancing ability to train effectively. They have considered matching their conditioning and capabilities to the skill demands of the planned training and they have developed the foundation of motor and motion patterns to spare the weaker links. They have considered the balance of strength around a joint and between adjacent joints, the balance of strength to endurance and the range of motion required by the task and whether their motion capability is appropriately matched. Now they are ready to seriously focus on enhancing strength.

Training motor units

The story of Bill Kazmaier's imagery for strength exertion preparation was described in the previous section. While this example illustrates the importance of the mental component, it must be coupled with contraction exercises. An example of how one can train to activate all motor units within a muscle is provided using a moveable fulcrum approach. As a result of our efforts to maximize the back extensor recruitment, we use the following back extensor exercise.

While the athlete is lying prone on a bench with the torso supported on a movable stiff pad, place weight in one hand. The edge of the pad is placed more cranial (or closer to the head). The cantilevered portion of the spine is slightly flexed (Figures 13.1 and 13.2) and then extended, combined with a very slight twist back to neutral. The spine never extends past neutral. After a set, place the weight in the athlete's other hand and have the athlete repeat the exercise. Then move the pad downward so that a greater portion of the torso is cantilevered. Have the athlete repeat the sets. Move the pad farther down the athlete's body, leaving more of the torso cantilevered, and have the athlete repeat the entire process. The goal is to challenge every motor unit within the muscle. To successfully complete this goal, up to 7 or 8 re-placements of the pad may be necessary. Loads in the hands are typically not large initially since the objective is to focus on the ability to sense the different section of the muscles and activate them – mental imagery is most important here. Similar exercise approaches can be accommodated with a movable surface such as a gym ball (see figure 13.3). Then, once the motor patterns are established, larger resistive weight can be employed.

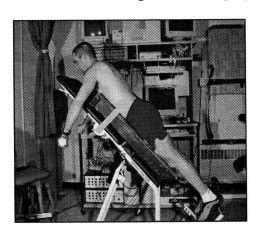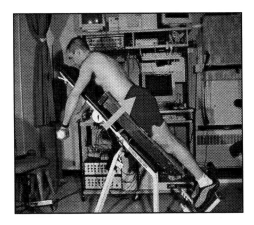

Figure 13.1 The moving fulcrum during back extensor exercise is a philosophical approach to train different motor units within a muscle. To train the back extensors, the fulcrum is systematically moved along the torso, slightly changing the mechanical demands with each positional change. This systematically challenges each section of the extensor motor unit pool. Imagery enhances the activation of every available motor unit.

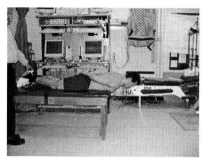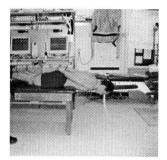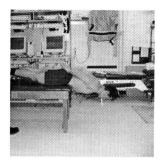

Figure 13.2 A variation of the "moving fulcrum" to practice activating all motor units within the torso extensors. The upper body is cantilevered out in stages.

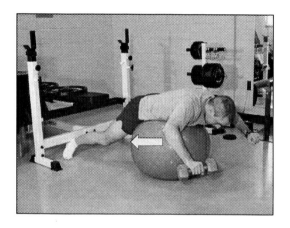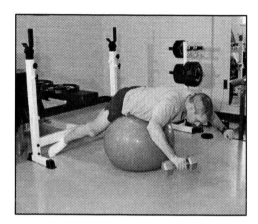

Figure 13.3 Moving a gym ball under the athlete in this extensor exercise helps to activate a greater proportion of the motor unit pool in the extensor musculature.

Bodyweight resistive exercises and surrounding the dragon: Tips for exercises for the upper and lower body

Ultimate back performance requires ultimate performance from joints above and below. Incorporating body weight as a resistive load has been recognized for centuries as an effective training approach. Unfortunately, and to the detriment of too many athletes, the invention and marketing of machines has created the impression that they provide superior opportunity for challenging athletic talent. Many progressions are shown in the next chapter that document challenges to integrate the torso. Several principles with supporting evidence are provided here to guide the reader in their decisions when formulating training programs.

Training with bands and cables has already been introduced. The simple pushup is a wonderful exercise to integrate the abdominal musculature, but the pushup can be enhanced with hand placement. Staggering hand placement, with one forward of the shoulder and the other behind, not only changes the shoulder activation patterns but also enhances the abdominal activation levels and stability further (see Freeman et al 2006). Note that individual differences are quite variable with this variation of the exercise based on actual hand placement and effort (see figure 4.4). Performing pushups with one hand on a medicine ball enhances both rectus abdominis and oblique activity, usually only on one side of the torso. Placing both hands on medicine balls activates the rectus and obliques on both sides of the torso to levels usually over 75% of MVC! (see figure 13.5) This is an exceptional level for abdominal integration and stability training for high performance tasks.

Figure 13.6 enhances the concept with lower load pull-down exercises. One armed cable pulls can be particularly helpful for shoulder range of motion together with elongating the spine musculature over the lumbar and hip region (see figure 13.7). This is a wonderful therapeutic exercise for some. This progression continues with the pullup (see figure 13.8). Tremendous gains can be obtained here with proper training methods. First, unfortunately many people simply perform pullups until they tire never making gains. Instead, if a person is able to perfom 8 pullups then only perform 2 in each set. The pull begins by centrating the scapulae (see figure 13.9). From this powerful posture the core and hip muscles pre-tense and burst as the individual performs a maximal explosive effort in the pull. Repeat for a second rep and release the bar. Relax but tilt the torso back and achieve the "fat tongue" (this means relaxing the tongue in the back of the throat and letting the arms dangle). Olympic weight lifters relax to prepare for the next explosive lift this way. Then rack onto the bar for the next set of 2. After a few sets the individual will feel facilitated rather than fatigued – a better way to train performance. Using straps for pushups creates a labile environment and challenges shoulder and torso control together with the entire anterior system (see figure 13.10). A similar philosophy can be employed for the posterior/extensor system with the reverse pull-up exercise (see figure 13.11).

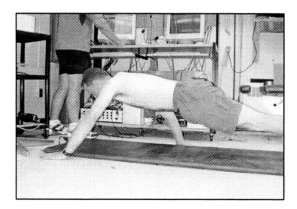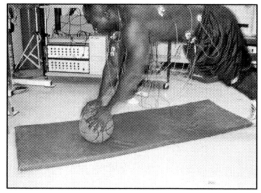

Figure 13.4 Progressions of pushups to facilitate abdominal activation for stability. In particular, moving the typical hand placement to a staggered position, with one forward and the other beside the lower ribs (left panel), and using a ball under the hands for lability are excellent techniques. Focus is on lumbar control with the rib cage locked to the pelvis.

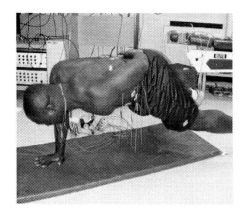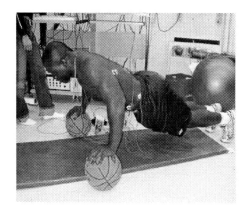

Figure 13.5 Other examples of using the pushup to challenge the torso flexion mechanism includes the one-armed pushup (creating 5847N of lumbar compression in this case) and a bilateral labile ball pushup resulting in 2841N of lumbar compressive load. The one-armed pushup requires the support of the additional twisting torque which involves many more muscles accounting for the much higher spine load. Choose the exercise to match the objectives while staying within the athlete's tolerance.

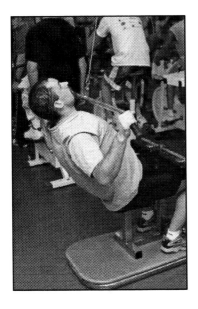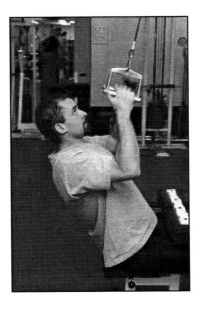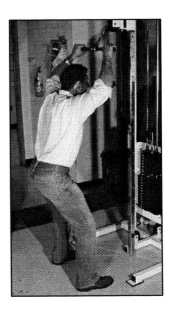

Figure 13.6 Pulldowns in front of the chest are a good way to challenge latissimus dorsi, trapezius and rhomboids. Some athletes perform pulldowns in the standing posture. For example, some basketball teams have pulldown machines built 8 feet off the ground to facilitate "playing position".

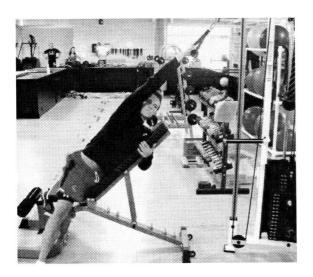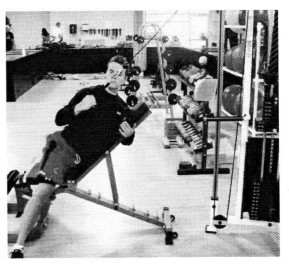

Figure 13.7 One arm cable pulls combine stretch and range of motion during shoulder work that emphasizes latissimus dorsi but also includes the lumbar region and hips. Focus on centrating the scapula first, then pull the cable down.

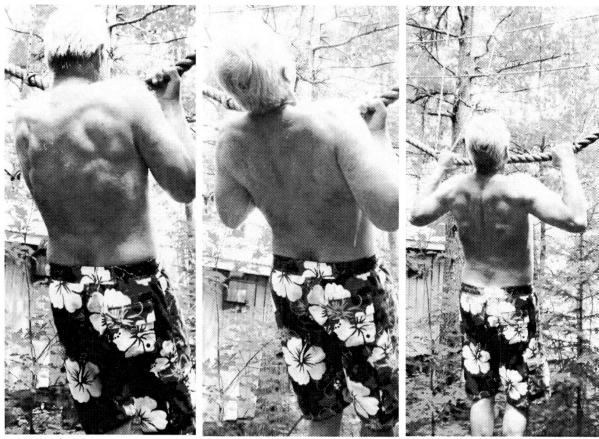

Figure 13.8 Pullups should be a goal of any strength/function program. Undergrip variations include the traditional pull and a pull to chest. Overgrip places more emphasis on brachioradialis and balancing grip athleticism. The old boy still has it to train but is too old to shave his back - my daughter tells me it's gross.

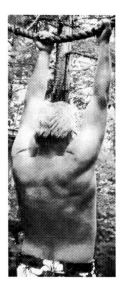 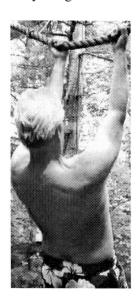

Figure 13.9 Begin pull-ups by first centrating the scapula, then stiffen the gluts and abdominals and pull up explosively. Stop before fatigue sets in. Train in short explosive sets to facilitate training rather than becoming fatigued. Gains will come faster this way.

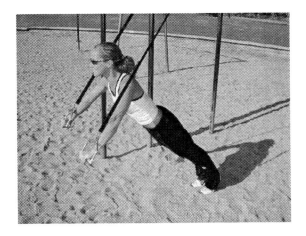

Figure 13.10 Straps create a labile environment for abdominal activation and torso control during a "pushup". This is an excellent trainer of the "anterior system"

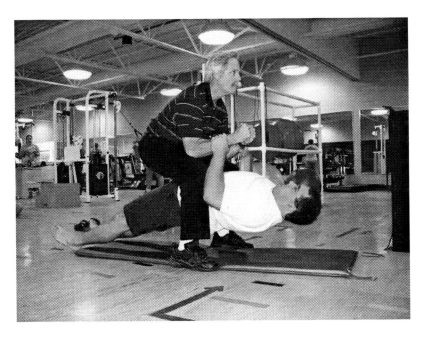

Figure 13.11 Reverse pull-ups train the entire posterior/extensor/stabilization system. This is also a great stiffening training exercise for the partner!

Dumbbells versus barbells

In many approaches, the mainstay of free resistance training is provided with barbells, yet very few tasks or events have the hands tied together with a bar – they move independently. Dumbbells (kettlebells in many cases are preferable) better mimic the environment of real sporting competition. A more attractive natural consequence of using a dumbbell in just one hand is asymmetric loading of the torso. This challenges the torso stabilizing mechanism to train optimal force transfer from the upper and lower body. Several progressions in this book utilize this approach to train the back to ensure ultimate performance. A variety of traditional barbell exercises have been adapted with a dumbbell to better challenge the torso with flexor/extensor, lateral bend and twisting torques (see figure 13.12).

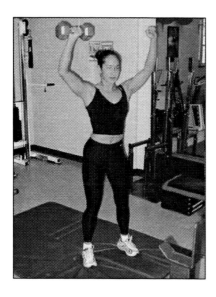 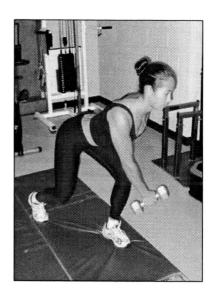

Figure 13.12 Several traditional barbell exercises may be adapted for a dumbbell to challenge the torso in order to stabilize torques about the flexion/extension, lateral bend and twist axes.

Cables: For multidimensional strength

Traditional weights operate under the influence of gravity in that their resistive force is downward. Furthermore, the traditional exercises using bars tend to challenge sagittal plane strength. Many strong squatters and lifters, for example, do not have matching strength in torsional modes – pull on one sleeve and they are relatively weak. Thus training for all resistive forces in sporting tasks that include vectors in all directions is important. These types of resistive challenges can be mimicked with cables.

Cables can provide the opportunity for training whole body motion. For example, compare those who train exclusively with the bench press to develop the ability to fend off an opponent. Fending requires skilled footwork to optimize the projection of force to the ground and allow the strength developed in the chest, shoulders and arms to be maximally productive (see figure 13.13). Those who emphasize bench press training may not be able to transfer their force when standing or moving. Certainly, there is better integration of the torso stabilization musculature during the cable press (Santana, Gray and McGill, 2008) (see figure 13.14). Compare a massive bench presser in their ability to perform standing cable pushes while moving in a star pattern with the feet. Bench press score has little correlation with this task! One good use for the bench press is to build shoulder and pectoralis mass, if desired. For example, in some specialized events such as Olympic lifting, the hypertrophied pecs form a "shelf" to place the bar upon following the clean phase of the lift. As the bar rests on the shelf, the athlete performs rhythmic vertical motions in tune with the bar which is bending elastically prior to initiating the jerk phase. Then the shelf is used to initiate the drive of the bar overhead.

Cables facilitate several important progressions where powerful hand motions follow sweeping trajectories. The "wood chop" progressions together with throwing progressions are excellent mimics of many sporting situations and can be accomplished with cables with movable blocks (see figure 13.15). High level cable exercises can be accomplished with a cable in each hand - one pushing and another pulling (look ahead to training the martial artist in chapter 16). These special cable machines accommodate high acceleration without blowing to the top of the cable weight stack. Be sure to qualify each athlete with torsional tests such as the one shown in chapter 8 if they have a history of back troubles.

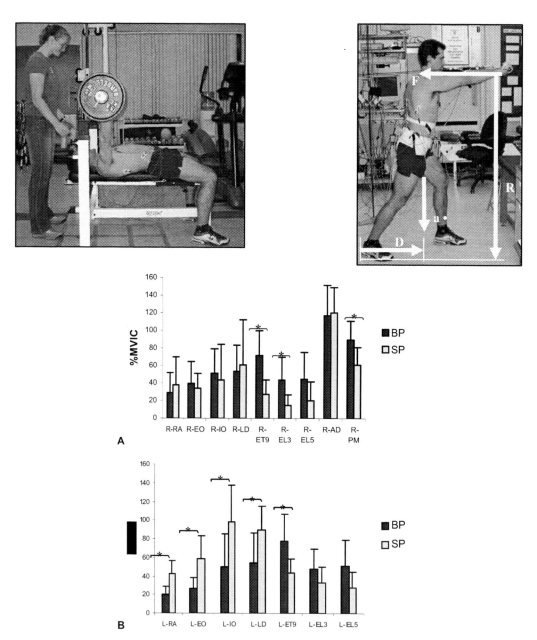

Figure 13.13 Muscle activation during the one arm cable press (SP) and the bench press (BP). "Core" integration is much higher during the cable press together with the requisite torsional control from the abdominal muscles and latissimus dorsi.

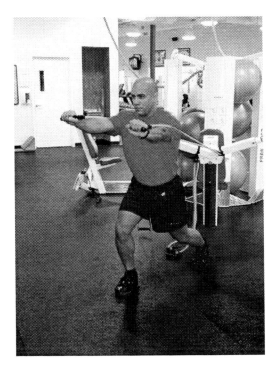
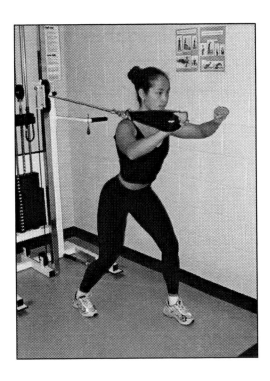

Figure 13.14 J C Santana shows a standing cable press with a walkout (left panel). "Fending" drills are assisted with cables (right panel). Footwork can be added. For standing presses it does not matter what you bench press as this ability is limited by the strength of the core (Santana, Gray and McGill, 2008). An athlete who bench presses must push press in a standing posture to enhance upright pushing ability.

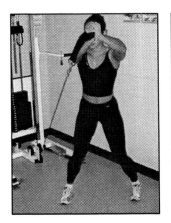
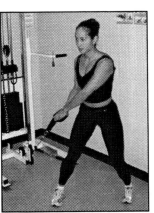
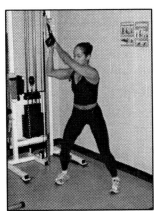
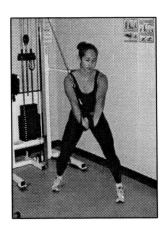

Figure 13.15 Wood chop cable progressions with the block in "top" and "bottom" positions. Spine load is largely determined by the perpendicular distance from the cable to the lumbar spine – closer is lower load, but lower muscular challenge. Motion is at the hips – not the spine.

Choosing the cable load

Choosing the load with cables is different than when choosing a traditional weight resistance. Cable pulling technique has great influence on the resultant joint challenge and general loading on the torso. A recent study that we performed quantified loads on the lumbar spines of firefighters, and on naïve workers (graduate students) while they pushed and pulled resistive loads provided by cables (Lett and McGill, 2006). The firefighters pushed and pulled more cable load with lower spine loads. They used technique to lean their bodies, creating driving forces and then directing the cable forces through their low back. In contrast, the naïve workers did not optimize the driving forces generated in the legs by leaning the body into the cable resistance. Further, they tended to not direct the pulling/pushing forces through the low back. The firefighters were excellent occupational athletes and wonderful examples of how technique influenced the choice of training load. Thus the load on the back is heavily influenced by the direction of the cable force and its distance passing by the spine, not by the amount of tension.

Bands

Elastic bands (and springs) have been used since the early 1900's to provide resistance but they have not been used to enhance high performance training until quite recently – at least in the West. The Russians used them and documented their success in books like those by Verkhoshansky (1977). Bands can increase the range of movement over which high resistive forces can be created, particularly for high amplitude body motions. While the use of bands in rehabilitative therapy is common, the focus here is on their use in conjunction with other resistance approaches – namely barbells.

Lability under the athlete, between them and the floor, has been popular for years. The real asset of bands for training the back is when they are combined with bars to create a "labile" load environment (see figure 13.16). An example of this approach is while performing squats with a barbell on the shoulders, have elastics on the ends of the bar and anchored to the floor. Dumbbells can be suspended from the elastics and allowed to swing. This produces a lability to the bar which requires much more control on the part of the lifter to maintain balance and joint stability. Muscles are facilitated throughout the linkage. In fact, the stabilizing mechanism of the spine is enhanced and challenged with the addition of the bands to a lighter load on the bar. Interestingly, this was a Russian "trick" to greatly accelerate squat performance training.

Others have discussed the notion that bands assist in pulling the load down and augmenting the eccentric phase of the exercise. From this perspective, it is recommended to decrease the volume of work once bands are added to the regimen.

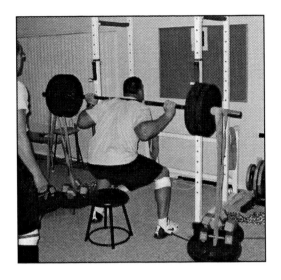

Figure 13.16 Bands add lability to the load, facilitating muscle activation throughout the linkage, in particular the torso muscles.

Chains

Chains have been popularized by Westside Barbell recently in the US. When used in a similar manner to the bands described in the previous section, chains better match the resistance to the strength curve. Typically, the chains are draped over the ends of the bar dangling to the ground. As the chain links land on the floor, the total bar/chain weight is decreased (see figure 13.17). The unloading as the weight is lowered can be controlled and changed by choosing different gauges of chain. For example, chain can be selected that weighs 2Kg per foot of length or 5Kg per foot. Several loops of chain can be used to double and quadruple the load-off. Once again they not only assist in lightening the resistance in the "weaker" body positions, but provide another valuable asset – lability of the load to challenge balance resulting in better utilization of the newfound strength.

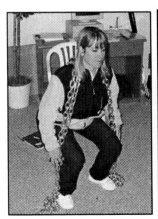 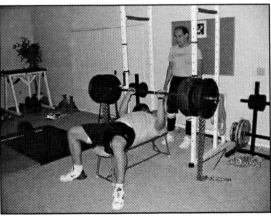

Figure 13.17 Chains, like bands and other devices can be used creatively. Here, an individual is grooving a basic squat pattern with chain resistance with load-off as the squat deepens. Chains in the bench press produce some bar lability together with a load-off as the bar is lowered.

Abdominal strength

Abdominal progressions continuing from the "big three" introduced in the previous chapter may include gym balls. Several variations of the "walkout" (see figures 13.18 and 13.19) challenge abdominal strength and control. Hanging leg raises with bent knees generate about 80Nm of flexion torque in the average male with over 3000N of compression. Nonetheless, this exercise requires abdominal buttressing forces with simultaneous hip flexion challenge. Emphasis is placed on maintaining a neutral spine for most athletes – some will want to allow lumbar flexion but under great control. This progression finishes with "stir the pot". An outstanding exercise to integrate the entire anterior chain with torsional control – an essential exercise for our MMA fighters! (see figure 13.20).

Eventually the athlete will want to progress to standing postures. Overhead cable pulls (see figure 13.21) are excellent abdominal exercises. For many athletes, even better are the progressions that involve a one-legged stance and even labile surfaces under the feet.

Finally, medicine ball tosses are an excellent progression to power and speed strength. They may be performed while the athlete is supine over a ball, or in a standing posture (see figure 13.22). A major objective is to train the storage and recovery of the elastic energy mechanism of the abdominal wall. The abdominal wall functions as a spring and should be trained this way. Emphasis is on minimizing torso motion as the abdominals check twisting and focus the explosive action from the hips. This is accomplished by very quick catches and throws rather than large arm trajectories that would increase the range of motion but slow the muscle contraction rate. One may consider this short-range plyometric training for the abdominals and the same care must be taken to observe extended recovery periods. The game of "hot potato" where minimal time is spent with hand-ball contact, can enhance the plyometric approach.

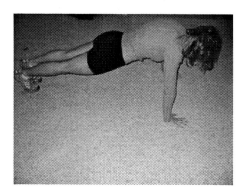 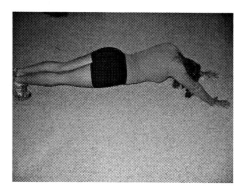

Figure 13.18 The "walkout" from a pushup position trains the abdominal mechanism with flexion and torsional isometric challenge.

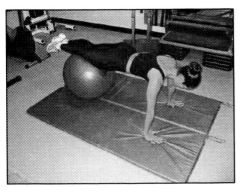
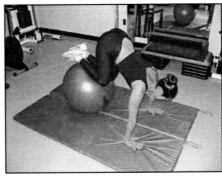
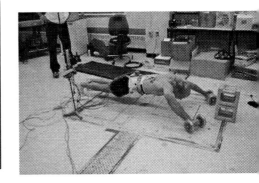

Figure 13.19 The "walkout" with a gym ball is an excellent exercise for challenging abdominal and hip moment with balance and control. The rollout takes it up a level in challenge and load.

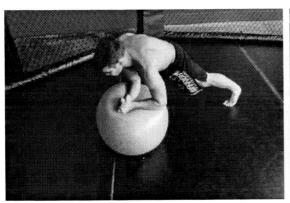
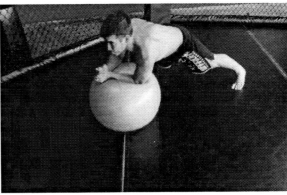

Figure 13.20 "Stir the pot" is the ultimate exercise for the ultimate fighter! Discipline is required for minimal spine motion but maximal shoulder motion.

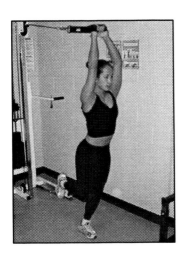
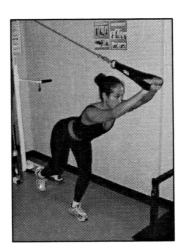
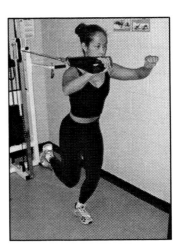

Figure 13.21 Overhead cable pulls are a whole body exercise integrating the abdominals. Focus is on abdominal bracing and a neutral spine.

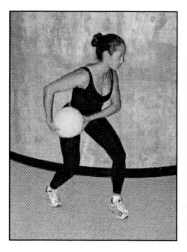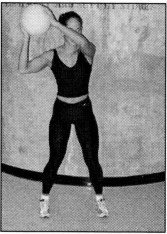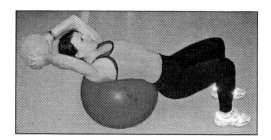

Figure 13.22 Medicine ball tosses are an excellent progression to power and speed strength. They may be performed while the athlete is supine over a ball or in a standing posture. Quick catch and throw "hot potato" sequences are a form of plyometric training to enhance the elastic energy storage and recovery system of the abdominal wall.

Training hip flexion strength and power

Sprinting and other power running events, such as those performed by football players, require hip flexion power. Top-end speed for most sprinters is limited by the recovery of the leg in flexion (hip flexion), not a lack of hip extension power. Thus, many train the psoas according to the power philosophy — but end up with a bad back. Large psoas contractions place high loads on the spine and the (usually) highly repetitive exercises only compound the problem. The general rule of thumb for power-psoas training is to ensure athletes maintain spine stability, specifically being conscious of the braced and neutral spine during hip flexor training for sprinting events. The 5 stages of training emphasized in this book are the essential requisites for injury avoidance and ultimate performance.

Several exercises already shown in this chapter may begin the athletic progressions for hip flexion strength and power. For example, exercises like the "dead bug" and the hanging leg raise all challenge the hip flexors. The various bounding progressions produce excellent results but will break down the athlete who cannot tolerate the forces associated with ballistic hip flexion (see figures 13.23 and 13.24). Locking the spine in neutral is one strategy that is used to enhance the tolerance of these progressions.

The standing one-legged squat progressions can be extended into good hip flexion exercises using the principle of dynamic correspondence. For example, in the one-legged squat, as one hip extends, the other is flexed. Speed can be increased to enhance the torque and balance challenge. Finally, some of the Russian progressions are very effective. They begin with various one-legged squats, and then add some external load to the free leg as it is pulled in hip flexion. An example with resistance provided by a cable band around the ankle is illustrated (see figure 13.25). Again this is an excellent exercise in those who can tolerate it, but many athletes will develop back troubles performing it. Discipline to lock the lumbar spine and lumbo-pelvic junction is the key to the avoidance of back troubles here. Finally, hanging flexion requires discipline and spine position control for safety and effectiveness (see figure 13.26).

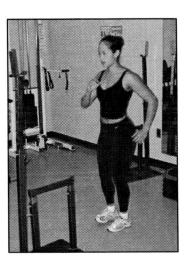 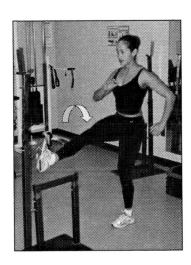 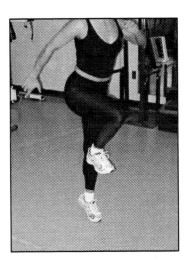

Figure 13.23 Bounding progressions produce excellent results, but sometimes break down the athlete's back. The prevention strategy is to maintain a torso that is braced and locked in neutral.

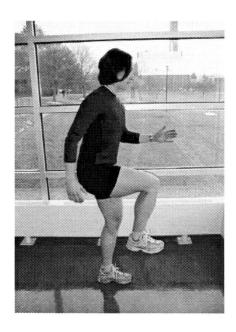 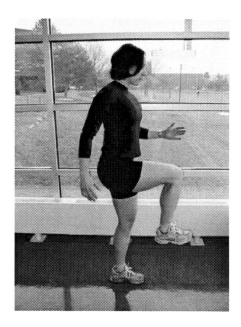

Figure 13.24 Poor form (left panel) illustrates the track exercise of A's and B's where hip flexion is accomplished with spine flexion – this leads to poor performance and back troubles. The torso is correctly braced and stiffened in the right panel.

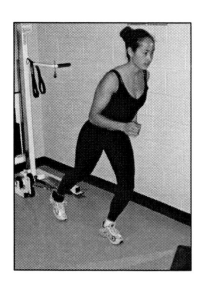 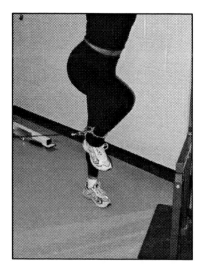

Figure 13.25 The Russian exercise of one-legged squats with cable resisted ipsilateral hip flexion.

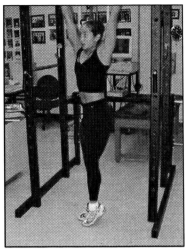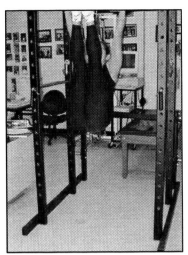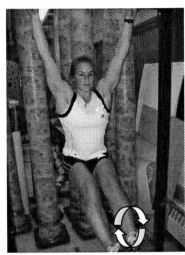

Figure 13.26 Hanging leg flexion can be a strength and power exercise but requires spine control. Large leg circles (left and middle panel) and small leg circles (right panel) cause high spine loads but the spine has enhanced tolerance being in a neutral posture.

Building squat performance

The pillar of most leg strengthening programs is the double-legged squat with a barbell on shoulders. Data in previous chapters showed that this traditional form is really training the quadriceps until deeper squats are achieved. Moreover, this style of squat fails to adequately train any athlete who needs strength but also runs, jumps off one leg, and changes direction. These tasks require ultimate hip extensor, abduction/adduction, and flexion torque strength. Optimal leg strength requires the simultaneous training of balance, like single leg challenges with appropriate corresponding actions in the non-support leg, in a way that spares the back. For these reasons, one-legged squats are superior in many ways where body weight is used as the primary resistance. This provides a rich proprioceptive environment, particularly using the techniques introduced in the previous chapter.

For building squat performance for the sake of squatting more load (competition) we need to look no further than Westside Barbell in Ohio, who have cleverly adapted many of the Russian techniques for power lifting training. They understand and take full advantage of hip extension strength. When squatting, the feet are planted on the floor (actually we train lifters to "grip" the floor with feet exercises) and the athlete images hip abduction and external rotation (see figures 13.27 and 13.28). This is isometric work – once the feet are planted no actual hip external rotation takes place. These actions are then emphasized while squatting to fully recruit the glut medius and maximus (see figures 13.29 and 13.30).

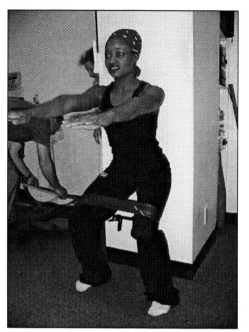

Figure 13.27 Bands around the knees are another technique to facilitate hip abduction during a squat. The hips are drifted posteriorly throughout the descent. Both of these techniques help to groove gluteal-dominant activation patterns for improved squat performance.

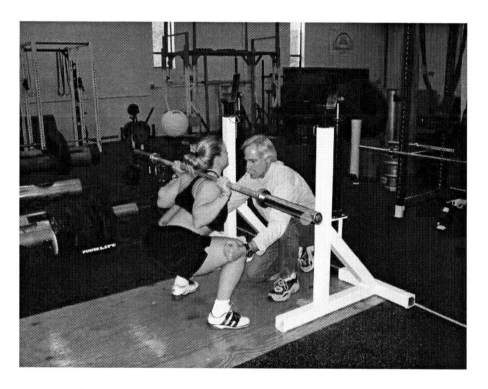

Figure 13.28 Facilitating gluteal integration by providing matched resistance to the knees during hip external rotation. The hands also guide optimal hip width and knee trajectory. This is simply grooving the pattern with an unloaded bar (with world champ Liane Blyn).

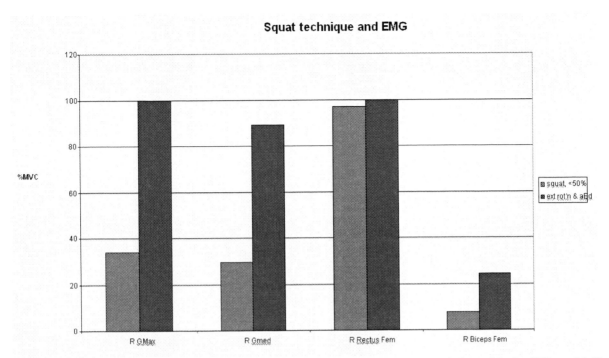

Figure 13.29 EMG data showing the additional glut med. and max. activity with the "Westside" technique of simultaneous hip external rotation and abduction.

Some other variations of functional squats are promoted by well-known gurus such as JC Santana and Mike Boyle. The one-armed, one-legged squat while pulling a load with one hand from the floor is an excellent example of a squat variation that requires full linkage integration with an overriding balance component (see figure 13.31). Using the kettlebell helps to spare the shoulder since the weight is actually behind the hand (figure 13.32). However, pushing the bell "upside down" teaches the "steering" and control of strength from the feet through the linkage to the hands – excellent! Emphasis is on spine posture and bracing with power developed at the other joints.

For some squatting athletes, squatting "back into the hole" without the low back flexing is a challenge. This inhibits performance and compromises injury risk. One "trick" to facilitate a deeper squat without "breaking the back" in flexion is to train hip flexion torque while grooving the squat pattern. This can be done with resisted flexion during the decent (see figure 13.33). Progressions for correcting the squat are shown in the DVD "McGill's Techniques"

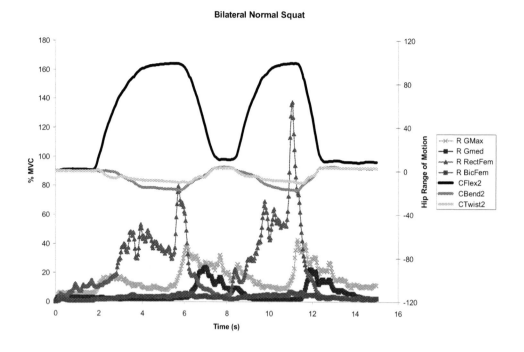

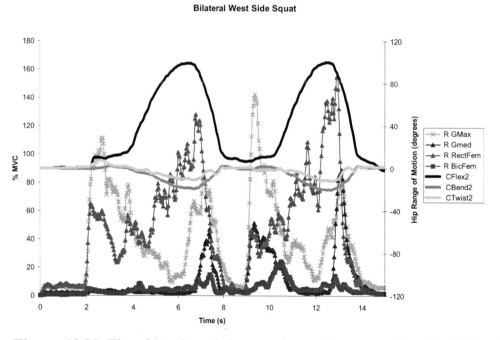

Figure 13.30 Time histories of the muscle activity comparing the "Westside" technique with the traditional squat. The Westside technique produced much higher gluteal integration.

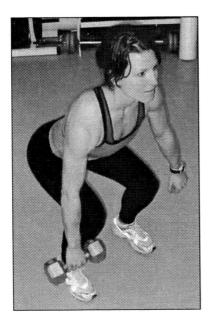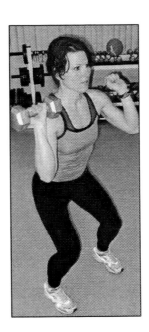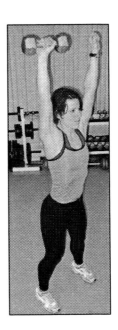

Figure 13.31 The one-armed, one-legged squat (left leg is off the ground) while pulling a load with one hand from the floor is an excellent example of a squat variation to integrate the linkage in a balance environment.

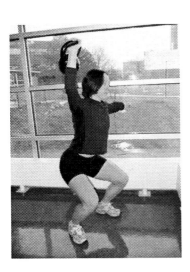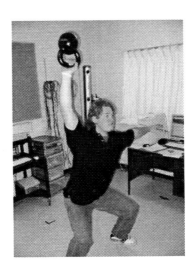

Figure 13.32 One-armed kettlebell squat trains "steering" the strength, challenging refinement of control. Another excellent attribute of the kettlebell is the mass distribution which in this case allows sparing of the shoulder since the kettlebell can be "balanced" without forcing the shoulder into full extension (left panel). The kettlebell is held upside down and "steered", training control of strength (right panel).

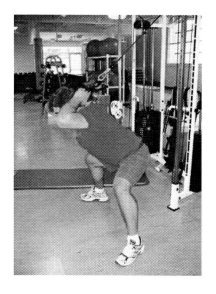

Figure 13.33 Squatting with flexor resistance provided by a cable trains hip flexion. This helps to squat back "into the hole" through the hips to eliminate lumbar flexion.

Building back and hip extension strength and performance

Assuming the foundation has been laid from following the progressions in the previous chapters, building extensor strength in the back and hip usually goes together. More advanced back bridges (see one-legged back bridges in figure 13.34) further groove the gluteal patterns established during stage 1, which will be needed for successful performance.

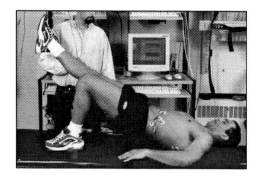

Figure 13.34 One-legged back bridges reinforce the glutual patterns established with the exercises shown in stage 1 of the training progression. Focus is on continual gluteal activation as the pelvis is raised and lowered.

Here is a nice sequence to begin strengthening the back and hips. This approach grooves some desirable motion/motor patterns while remaining in the lower end of the spine loading spectrum: the overhead hand push two legged squat (figure 13.35); single leg good morning, then with load (figure 13.36); and finally one armed lift and farmers walk (figure 13.37). Pay close attention to the mechanics and all important muscles of the back and hips will be challenged.

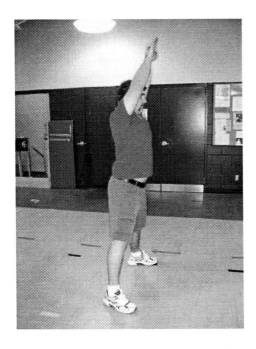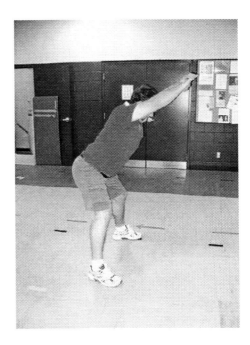

Figure 13.35 First, press one hand into the other. Employ a full "floor grip" with the toes and heel and then "spread the floor" emphasizing the hips. Stiffen the torso and hip hinge. Reverse hand position and repeat. This should be exhausting when done properly.

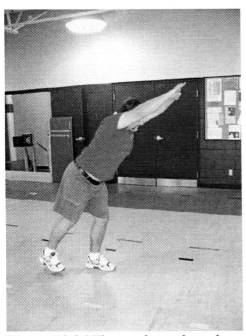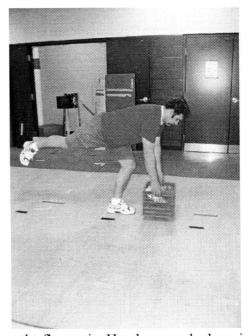

Figure 13.36 The one legged good morning employs the floor grip. Hands are pushed one into the other. Emphasis is placed on the hamstrings and gluteal complex to "hip hinge" up and down. Now try lifting a load.

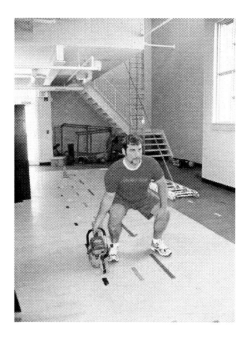

Figure 13.37 One armed lift and farmers walk is an outstanding torso conditioner. Emphasize the hip hinge for the lift, together with a stiffened torso using lattisimus dorsi and quadratus lumborum. Remember to emphasize the hand grip to facilitate the shoulder rotator cuff.

Consider the kettlebell "swing" (figure 13.38) where the emphasis is placed on hip extension. The spine is braced in a neutral posture and quite dynamic hip extension activation can be trained. It is also an exercise where the entire posterior chain is "balanced" in all aspects of performance back fitness.

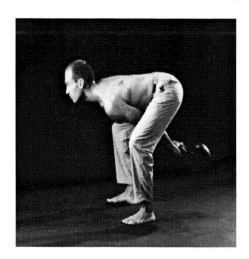
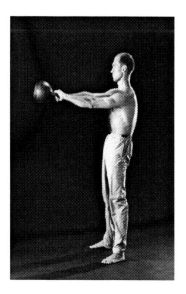

Figure 13.38 The kettlebell swing is an example of a high-level therapeutic extension exercise as it "balances" the torque distribution throughout the body linkage. Pavel Tsatsouline has the strongest pound-for-pound core I have ever measured – his approaches work!

Some of the specialized machines that have been developed need a cautionary note here. For example, the hip extension machine (see figure 13.39) can produce large posterior shear forces on the low back, which can irritate some backs. However, the machine can be very effective in helping to develop hip extensor power; a modification to the posture can help reduce some of the risk (see figure 13.40). The same posterior shear forces on the back are created in the reverse leg raise (shown in figure 13.41) and should be avoided by most athletes. Cable pulls between the legs is an alternative that produces much more "physiological" loads on the spine (see figure 13.42). Finally, sled drags are wonderful for training the extension strength. Many machines can be replaced with this exercise, resulting in much lower back loads. The "stiff-legged" drag (see figure 13.43) accomplishes the same objectives as the hip extension machine but without the worrisome shear loads. Further, the full body linkage is enhanced, in a natural balance environment, with foot grip, etc. The forces from the cable follow a line of action close to the spine which minimizes the spine loads. Focus on excellent technique. Speed and cadence can be manipulated together with short "pops" or bursts of activity in the hip extensors to prepare for speed development (stage 5).

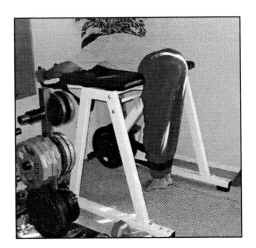 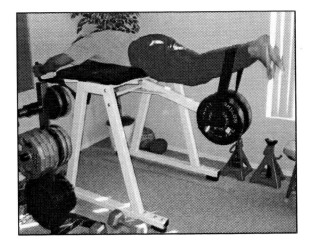

Figure 13.39 This hip extension machine is an excellent trainer for hip extension but can impose large posterior shear load on the back. It can create back troubles in some and its use requires qualification of the athlete. Focus on the elimination of spine hinging and the entire motion centered about the hip. Never sacrifice form and control to lift more weight.

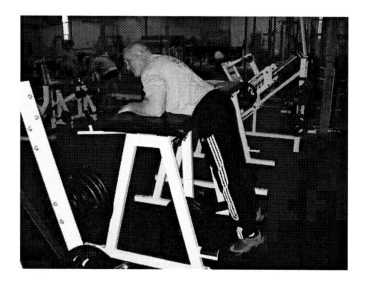

Figure 13.40 Art McDermott demonstrates a more spine conserving posture (supporting the upper body up on the elbows) while on the hip extension machine. This helps buttress and stiffen the torso/spine focussing the motion about the hips.

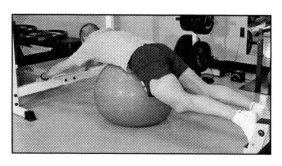

Figure 13.41 This reverse back/hip extension exercise once again causes very high posterior shear forces on the back – it is not recommended.

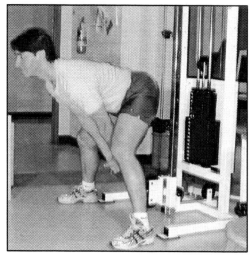
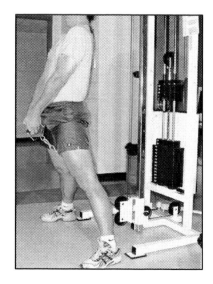

Figure 13.42 Cable pulls between the legs is a much safer alternative since anterior shear forces are imposed on the spine which are better buttressed by the musculature and the facet joints. The "hip hinge" motion is emphasized in this patterning exercise.

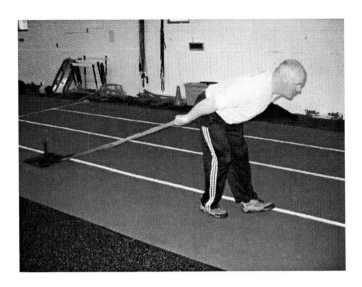

Figure 13.43 Art demonstrates the sled drag where knee flexion is kept to a minimum (stiff-legged drag). The line of action of the cable projects through the spine minimizing spine loads. This exercise can also be adapted for bursts of hip extensor activity as a precursor for the training in stage 5.

One of my favourite exercises for final transitioning into performance is the car push. Many variations of the technique can train tremendous functional strength, power, endurance and technique refinement. Functional feet must be developed to maximize grip on the ground – this is a very important aspect of performance. Then tri-planar strength is challenged and sticking points are overcome (see figure 13.44). Endurance is further enhanced by stopping the car – the athlete runs to the other end of the car and stops the motion – only to reverse the motion and complete the cycle. This is a tremendous "strongman" exercise. Another variation is to have a driver start and speed up the car as fatigue sets in to train more speed with endurance.

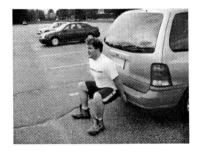 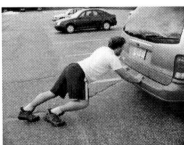 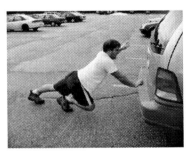

Figure 13.44 The car push is a fantastic "strongman" transition exercise involving all mechanisms from developing foot strength and control to grip the ground, to steering force through the linkage, and to final hand strength in multiplanar modes. Different techniques are trained to conquer "sticking points" and train the "tricks" of the successful strongman.

Training to power squat

Squats and power cleans are good exercises to develop power for athletic performance. The instructions from our perspective are very simple: Never sacrifice form for lifting more weight. Year after year I give this advice to young athletes, and year after year a substantial proportion will ruin their backs by not heeding this simple guideline. As the old saying goes, "it's amazing how much your parents learned as you grew older."

Very few people in North America can perform squats and power cleans with form that minimizes the risk and enables superior performance. The Eastern Europeans are technical masters; young Eastern European athletes spend years developing the form by lifting broomsticks. Only when the form is perfect is strength and weight increased. Generally, preserving the neutral lumbar spine will solve many of the safety issues. Some have found that placing the weight bar on blocks to raise the starting height improves the utility of this exercise. This way a lifter can accomplish a fast lift without the larger back loads associated with the crouched posture needed to pull from the floor. In this power exercise, speed is important. Participants are advised to "train slow to be slow, train fast to be fast". For those interested in these exercises, the actual weight kinematics for the full power clean and the coordination of the leg muscles, torso muscles, and those involved in the shoulder pull can be found elsewhere.

An interesting thought for consideration is the toll on the joints for many who continue to squat. They have to give up the exercise as they develop in their athletic career. This is why the following saying is heard – "maintain the squat but train the deadlift". This means an emphasis on the hip hinge while preserving a clean squat pattern.

What about box squats?

Given the discussions regarding "box squats", I will weigh in on the issue here. The basic intention is to enhance explosive extension and upward drive of the load. In terms of technique, the athlete sits "back" to the box (not down on the box), relaxes and then explodes up. During the seated relaxation phase the spine can be placed in peril as the muscles are needed for control to ensure stability. No spine motion can be permitted while seated. Further, some are unable to squat back to the box and sit without some spine flexion. The key is to keep the spine controlled in a neutral posture and stabilized with isometric torso muscle cocontraction. So the spine and torso are not relaxed – only the hips. This is the key for safety. Then the hips generate the explosive drive. Many athletes do not have the required hip flexion ability to accomplish the seated posture particularly when under this type of loading.

As we have seen so many times before, qualifying the athlete is extremely important. So the argument regarding the appropriateness of box squatting boils down to the suitability for the individual athlete. There are many other ways to accomplish similar goals. Hip explosive contraction training is discussed in the next chapter. The performance enhancing technique of optimizing hip hinging is found throughout this book.

Don't forget hip external rotation

Consider the athlete who runs and changes direction, or skates, or plants one foot, in other words nearly all athletes. Hip external rotation motion, strength and control is fundamental. Yet many strength programs based on sagittal plane exercises such as squats, power cleans, bench press, and Olympic lifts neglect this component as a single leg is never lifted. Begin this progression with hip airplanes (figure 10.45) followed by ballistic external rotation cable pulls (figure 13.45). Also consider bands around the mid foot while performing the monster walk as it really engages the hip external rotators with modest spine loads (Frost et al, in press) (see figure 13.46).

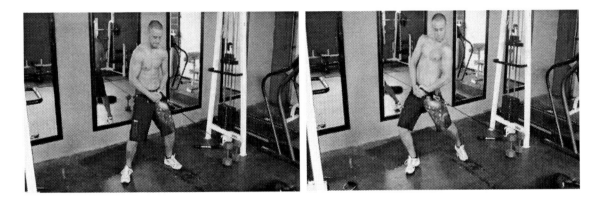

Figure 13.45 Ballistic hip external rotation cable pulls target this essential athleticism. Begin with the cable handle anchored to the front of the pelvis and progress to the hands in front – eliminate spine motion, only hip motion.

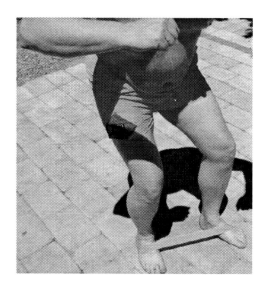

Figure 13.46 Monster walk with bands around the mid-foot optimize hip external rotation.

Don't forget Quadratus lumborum – essential strength

Our work with strongmen taught us that a strong core makes other joints stronger. We measured the hip abduction strength of a world ranked strongman to be 500 Nm yet 750Nm was measured as he carries the super yoke (McGill et al, 2009). Where did the missing strength come from to make the task possible? The hip was lifted to allow leg swing by the quadratus lumborum and obliques. This is optimally trained by asymmetric load carries. We realized then that every strength program should have elements of lifts, pushes and pulls and carries (see figure 13.47).

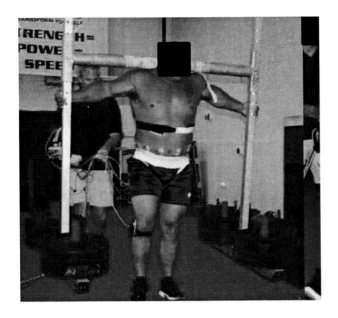

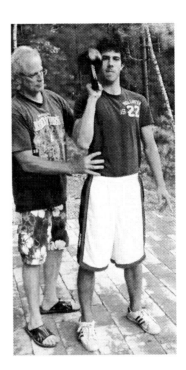

Figure 13.47 While the super yoke study revealed the essential contribution of QL more modest training methods include asymmetric carries. Carrying a kettlebell "bottoms up" teaches the discipline of steering the strength while challenging this important core capability.

Building torsional strength capabilities

Some activities that athletes or workers must perform require twisting and the creation of substantial torsional moments. The difference between the mechanics involved in twisting and the generation of torsional moments was discussed in chapter 4. The question is how to maximize stability and minimize the risk of injury during training for trunk torsion. It is unwise to train for torsion generation until the back is quite healthy. This is because, as previously noted, generating torque about the twist axis imposes approximately four times the compression on the spine as an equal torque about the flexion/extension axis. In summary, designing programs that challenge the back in all three planes should begin by training in the sagittal plane since this creates the lowest loads on the spine. Then move to the frontal plane (lateral torques) as the spine gains robustness. Finally add torsional challenges being cognizant of the high cumulative compressive load on the spine.

The technique we have found for producing low spine loads while challenging the torsional moment generators is to raise a handheld weight while supporting the upper body with the other arm and abdominally bracing (see figure 13.48) to resist the torsional torque with an isometrically contracted and neutral spine. Dynamic challenged twisting is reserved for the most robust of athletes. We would never recommend training on the torsional machines unless specific athletic performances were the training objective, and the individual must be made aware of the elevated risk of pursuing this approach.

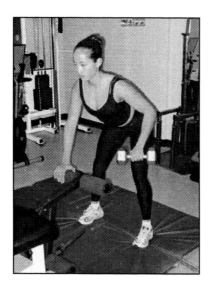

Figure 13.48 Beginning a torsional training progression is risky for some troubled backs. The most spine conserving approach that we have been able to document is the one-arm weight raise, where the abdominals are braced and the lumbar region is positioned in neutral.

Torsional progressions can be assisted with weights, bands and cables. For example, very useful and transferable twisting motion patterns are produced with the various cable exercises static cable holds then walkouts (see figure 13.49) and high pulls and low pulls (see figure earlier in chapter), together with the challenge to buttress high torsional challenges with a locked spine, if this is a desirable goal. Because of the lumbar compressive loads associated with these torsional torque challenges, we suggest discipline in bracing the torso in a neutral posture for less robust athletes. It would also be wise to consider the transmissible vector (the perpendicular distance between the cable force and the lumbar spine) when choosing the technique to control the torsional torque and resultant spine load.

The seated torsional machine found in many gyms is an example of an exercise that imposes very high spine loads throughout the range of motion. Some of the standing trunk torsional machines or resisted twisting motions are reserved for those who want to excel at very special tasks such as Olympic discus throwing. (I must add that some athletes with whom I have been associated do not perform these exercises because it exacerbates their back symptoms). Interestingly, one world-class discus thrower who has sought my advice removed twisting exercises from his regimen and his back troubles recovered to the point that he could compete and set more records. He did maintain training torsion but focused on it with an untwisted spine. The neutral position is the most robust posture to withstand the elevated spine loads; it is also the spine posture that is transferable to other activities that require torsional moments with the least risk of spine damage – even those such as discus throwing. Consider progressions such as lateral cable walkouts, then woodchops (see figure 13.42).

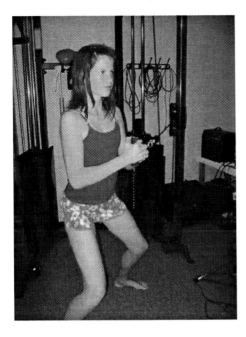 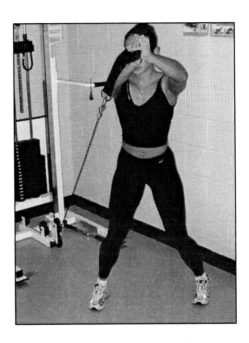

Figure 13.49 Static cable holds varying the hand/torso distance progresses to lateral cable walkouts, and progress to cable pulls. The spine is neutral and the actual "twisting" is generated by the extremities.

Very ballistic torsional training such as the "washing machine" and rapid twists with a ball in a sac bouncing on a wall to either side of the body can produce symptoms in some otherwise well-performing backs. The torsional and associated compressive loads on the spine are extremely high – again highly dependant upon the effort and vigor applied by the athlete. Recall the potent disc injury mechanism documented in chapter 3. Generally, we discourage this type of training except for rare cases (see figure 13.50).

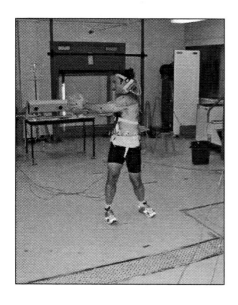

Figure 13.50 The "washing machine" shown here and the ball twist in a sac bouncing on a wall to either side of the body produces extremely high lumbar loading. The risk must be justified by the potential payoff in exercises such as this.

Various medicine ball tosses are encouraged, but only for the most robust of backs. Many will need to maintain strict bracing of the abdominals and locking the rib cage and pelvis together with no motion.

References

Behm, D.G., and Sale, D.G., (1993) Intended rather than actual movement velocity determines velocity-specific training response. Journal of Applied Physiology, 74:359-368.

Boyle, Michael, (2003) Functional Training, Human Kinetics Publishers, Champaign, Illinois.

Freeman, S., Karpowicz, A., Gray, J., and McGill, S.M. (2006) Quantifying muscle patterns and spine load during various forms of the pushup. Med. Sci: Sports and Exerc. 38(3): 570-577.

Lett, K. and McGill, S.M. (2006) Pushing and pulling: Personal mechanics influence spine loads, ERGONOMICS.

McGill, S.M., (2007) Low Back Disorders: Evidence based prevention and rehabilitation, Second Edition, Human Kinetics Publishers, Champaign, Illinois.

McGill, S.M., McDermott, A., Fenwick, C. (2009) Comparison of different strongman events: Trunk muscle activation and lumbar spine motion, load and stiffness, Journal of Strength and Conditioning Research. 23(4):1148-1161

Fenwick, C.M.J., Brown, S.H.M., McGill, S.M. (in press) Comparison of different rowing exercises: Trunk muscle activation, and lumbar spine motion, load and stiffness. Journal of Strength and Conditioning Research.

McGill, S.M., Karpowicz, A., Fenwick, C. (in press) Ballistic abdominal exercises: Muscle activation patterns during a punch, baseball throw, and a torso stiffening manoeuvre. Strength and Cond. J.

McGill, S.M., Karpowicz, A., Fenwick, C. (in press) Exercises for the torso performed in a standing posture: Motion and motor patterns. J. Strength and Conditioning Res.

Santana, J.C., Vera-Garcia, F.J., McGill, S.M., (2007) A kinetic and electromyographic comparison of standing cable press and bench press. Journal of Strength and Conditioning Research, 21(4): 1271-1279.

Verkhoshansky, Y.V., (1977) Osnovi Spetsialnoi Silovoi Podgotovki I Sporte (Fundamentals of Special Strength training in Sport), Fizkultura I Sport Publishers, Moscow.

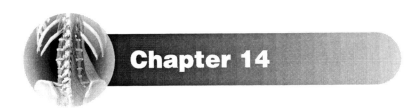

Chapter 14

Stage 5: Ultimate Performance with Speed, Power and Agility

As has been noted before in this book, developing spine power compromises both safety and performance. Power is developed in the extremities and transmitted through the torso. Power transfer through the torso requires spine posture control, spine stiffness and stability, as well as strength. The ability to repeat the transfer requires endurance. The athlete will have this foundation prior to power training. In summary, we don't train spine power, rather power development at adjacent joints is emphasized.

A note about the dead lift

Power in the torso is typically associated with power lifting – and the dead lift. The dead lift is not actually a power movement given the slowness of the task. Too many power lifters train slowly attempting close to maximum lifts but find very constrained progress. Instead, many see better performance gains by adopting true power training approaches. One example of power training for the dead lift would be to reduce the weight and lift at a much higher speed. This approach recruits a new population of motor units. The pull from the floor is problematic for many athletes, particularly those who train with dead lifts but are not competitive power lifters. For these athletes, safety can be enhanced by raising the bar and weights onto blocks for the initial pull. The athlete concentrates on the initial set position, imaging the motion and muscle recruitment. Focus is on the lumbar spine locked into a neutral position and the extensor stress is felt in the hips. Then on cue (or self-initiated by the athlete) exploding hip extension occurs, giving perfect vertical projection of force on the bar. The hip hinge is a power imaging task for many athletes (see figure 14.1).

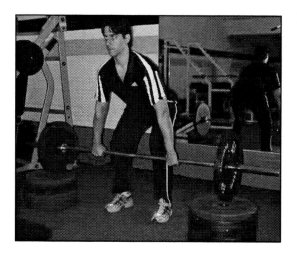

Figure 14.1 True power training with the dead lift can be facilitated by raising the bar onto blocks to raise the starting position of the bar. Many athletes are not "qualified" to attain the proper initial set position with the bar placed on the floor – thus the risk is too high. For those "qualified", the lift is performed explosively, recruiting a new population of motor units in the back extensors, gluteals and hamstrings.

Other power training for the back includes the family of medicine ball tosses, leaps, bounding and virtually any other whole body motion where focus is on the back as a link in the system (see figure 14.2).

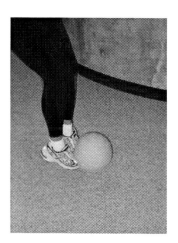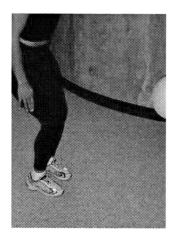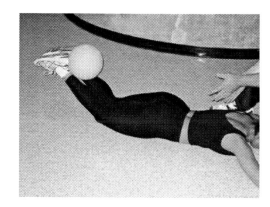

Figure 14.2 Medicine ball tosses using the feet. Hip flexion is trained as the ball is tossed with a "hop" - an excellent master level exercise. Knee flexion is challenged with the same philosophy – the coach rolls a medicine ball down the athlete's legs, who then powers the ball up off the heels. The torso is heavily braced.

Speed strength

Any person using EMG quickly comes to the realization that dynamic contraction recruits many more motor units than isometric efforts – even maximal efforts. The pioneering work of Carlo Deluca's group documented the different motor units involved with different types of muscle work and how many types of challenges are required to challenge all motor units, showing fast contraction was better at recruiting the most units. Further, the work of Behm and Sale (1993) showed that it was important to try and move the resistance as quickly as possible, even if in actuality that did not occur. Thus the effort, and intent, to move with maximal speed was important regardless of what speed was actually obtained. Speed strength training requires dedicated mental focus and discipline. The more mentally focused the athlete can be on sensing body segment trajectories, balance and attempting maximal speed, the more effective they will be. Having stated this, the emphasis is on training at a speed where the athlete is able to maintain excellent technique as opposed to training to be fast with movement flaws. Train "as fast as one can – not as fast as one can't".

An interesting discussion of speed is in the next chapter. Speed of limb motion cannot be accomplished with fully contracted muscle since the resulting stiffness hinders motion. A balance must be struck between relaxation and contraction. Failure to recognize this relationship results in too many athletes becoming slow due to their strength training.

Tips for speed strength

Most athletic tasks involve external cues to trigger the onset of speed strength. The sprint start or ball snap in football are the obvious situations. But think of the soccer goalkeeper who must react to the kicker to gain position and stop the ball. The best keepers read the biomechanical profile of the kicker and start to move even before the ball leaves the kicker's foot. This visual cue involves a different cognate process than an auditory pistol fire, or the perception of force or limb motion that a martial artist or wrestler would experience.

Integration of these triggers into speed strength training can be very important. Generally the triggers fall into three categories: auditory, visual, and tactile. These three types of cues form a continuum in terms of training difficulty with auditory being the easiest and tactile being the most difficult. The football lineman on the offensive team triggers to a verbal cue from the quarterback, as would a sprinter to a starter's pistol. Of course, training the explosion from the starting stance involves the coaching to achieve impeccable technique, but it is trained with auditory cues. A coach saying the word "hit" to initiate motion would be such an example. The way in which the word is spoken is critical. In this case, it is spoken very quickly – the best way to describe it is to have the coach try and say the word as fast as possible with nothing preceding or following the word – it is delivered with a punch out of the mouth. Exploding from a starter's block is the same motion each time, the objective being maximal forward acceleration. The defensive football lineman, on the other hand, reacts to visual cues – namely, movement of the opposing players. They have to cognitively process the visual cues and plan their motion, which may be to move forward, drop back or move laterally to the side. Training this cue can be accomplished with hand motions of the coach to fire out of the stance (see figure 14.3). The soccer keeper may adopt an initial posture that is balanced and neutral and initiate motion to the right or left based on the hand motions of the coach. Upward and downward hand trajectories can be trained in the same way to maximize speed and ball-stopping ability. Wrestlers are an example of a group that utilize tactile and proprioceptive cues to formulate a speed strength strategy. Training initiating speed movement with tactile input can begin with the athlete in the starting stance and the coach tapping them on the behind, the intensity of which will vary. A wrestler may setup for a lift drive and throw on a tackling dummy with a coach's touch cue. The techniques can be endless – but their consideration is important.

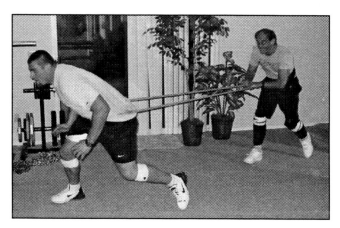

Figure 14.3 Football linemen use visual and auditory cues to fire out of their starting stance. These cues are trained together with resistive bands to stimulate more speed power.

A final notion regarding initiation of motion completes the discussion: Initiation of motion cannot be fast in an uninspired athlete. No Russian coach would place their hand on the shoulder of their athlete during speed training or competition. That naturally has a calming effect, inhibiting speed. Rather, they would square their shoulders to the athlete and whack them on the shoulders or chest usually verbally punching out a sharp loud word. "VEECH". This stimulates the speed athlete.

Agility

Training agility can involve many approaches depending on the athlete and sport. The focus here is to emphasize performing these exercises with a braced spine in a position of strength to enhance safety. It is nearly impossible to report spine loading during power exercises since the amount of effort and the resulting acceleration determine the loading. Only principles based on strong science, together with the wisdom that is developed in those who have worked in training high performance, can be used to guide the expert. Some of these exercises will greatly enhance performance in qualified athletes, while some backs simply will not tolerate these higher-demand exercises.

When designing agility workouts, we recommend that the "big three" (described in the previous chapter) be performed at the beginning of the workout to help groove and establish the stable motor patterns for the rest of the training session. Some trainers also like to finish the session with these exercises, sometimes taking the exertions to fatigue.

The exercise variations are endless and are outside of the scope of this book. However, several approaches are described here. Developing "quick feet" is a challenge that requires hip flexion and lateral moment ability, whole body balance and integration of the full torso. While there are many quick feet progressions, one involves the dynamic lunge/jerk. The athlete assumes a lunge posture and then quickly switches his stance and foot position (see figure 14.4). Mental focus is on imaging the motor units involved prior to the jerk; in addition, focus is directed towards balance both before and during the jerk. The objective is to switch the feet and land with no imbalance. Variations include lateral foot placement patterns as well. We use these drills for athletes such as soccer goalkeepers and volleyball players. Sometimes no weight is used, from which the athlete can make sudden lateral movements or transitions into the appropriate gait patterns of their sport.

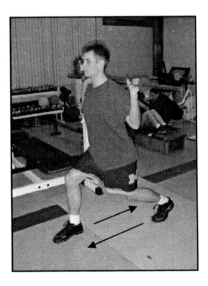 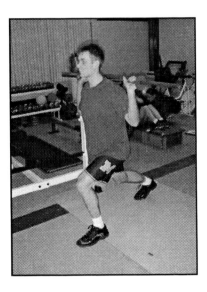

Figure 14.4 Quick feet exercise where the focus is on speed, balance and imaging motor units for optimal performance.

Progressing into plyometrics

There are many good sources for information on plyometric

training. Only a few back and spine issues need addressing here. As with all training approaches, plyometric training must follow a progression. For example, any sort of jumping or leaping performance requires a very stiff torso to allow the explosion of hip extensor torque to transmit through the body linkage without energy losses. This training is begun with a modified birddog. The posture is assumed and the torso stiffened with abdominal contraction as very quick bursts of hip and shoulder extensor activity are created. All motion is about the shoulder and hip as no motion must occur in the spine (see figure 14.5). Then jumping training can proceed.

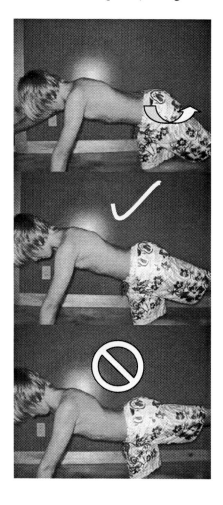

Figure 14.5 Very quick bursts of extensor activity are performed at the shoulder and hip. No spine motion must occur. In the starting position, the torso is stiffened with abdominal contraction (top panel). Excellent technique is shown (middle panel) together with poor technique (bottom panel) where spine motion increases the injury risk and compromises performance with energy losses.

Mike Boyle, for example, provides excellent progressions for hopping and jumping, where first the takeoff mechanics are perfected followed by specific emphasis on landing mechanics. Several tests are used to ensure the athlete possesses the required eccentric strength to avoid injury and optimize the elastic energy mechanisms. Generally, the motion is about the hips and knees – not the low back, at least for hopping and jumping. The spine is in a neutral posture and stabilized with abdominal co-contraction. The exercise of hopping on one leg from one square to another is an excellent beginner's exercise to start plyometrics while the effort is controlled and the forces "steered" (see figure 14.6). Simple hopping on to a box is added, but lateral motion is often neglected at this stage (see figure 14.7). Abdominal plyometric exercises were introduced in the previous pages with medicine ball tosses. Observe the extended recovery times needed to avoid back troubles with this type of training. Additional torso plyometric exercises include the deadbug adapted for plyometrics to enhance torso, hip and shoulder dynamics. The "clapping" pushup is a plyometric exercise that challenges the entire stiffening mechanism – the contrast between excellent technique and performance with average performance is seen in figure 14.8. More short-range abdominal stiffening under plyometric conditions can be accomplished with the "1 inch punch" (see figure 14.9). Some record-setting lifters actually engage the "springs" by setting their hip and torso posture with the hands not able to reach the bar. Stiffening of these joints is the focus. Then a rapid descent to grab the bar followed by the lift is performed. I do note that this is a very controversial technique and may cause unnecessary risk.

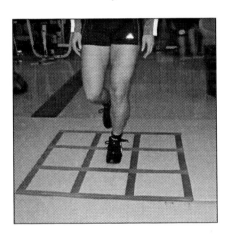

Figure 14.6 The athlete stands in the middle square and then "hops" into each other square and back to the middle. This teaches "steering" force and emphasis is on control of both balance and spine stability. The squares are about 1 foot each.

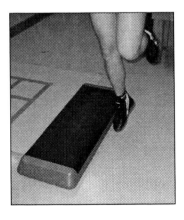

Figure 14.7 Lateral "hops" onto a box assists in optimizing the plyometric progression. Ensure that these progressions are well established prior to incorporating landing exercises. (The athlete is in mid-air here).

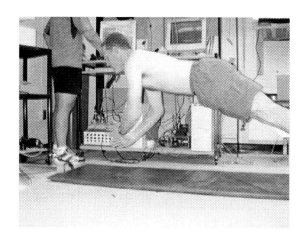

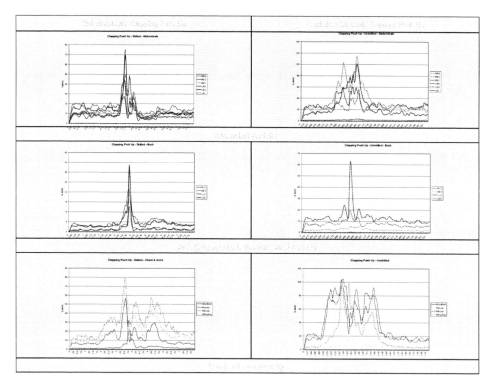

Figure 14.8 The clapping pushup is an excellent plyometric exercise building short range stiffness. Technique is important, as seen in the left panels of a professional athlete demonstrating coordinated muscle contraction with perfect timing of the activation burst resulting in superstiffness (see next chapter). In contrast, an "average graduate student" (right panels) is replicating the exercise but simply can't achieve the level of coordination, the speed of muscle activation and deactivation needed for high performance.

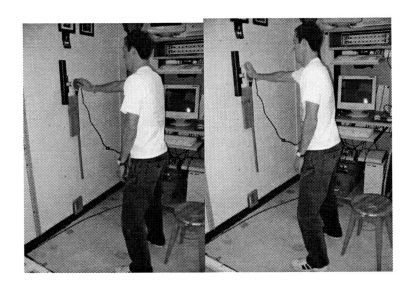

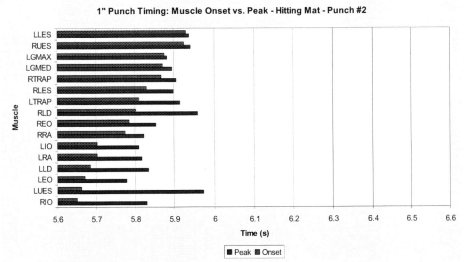

Figure 14.9 The "one-inch punch" made famous by Bruce Lee contains an element of plyometric contraction. Muscle onset times together with the peak forces which occur later, show how the peak forces align more tightly in time than do the muscle onsets. Note that the peak force is important for performance, not onsets. Some mild pre-coactivation to stiffen the elastic components of the muscles usually results in a more precise alignment of the peak torso forces – and a more devastating punch.

Final thoughts on program design

There are all sorts of sport-specific manuals that discuss training and program design to suit a particular season of play. There are specific plans to peak and taper performance which are a most important component of program design. This book has added another important approach for your training toolbox. Begin with the establishment of basic motion and motor patterns. Moving to stability and endurance builds a foundation for ultimate strength and power training. Progressing from exercises that utilize body weight through to external resistance is another general approach. Beginning with floor exercises and stable surfaces and progressing to various types of labile surfaces and labile loads helps to develop the supreme performer.

Speed was discussed at several junctures in the book. Many athletes impede their speed-strength development by designing their training regimens around "heavy" and "light" training sessions. This usually results in the same old exercises in a mixture of loads to challenge strength and endurance. This produces an average or poor performance outcome. Light sessions usually result in exhaustion and reflects a body-building philosophy rather than a performance philosophy. In contrast, performance would probably be enhanced by switching to a "fast" and "slow" session design. Slow training with large resistances will build the musculoskeletal and neurological capacity needed for dense contraction. Fast training with different exercises will enhance performance.

Another theme of the book was to thoughtfully dissect the demands of the athletic task and train for them. Catalogue the athletes' performance for athletic demands and train for them. As a Russian hockey star replied to a North American trainer telling him to warm up on a bike, "when the NHL puts bikes on the ice I will ride one". My colleague Jon Chaimberg catalogues his fighters fights for demands such as isometric holds, explosive strikes and escapes, changes in levels from standup to on the ground, changes in direction, etc. He organizes the training sessions the same way – no jogging for his athletes. Resist the urge to follow traditional "strength" programs but make them sport or activity specific. There are no rules – only guidelines. Use training time wisely by choosing exercises that accomplish several goals at once, such as enhancing balance, stability, strength and power. Train the motion – not the muscle.

A summary of considerations for developing general progressions:
1. Peak and taper according to competition schedule.
2. Corrective exercise to performance training.
3. Basic motion/motor patterns to stability/mobility to endurance to strength to power.
4. Body weight to external resistance.
5. Stable surfaces to labile surfaces to labile loads.

6. Combine "fast" and "slow" exercise sessions, not "heavy" and "light".
7. Resist designing programs around areas of the body, rather, think of a push, a pull, a carry and a lift.

References

Behm, D.G., and Sale, D.G., (1993) Intended rather than actual movement velocity determines velocity-specific training response. Journal of Applied Physiology, 74:359-368.

Boyle, Michael, (2003) Functional Training, Human Kinetics Publishers, Champaign, Illinois.

Freeman, S., Karpowicz, A., Gray, J., and McGill, S.M. (2006) Quantifying muscle patterns and spine load during various forms of the pushup. Med. Sci: Sports and Exerc. 38(3): 570-577.

Lett, K., and McGill, S.M., (2006) Push and pulling mechanics and implications for low back load. 49(9): 895-908.

McGill, S.M., (2007) Low Back Disorders: Evidence based prevention and rehabilitation, Second Edition, Human Kinetics Publishers, Champaign, Illinios.

McGill, S.M., Karpowicz, A., Fenwick, C. (in press 2009) Ballistic abdominal exercises: Muscle activation patterns during a punch, baseball throw, and a torso stiffening manoeuvre. Strength and Cond. J.

Santana, J.C., Vera-Garcia, F.J., McGill, S.M., (2007) A kinetic and electromyographic comparison of standing cable press and bench press. Journal of Strength and Conditioning Research, 21(4): 1271-1279.

Verkhoshansky, Y.V., (1977) Osnovi Spetsialnoi Silovoi Podgotovki I Sporte (Fundamentals of Special Strength training in Sport), Fizkultura I Sport Publishers, Moscow.

Chapter 15

Final transitional training - Ultimate performance with the techniques of Super Stiffness, and other tricks

The foundation for performance has been laid with the 5 stages of back training described in this book. The best performers in the world use techniques to best utilize their strength and speed. They are able to conquer the "sticking points" during a lift or eliminate "energy leaks" during a jump, takeoff or throw. They redirect neuronal overflow into the desired region of the body for extraordinary effect. They employ the muscle/fascia binding effect from coordinated activation of families of muscles. There is no question that every world record holder is biologically gifted but they are technique masters as well. Many training gurus and therapists understand how to build a foundation but often fail to complete the final transitional training, taking the athlete to their ultimate performance. This chapter is intended to reveal some of the components to enhance the transition to optimal performance.

Principle #1 – Rapid contraction and then relaxation of muscle

I have measured muscle contraction in many top athletes. Their ability to rapidly contract muscle is astounding, but even more astounding is their ability to rapidly relax the muscle. Too many coaches train for speed with more strengthening approaches, actually slowing the athlete down. True speed requires rapid reciprocating limb motion. Rapid limb motion requires rapid transitioning between compliant muscles for speed but very active and stiff muscles for force and joint torque production. A muscle that cannot relax quickly will slow the athlete. Consider a world class sprinter: In the starting blocks they are relaxed. They are not "primed" with substantial muscle activation because the resulting stiffness would slow any subsequent motion. Then, upon the gun, an impressively rapid contraction transpires to generate speed. But, an equally impressive rapid deactivation of the muscle occurs to maintain the speed. The muscles then activate to prepare for the next leg cycle. All this occurs in the first step out of the blocks! And this happens in each stride (see figure 15.1).

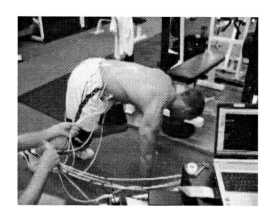
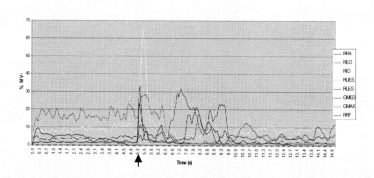

Figure 15.1 The muscles contract at an astounding rate at the sound of the gun (arrow); equally astounding is the rate of deactivation to allow speed. The elite athlete shown here is simply reacting to the gun and then falling forward to practice contraction onset/offset.

In this way, super stiffness is used by the best football hitters, golfers, martial artists and weightlifters. Consider the hit in football where maximum speed of approach requires the combination of sufficient stiffness and compliance. At the instant of impact, a total body stiffness is generated by rapid contraction of all muscles. This is what makes the impact so devastating by some. We has measured some of the great UFC mixed martial arts fighters recently who create a double pulse that results in impressive strike speed and power. World Champ Georges St Pierre shows the form (see figure 15.2). The first pulse initiates the foot or fist motion. Then some core muscles relax as speed increases while the hand/foot close the distance. Then the second pulse is timed to impact which stiffens the entire body. This is known as "effective mass" where the body is instantaneously turned to stone and the impact has the full weight of the fighter behind it. Rapid relaxation allows for a quick return to a defensive posture. Pavel shows a kick and his erector spinae EMG signal highlighted. He hits fast and hard – as a side note he has the strongest core, pound for pound we have ever measured. Add speed to this ability and awesome kicks result (see figure 15.3). The professional golfer who has a relaxed backswing and initiation of downward club motion, but rapidly obtains super stiffness at ball impact, is the one who achieves the long ball (see figure 15.4). The one who tries to swing too hard with muscle activation too soon actually decreases speed of movement. This is why trying to "kill the ball" only results in a shortened distance. The axeman splitting wood uses the same technique. Muhammad Ali, Bruce Lee and Vasily Alexeyev all knew the secrets of Superstiffness. Understand the relationship between speed, compliance and stiffness and you will be achieving ultimate performance. I recommend Pavel's "Fast and Loose" DVD here.

The beat: "Boom - Boom"

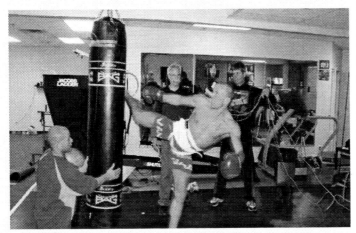

Figure 15.2 Georges St Pierre shows the "stiffening" at impact from the second pulse. The EMG electrodes are measuring the torso and hip muscle activation while other instrumentation measured spine motion. There is a "beat" to the motion and he is conscious of the two pulses – one to initiate motion and the second for impact with a relaxation phase for speed between them.

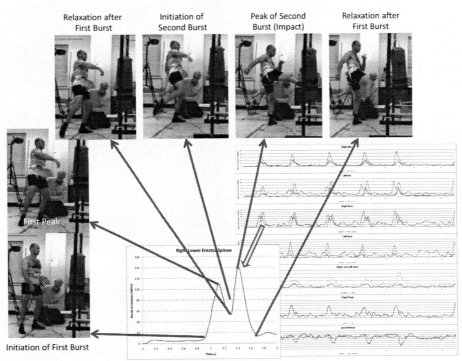

Figure 12.3 Pavel shows the first pulse (low back extensors) initiates foot motion but relaxes as the foot leaves the ground. The second pulse is timed to impact – resulting in a devastating kick.

Good Swing - Torso Muscle Activation

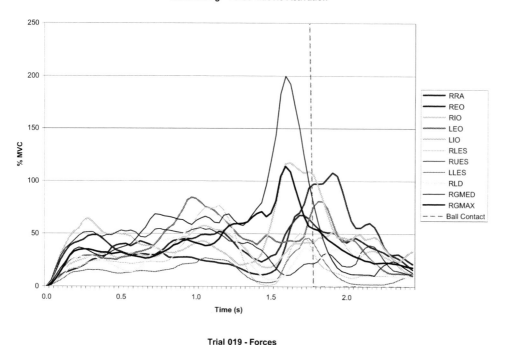

Trial 019 - Forces

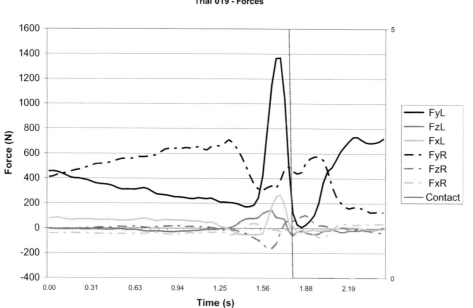

Figure 15.4 This elite golfer illustrates the burst of muscle activity just prior to ball contact to stiffen the linkage (upper panel). Too much activation either before or after contact would slow the swing. Too little activation at ball contact would thwart superstiffness and allow energy leaks. The lower panel shows the three-dimensional foot forces (y axis is vertical, x is lateral, z is anterior-posterior) and the massive stiffening down the left leg (emanating from the hips and torso) just before ball contact, followed by complete unloading.

The implication of this phenomenon is that the neuromuscular system must be trained for rapid muscle contraction, but equally as important is the training for rapid muscle relaxation. This is difficult and requires the athlete to look for opportunities within their motion repertoire. For example, the boxer or martial artist can train being "light on their feet", the Ali "float and shuffle" if you will, exuding relaxation. Then very rapid arm motion is initiated with a rapid "snap" halting hand motion. This exercise is to simply train the muscles to "pop" ON and OFF. The exercise then transitions to a total body contraction, initiated in the hips and core, upon fist impact ensuring super stiffness. Technique is enhanced to ensure proper line of drive of force throughout the body linkage.

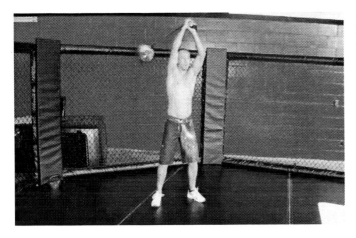

Figure 15.5 Mark Hominick shows an exercise we use with MMA fighters to create endurance with isometric contractions but "pulses" are overlayed for speed. As the ball passes 12 o'clock the athlete pulse-stiffens the body. Then switching to other times such as 3 o'clock trains neurological dexterity. The emphasis is on rapid contraction and relaxation.

Other exercises can include, for the hip extensors, performing the one-legged squat while "popping" the gluteal muscle on the leg held out behind at the beginning of the motion (see figure 15.6). The medicine ball exercises shown in the previous chapter are adapted to focus on "popping" the hip and back extensors during a double underhand throw, or the flexors with a double overhead toss. Again the focus is on rapid muscle activation and deactivation. Any of the stabilization exercises shown earlier can be adapted to train this neural ability to enhance short range stiffness. For example, the "dead bug" can be adapted so that the hip and opposite arm are "popped" in unison at just a short distance (see figure 15.7). However, such an example leads to the discussion of "tuning" of the abdominals.

Matveyev (1981) proposed that an efficient way to train speed of relaxation was to release an isometric contraction. Using an example with the fighters, we have them take a "ready position". They over-emphasize the isometric contraction. Then they try to release the stiffening contraction upon rapid arm motion such as with a strike. Once this is mastered an impact with a bag is introduced to encourage the second pulse. Consider the superstiffness concept of pulsing for speed in all sorts of performances.

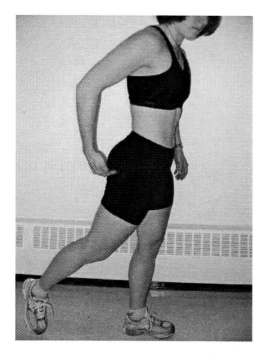

Figure 15.6 Starting relaxed, the athlete "pops" the gluteal muscles by quickly activating, then relaxing, them. This "control" for rapid contraction onset/offset can be trained in many postures.

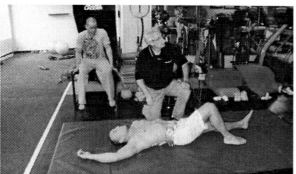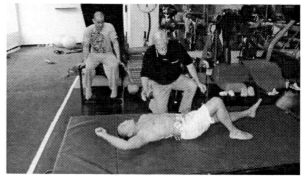

Figure 15.7 Denis Kang shows the pulse to train rapid contraction then relaxation of muscle. The arm and opposite leg are twitched at the shoulder and hip. Very little motion takes place – the emphasis is on neurological speed of contraction the relaxation.

Principle #2 - Tuning of the muscles

Consider the abdominal wall, which has been shown earlier in this book to act as an elastic spring for many athletic endeavors. The thrower, kicker, runner or golfer all employ the abdominal spring. Storage of elastic energy in a compliant spring, or a soft spring, is rapidly dissipated or lost. This happens if the muscle is not activated to a sufficient level. If the spring is too stiff, elastic energy storage is hampered because there is minimal elasticity and no movement (for the biomechanists, this is because the integral of the force-displacement curve is compromised). So, the pre-contraction level of the muscle just prior to the loading phase is extremely important. Another phenomenon is linked with this process. Interestingly enough, the contraction level and the resulting stiffness and stability forms a non-linear asymptotic function. In other words, a lot of stiffness and stability is achieved in the first 25% of the maximum contraction level (see Brown and McGill, 2005 for an example from core muscles). From our work examining several different rapid loading situations, it appears that a pre-contraction level of about 25% of MVC creates the amount of muscle stiffness for optimal storage and recovery of elastic energy in the core muscles (at least in many situations). Less than this results in a spongy system while more than this creates stiffness that impedes energy return and also unnecessarily crushes the spine and joints.

Principle #3 - Muscular binding and weaving

When all muscles at a joint stiffen together a "super stiffness" phenomenon generally occurs. The total stiffness at a joint suddenly becomes more than the sum of individual muscle stiffnesses. Consider the abdominal wall in creating "core stability". The three layers of the abdominal wall have fibres that run in different directions. This architecture is similar to that of plywood, where one layer has the wood grain running north and south while the next layer runs east and west. The layers are bound by glue forming a composite material. The properties and features of similarly constructed composites include light weight and stiffness. Rectus abdominis, external and internal oblique and transverse abdominis form a composite when activated together. They appear to bind together when all are active to create a super stiffness that is higher than the sum of each individual muscle (see Brown and McGill, 2009a, 2009b). For those activities that demand high core or torso stability, all muscles must be activated – never isolate one. This superstiffness may be maintained for a substantial amount of time, such as a weightlifter needing high stability to prevent spine buckling. A golfer may create superstiffness temporarily just at ball impact with more compliance pre and post ball contact to ensure maximal swing speed.

The training suggestion here is to simultaneously contract all layers of the abdominal wall, or all components of the back extensors, or any other muscle group. For some reason, some coaches and trainers have adopted the notion of training just transverse abdominis or multifidus in an attempt to train core stability. This is pathological in that muscular binding will be compromised. The fascial raking techniques described previously are helpful techniques to optimize binding. Consider the hanging kip exercise, where substantial performance improvements are seen with proper contraction of the complete abdominal wall.

Principle #4 - Directing neuronal overflow

The phenomenon of strength training one arm, but not the other, with subsequent strength gains in the untrained arm is well known. Of course, there will be some enhancement in motor patterning, but there also appears to be neuronal overflow to the unexercised arm accounting for some of the enhancement. Rehabilitation clinicians use the phenomenon to enhance strength at a compromised joint. In principle, contraction at other joints is utilized to "squeeze" the neural drive back to the joint where enhanced performance is required. Here is a well-known, and graphic example of the phenomenon. Shake a partner's hand, and squeeze as hard as possible. Then, repeat the task after doing the following. Use the techniques previously described to prepare for a competitive squat – grip the floor, preactivate the gluteal muscles, stiffen the core and make a fist with the other hand while co-contracting the "other" arm. Now repeat the squeezing handshake. You should experience a much more robust contraction. This is one of the principles to get through the "sticking point" experienced during many strength tasks and is described in the next section. Another example to illustrate the enhancement of strength performance is to stand on a bathroom scale (or forceplate) and hold out the arms in an Iron Cross posture while pushing down on supporting objects. Measure how much of your body weight is supported off the scale. Then cocontract the abdominals with all of the techniques (described above) optimized. Some individuals will see a 30% increase in the amount of weight they can lift off the scale. Look for this opportunity in your sport-specific training. Some simply practice stiffening against immovable objects; a park playground offers all sorts of opportunities (see figure 15.8).

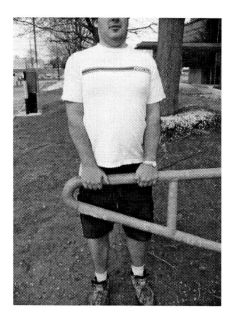

Figure 15.8 Isometric whole body stiffening exercises can be performed at a playground against bars or racks. In this example, the athlete stiffens all joints while pulling up on the immovable bar although the mental image is directed to pushing the ground down. **Special Note:** The idea is not to crush the joints with maximal effort, rather, it is to train the neuromuscular system to create whole body stiffness.

Principle # 5 - Eliminate energy leaks

Several techniques are necessary to eliminate energy leaks and ensure ultimate performance. At a gymnastics or martial arts meet, or at a weightlifting competition, listen to the coach's advice to the athlete – *Stay tight*! This means to maintain stiffness. Being stiff ensures minimal energy losses, as forces are transmitted through the linkage, and that joints will not buckle and injure. Of course, knowing the difference between when to be stiff and when to be compliant is the key. Bruce Lee was a master from the perspective of employing this principle for martial arts performance. His analogy of water was appropriate, which is extremely hard when hit quickly (it stiffens) but "gives" and flows when pushed slowly (to dissipate energy). Structural engineers work to minimize energy leaks in mechanical systems by enhancing stiffness. Consider an expensive bicycle frame, which is stiff. As one pushes on each pedal the forces are transmitted to the wheels – a compliant frame allows flex which results in energy losses with each foot exertion. Optimal and efficient transmission of force through a linkage requires joint stiffness. Whole body stiffness is important for certain tasks such as lifting, or for some of the "strongman" competitions to avoid injury and work through the compromised joint "sticking points"(see discussion in previous chapter, McGill et al, 2009). Read "The Naked Warrior" by Pavel (Pavel Tsatsouline, 2003), to see the tests and training for super stiffness in sustained contractions – his technique of using a stick to whack and prod looking for "soft areas" when performing a pushup is an excellent example. It is not for the faint of heart.

Energy leaks are also eliminated with technique so that concentric contraction at stronger joints does not force unwanted eccentric contraction at weaker joints. Consider the leaper in basketball. The planting foot is flat on the ground and the power source is primarily the hip. The hip is so powerful in rapid extension that if the foot plant was on the ball of the foot, the foot would be forced flat to the floor and the ankle extensors forced into eccentric contraction, resulting in lost energy. (This is why I am continually puzzled by coaches who train ankle extension with ankle/heel raise exercises in their leapers). Once again, many martial arts techniques employ this principle to stiffen weaker joints, thus allowing the more powerful joints to efficiently transmit their force (for example, the stiffened fist with wrist pronation stiffens the wrist and elbow to transmit power generated at the shoulder). In a similar way, a fast runner stiffens the torso including the pelvis to allow the efficient transfer of force between the arms and the legs – there should be no moving joints in between the hips and the shoulders. Training to stiffen the core will enhance speed in these athletes.

Stiffness is also enhanced by positional techniques within the body segment linkage where one segment can be stiffened against another – for example, stiffening an arm against the torso. Body checking athletes employ this technique.

Principle #6 - Get through the "sticking points"

In many strength tasks, there is a "sticking point", a compromise of joint torque or strength, which results from the biomechanics linked to muscle architecture. For example, the force generating ability of the muscle itself is constrained by its force/length and force/velocity relationships, determined by morphology. These relationships are further modulated by angles of adjacent joints, given that many muscles span more than one joint. Muscle lever arms, with respect to the joint fulcrum and angle of pull, also change as a function of joint position. However, these mechanics can be cleverly altered to reduce inherent weakness.

The techniques involved in "superstiffness" can shift some of the demand from weaker joints to stronger joints. Consider the strongman competitor who is lifting the huge earth mover tire. Usual technique is to grip the edge of the tire, dead lift until the tire will move no further as elbow flexion is maximal, but insufficient. The athlete is stuck. Superstiffening the entire body at this moment drives the hands higher. More power from the hips is transmitted through the linkage this way. This occurs in the Olympic lifter just as the initial drive is completed with transition into the catch.

Consider the bench presser who is stuck at the mid point of the lift. Bench pressing should be a total body stiffening effort. Consciously trying to "spread the bar", and "bend the bar", through the handgrip is an example of stiffening to alter the mechanics and drive through the sticking point.

Principle #7 - Optimize the passive connective tissue system

For years, coaches and trainers have been ruining athletic performance with inappropriate stretching. Consider elite runners: They are elite because they run, to a large extent, on passive tissue, not muscle. They are kangaroos! In fact, they are able to stiffen their passive tissues further with muscle activation given the many ligamentous and fascial connections. This ability is enhanced with plyometric training (which is often accomplished by simply performing the actual task) but is compromised with stretching. For example, a general guideline is to never stretch a runner beyond the joint angles utilized in running. Keep them tight to engage the springs with each stride. This is a form of superstiffness. Stretching should only be considered to correct asymmetries between right and left sides of the body. Once again, this should be in conjunction with core stiffening and reciprocal stiffening. This requires high expertise and consideration of the individual – it is a key component of my consulting with elite athletes. Thank goodness the good coaches are realizing the interaction of the passive systems with the neuromuscular system, and the effects of stretching vs optimal stiffness.

Principle #8 – Create shockwaves

Creating shockwaves through the body linkage, with appropriate stiffening, is a tremendous technique for performance enhancement. Consider a one-armed dumbbell or kettlebell military press. Use a weight that is too heavy to simply press it up. Then try the following: Stiffen the body linkage all the way through to the gripping muscles. Then with the knees and hips create a rapid, but very small amplitude "dip". This initiates the shockwave. The body must be very stiff to transmit the wave upwards to the load. Then the load will start moving and the press will be successful. Insufficient stiffness is akin to tying to push a rope. But a stone can be pushed. Turn the body to stone.

Another example is used by some benchpressers – particularly the Russian trained competitors. As the bar is lowered to the chest, the heels of the feet "stomp" to initiate the shockwave which then travels up through the stiffened torso to initiate the drive on the bar (see the writings of Pavel Tsatsouline).

This is an effective technique used by many world record holders in all sports.

Consider the concepts of superstiffness. If they are harnessed correctly, performance will be enhanced and the risk of injury reduced.

References

Brown, S.H. and McGill, S.M. (2005) Muscle force-stiffness characteristics influence joint stability. Clin. Biomech., 20(9): 917-922.

Brown*,S., McGill, S.M. (in press 2009) An ultrasound investigation into the morphology of the human abdominal wall uncovers complex deformation patterns during contraction. Eur. J. Appl. Physiol.

Brown, S., McGill, S.M. (2009) Transmission of muscularly generated force and stiffness between layers of the rat abdominal wall. SPINE, 34(2): E70-E75.

Matveyev, L., (1981) Fundamentals of sports training, Progress Publ. Moscow (English).

McGill, S.M., McDermott, A., Fenwick, C. (2009) Comparison of different strongman events: Trunk muscle activation and lumbar spine motion, load and stiffness, Journal of Strength and Conditioning Research.

McGill, S.M., Chaimberg, J., Frost, D., Fenwick, C. (In press, 2009) The double peak: How elite MMA fighters develop speed and strike force.

Tsatsouline, P., (2003) The Naked Warrior, Dragon Door Publications Inc, St Paul, Mn. USA.

Chapter 16

Putting it All Together: Case Studies

As has been noted earlier, some of the best athletes are not only physically skilled mutants, but mentally skilled ones as well. While they have worked to develop their skills, they also possess special gifts. Even so, it is surprising to find there is often potential remaining to be exploited for even higher performance. Of course, our interest is to find this potential and harness it in a way that compliments additional objectives to either reduce existing back symptoms or prevent new ones from occurring. Here is a sampling of some of the interesting cases from athletes who have asked for our opinion and expertise, and how we attempted to assist. Each case is different and may not be suitable for other similar athletes. Some details, not relevant to the back exercise issue, may have been changed to protect the identity of the athlete.

Enhancing the agility of a soccer goalkeeper

One of the gifts/strengths of elite goalkeepers is superb anticipation skills – specifically anticipating where the ball will be directed. In fact, the keeper will begin moving in a direction even before the ball leaves the offensive kicker's foot. The keeper makes a bet based on their perception of the kicker's leg trajectory, foot-ball contact angle and then attempts to get to the anticipated target. The best offensive players in the world are masters at giving false cues – at the last instant they can change the angle of their foot and redirect the ball in a direction most confusing to the keeper.

We have the challenge of further developing the agility and "speed off the mark" of a keeper – moving in any direction but mostly laterally. While this keeper had not had serious low back injury concerns, the subsequent training required to develop agility is a "back" concern. For example, supremely "quick feet" are required, and these impose elevated hip torques and back loads, resulting in a high risk for subsequent back troubles. Hip flexion power is tricky to train without producing back symptoms in those so inclined. Psoas loading is a concern and is often problematic.

Before we began training agility, in particular "quick feet" we had to develop the foundation of excellent motor patterns and a highly stable spine. The keeper had excellent spine position awareness and spine movement and conserving skills. Training consisted of taking the keeper through training to the highest challenge level of the Big Three, fusing challenged breathing and one legged-squats with dynamic correspondence of the opposite hip, etc. Only then would we take the risk to develop supremely quick feet and "speed off the mark".

"Quick feet" began with the athlete taking a lunge position with a light barbell "shelved" on the trapezius behind the base of the neck. Mental training, specifically imaging, was integrated to optimize the concentrated focus of recruiting the maximal number of motor units in the hips and torso while maintaining standing balance. The athlete focused on remaining balanced and still, and then on the upcoming movement. The task was to quickly reverse the lunge, with the feet changing position, and was to "stick" the landing with no further movement of any body part. Mental focus was directed towards perfect balance and once achieved, was then directed towards the next repetition of lunge reversal. Imaging is focused on the hip torques to switch the legs at the highest velocity possible, the "stuck landing" and the held position. Minimal spine motion with robust torso muscle bracing was emphasized throughout.

Once the sagittal plane lunges were mastered, the next stage was to begin lateral lunges where the feet cross over upon landing. Once again, mental focus was directed toward balance, "stuck landings", minimal spine motion and torso bracing patterns. Additional stepping patterns were also developed and practiced with no resistive weight – pulling quickly to the right and left, perfecting and integrating the newfound power and speed. Leaping drills to height with projections to both sides enhanced the process. The dynamic motions were filmed and reviewed with the athlete following the optimal movement principles introduced in chapter 7.

The final stage was to integrate the relevant stimulus – in this case, it was a visual cue perceived by the keeper, based upon the kicker's kinematic patterns. To complete the preparation, the coach stood in front of the keeper, who was in the "quick feet" lunge position. Using the coach's hand signals only, the keeper reacted by performing the appropriate feet switch. Be very aware of the hip torques demanded in this exercise and the superb preconditioning required to minimize the risk of back troubles. If done well, the "speed off the mark" in any direction will be enhanced.

Re-grooving the chronic back of an elite golfer

It is not uncommon for all levels of golfers to have their careers shortened by back complaints. Such was the case with a pro golfer whose symptoms prevented both sufficient practice and competitive play. After measuring his three-dimensional range of lumbar motion, it was clear that his full spine motion used in the swing prevented any hope for recovery. The only option was to remove the cause – specifically, shorten the backswing and reduce the "lateral crunch" associated with the instant of ball contact. The great golfers also have a distinct "pulse" of muscle activity that corresponds with ball contact. Work to time the pulse when the spine is in a more neutral posture. Those with painful backs often have the pulse mis-timed such that it occurs when the spine is still deviated. Reducing these three parameters a small amount stopped the spine from slamming into the passive tissue "stops" to motion. Symptoms were reduced. To re-groove a golfer's swing is challenging since it is a pattern that had been reinforced for most of their life.

We began this motion pattern process at the fundamental level. This comprised of teaching the abdominal brace together with minimizing lumbar motion and locking the rib cage onto the pelvis. We started on the wall with the wall roll (chapter 10), correcting the technique until all lumbar motion was eliminated. Then we moved to easily swinging the club while keeping the rib cage locked on. Slowly the transition was made to hitting a few balls – focusing on the torso motion and motor patterns, not on ball performance. Timing the muscle pulse at ball contact and focusing on an neutral spine at this instant also greatly assisted. Eventually, the full swing was practiced and the reduced swing habituated at low speed. The swing range of motion was not dramatically reduced – the critical accomplishment was to avoid 100% of full range of motion and the resultant irritation of the associated passive tissues. Final training continued with the integration of "superstiffness" at the moment of ball contact, as described in the previous chapter.

The rower who had to continue

As the lumbar range of motion was reduced in the previous example, the same strategy was necessary for a competitive rower. She was showing the classic rower's back. Rowers rise early in the morning to row on flat water before weather and other boats cause conditions to deteriorate. This regimen of early morning bending elevates their risk for disc herniation. The risk is further elevated with high repetitions of full lumbar flexion and with spine compression. It's no wonder that herniations are known as the "rower's disease".

Analysis of her rowing technique revealed that the catch (the reaching phase of the rowing cycle) involved her fully flexing the lumbar spine. Her flexion exacerbated symptoms simply would not resolve unless this was avoided; the only option was to reduce lumbar flexion. Torso flexion can be achieved with lumbar and hip flexion. Video analysis revealed there was reserve hip flexion available. Hip mobility was challenged with lunge exercises and hamstring stretches. More hip flexion required an emphasis on hip extensor power. Interestingly, the original lumbar emphasis for motion was probably the result of poor hip power, transferring the active torque responsibility to the lumbar extensors.

Prior to hip extensor training, spine stability work was accomplished with the Big Three, working through the progression to the highest of athletic challenges. Then gluteal patterning began with isolated motor patterns in the gluteus medius and then maximus (see chapter 10). The squat motion pattern was slowly progressed from the potty squat through to one-legged squats (chapter 10). Leap training and back extensor medicine ball tosses vertically completed the power training.

A final note regarding "sweep" rowers is in order here. Our most recent data shows that flexion with some motion bending to one side causes the herniation to progress to the opposite posterior quadrant of the disc. Sweep rowers row on one side of the boat with a lateral bend to one side. We hope to confirm our suspicions shortly that the side of the disc bulges are associated with the sweep rowing side. If this is true, we will have to look seriously at the strategy of switching boat sides. Many elite rowers are able to row both sides, but others cannot as they have noticeable performance deficits on the poor side. I suspect that re-grooving the rowing patterns to the opposite side may be the key to salvaging some careers.

The washed-up baseball catcher

A baseball catcher requested a consult because they were unable to continue playing due to debilitating back troubles. The component of play that was most painful and disabling was rising from the crouch and throwing the ball to second base to check the runner trying to steal. This was performed numerous times in games and during practice. Measuring the lumbar motion during the throwing task revealed motion requiring most of the available range – provocative testing proved this was indeed the motion that produced the symptoms. The program began with motor/motion training, teaching the abdominal brace together with locking the rib cage onto the pelvis, similar to the golfer case study above. The catcher was able to then rise from the crouch with a braced torso and reduced spine motion. Interestingly, the superb athleticism of this individual in the forearm and wrist still produced the majority of the "zip" on the ball, but nonetheless some speed was sacrificed. We needed to find more potential. Not being a professional baseball catcher myself, I resorted to the complex movement partitioning and analysis process outlined in chapter 7. Rising from the crouch began with a squat pattern which transformed into a lunge pattern as the throw progressed. Overlaying the lunge was a push pattern (of the hand-arm linkage through the shoulder), together with a twist pattern (the shoulder twisting relative to the pelvis). The squat, lunge, twist and push were developed in a progressive manner using cables. First, slow motion patterning progressed by speeding up the motions. They were then put together in combination with special focus on the torso bracing motor pattern and the lumbar restricted motion pattern. A few more critical miles per hour were added to the throw, using the superstiffness technique without symptom exacerbation.

The CEO who had painful "midnight movements"

One thing that I have come to appreciate is a trait shared by many elite and successful business personalities and the best athletes in the world: The demands they place on themselves and the ability to solve problems and complete the task at hand. I have enjoyed working with these business celebrities and can frankly state that I have learned a lot from them. One of the first who asked for a consult had chronic back pain and couldn't sit through business meetings, or plane travel and was unable to enjoy the midnight movement with his wife. I began with an interview and examination to determine the exacerbating motion/motor patterns through interview and provocative testing. I began giving him my opinion by stating all of the things that he was currently doing and should remove from his daily routine. I saw his face grow impatient as he repeatedly interrupted asking "so what should I do?". A lesson for me – I always try to link every contraindicated activity with a recommended task. Gifts come when least expected!

Clearly, this man had discogenic back pain that we were able to control almost immediately with motion patterning to avoid a flexed spine. He also showed an instability catch (documented in chapter 9) which we were able to identify. We taught him the appropriate bracing pattern to remove the catch as he moved and minimized the pain. This process involved spine position awareness training during which the "light went on". He blurted out, "This is why sex with my wife hurts so much!" The second lesson he taught me. Much time in the clinic can be saved in lumbar and pelvic motion patterning with these types of patients by having them roll their pelvis in the "midnight movement" and then show them that this is exacerbating. Painless technique requires that the motion comes from elsewhere. The delightful part of the story comes from my seeing a voluptuous French Canadian woman – suffering the same discogenic back troubles. I was clearly embarrassed to show her the concept of lumbar flexion motion via the midnight movement but I bravely proceeded nonetheless. Finding the courage, I lowered my voice and said how this is replicating the midnight movement – to which she smiled and said, with that accent that only a French lady can have, "Oh you mean afternoon delight!"

So from then on, our discogenic patients have become conversant with the "delightful" concept of spine sparing motion!

Building the power lifter

There is no substitute for a "lifting clinic" to perfect technique, and good technique cannot be obtained from reading a book. Nonetheless, here are a few items to spare backs and enhance performance. There are many lifters with disc bulges and herniations who compete at high level. Typically, those with herniations can tolerate compressive loading but not flexion bending. There is a message here for those who have no injury history: The spine must not bend when under load; only after the back is pain-free should training resume. Flexibility must be present in the hips and ankles to achieve the starting position (test and/or develop the motion with the potty squat, chapter 10). Begin with an unloaded bar. When in the starting position, tension the abdominals and back muscles together with latissimus dorsi to brace the lumbar region. Some specific coaching and conscious effort may be necessary to develop the preparatory pattern. Stroking the muscle and "raking" the abdominals with a wide grip using the thumb and index finger into the muscle are techniques used to maintain the stabilizing activation. Prior to tensioning the muscles the lifter should inhale, filling the lungs to an almost full level. This pressurizes the thorax and abdominal cavities, stabilizing the spine in concert with the subsequent muscle tightening. The torso now acts like a block of cement. The neutral curve (or even slight spine extension in some lifters) is never compromised. One is only as safe as the ability to maintain this neutral and braced spine. Groove the motion with impeccable form. Do not wear a belt at this stage; belts are used to win competitions. Consistent with the 5 stage program outlined in chapters 10 and 11, this forms a component of the first stage which is grooving the motion and motor patterns.

Let's assume that the motion and motor patterns are in place, the gluteals are contributing as they should, and the athlete is neither over nor under trained. The foundation is laid. Let's focus on a common shortfall of the powerlifter whose objective is to maximize deadlift performance. While specificity of training has been discussed before in this book, here is a case where we will violate this principle. Specifically, optimal performance will be achieved by not replicating the athletic performance. The deadlift involves slowly raising the weight from the floor – slow when compared to the Olympic lifts. The mistake of too many power lifters is to focus on the maximal effort lift – here we take a cue from Vasili Alexeyev, the great Soviet lifter. Alexeyev lifted to perfect technique and develop speed strength. He practiced by lifting a lighter, non-competitive weight at the highest speed possible. Some lift with ultimate speed and power and toss the bar into the air which lands behind (I mention this only to illustrate a point and recommend that this NEVER be attempted – it can kill you). The powerlifter must train all available motor units and they are only recruited at speed. Generally, we begin by placing blocks under the weights of the bar to raise it off the ground so the bar is about knee height or even higher to begin the pull. The athlete then sets the initial position and mentally images lifting form and maximal motor unit recruitment. The light weight is lifted at the fastest rate possible. The bar may be lifted from the floor using the same philosophy once the box lifting technique (speed training) has been mastered. Emphasis is on technique here to ensure the training builds tissue rather that tearing it down. Care is also taken to monitor the athlete. There are many good athletes who simply cannot train this way as they are unable to recover.

Common mistakes that lead to sub-potential performance and back injury include failing to "set" the back into a locked posture with the extensors, abdominals and latissumus dorsi, and failure to achieve a "hip hinge". Driving too early in the lift, with the knees, causes energy leaks (see figure 16.1) and higher back loads. It is a shame that too many lifters ask for my advice after a back injury. Nonetheless, by never sacrificing form, many are able to lift again to break their previous best records.

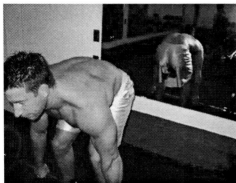 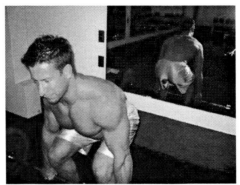

Figure 16.1 Driving with the knees usually causes the back to "spring" with an energy leak (left panel) together with a larger load moment arm, causing unnecessary low back loads. Better technique is to squat "back" to allow the bar to clear the knees, with nearly all motion occurring at the hips (right panel). Two "lifting cams" are used – hip external rotation and abduction to fully activate the gluteal muscles, together with bending the bar in shoulder external rotation engaging the latissimus dorsi.

Squat performance can also be enhanced using elastics on the bar (Westside squat) during slower lifts, described in chapter 13. Never sacrifice form to increase the training load – in fact the optimal motor patterns are achieved by grooving perfect technique first with lighter loads.

A final note on the third event for the powerlifter, the bench press: Here, many athletes can increase their best lift by understanding how to optimize their back and torso. The shoulders are squeezed posteriorly so the shoulder blades (scapulae) form a rigid platform to transfer load to the bench. The shoulders are depressed with latissimus dorsi, the torso is stiffened, as are the legs, including the gluteals about the hips. The feet grip the ground similar to the squat foot grip (see figure 16.2). This total stiffness technique is exhausting. The weight is not lowered in a vertical track but down an imaginary "ramp" towards the lower part of the sternum. The bar is "bent" with external rotation through the shoulders and latissimus. This is part of the "steering" of the bar with the hand gripping musculature. The bar is "spread" through the sticking point.

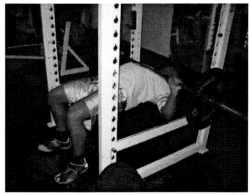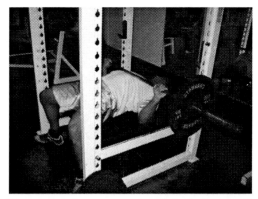

Figure 16.2 A good bench presser with so much more potential (left panel) that remains wasted. Performance enhancing technique (right panel) includes a wider and purposeful foot grip, leg and hip stiffness, more stiffness through the abdominals and latissimus dorsi, stiffer link between the scapulae, pelvis and the bench, a bar trajectory lower down the chest, and "bending" and "spreading" the bar through the sticking point.

The misguided football lineman

I recall consulting for a team and eavesdropping on a conversation among some linemen. They were discussing the perfect elbow curl technique and how standing against a wall to lock the elbow is probably a good idea. I knew that I had a lot of work to do. Holding the bar for a bicep curl with a supinated grip is purely a body building exercise. It is designed to isolate biceps by taking out brachioradialis, but functional performance needs every available muscle about the joint. Clearly, the linemen benefit from size and bulk but only if they are trained to direct their strength through the linkage to the ground, and conversely to develop leg drive and transmit it to the upper extremities. Analysis of the movement revealed dominant patterns involving the lunge, the rip, quickly changing feet position and projection of force on a moving target (the opponent). Using a dumbbell, with a hammer grip and flexing both at the elbow and the shoulder, is a motion much closer to the "rip" used on the field.

First, the perfect curl was grooved with a dumbbell ripping out of the lunge. Squat and lunge postures with push/pull cable "punches" continued the progressions. Then quick-stepping was added to the complex training task.

Training a sprinter

A sprinter is a speed machine. Ultimate acceleration and top-end speed are the objectives. While the "engine" will be built through exercises explained in the next paragraph, the mechanics of running speed need a brief review. They form the training objectives. You are encouraged to re-familiarize yourself with the fundamental principles of movement from chapter 7. Ultimate performance requires a highly developed "steering mechanism". Every force is steered toward the performance objective. The starting posture begins with the feet slightly less than shoulder width to minimize force being directed laterally – clearly the forces need to be projected posteriorly to maximize forward thrust. The gluts and pelvis are never lower than the head since the inertial drive of the torso would be directed over the foot-ground contact point (the body fulcrum when exploding from the blocks) rather than directly through it. Many other posture details are important, all in the effort to steer the musculoskeletal forces toward optimal driving force on the blocks. As noted in the previous chapter, the best sprinters are astoundingly relaxed while in the starting posture. The rate of force development upon the gun is equally astounding, as is the rate of relaxation for the speed phase of each reciprocating segment motion. The gift of speed boils down to the ability to optimize stiffness and compliance.

The explosive start incorporates techniques to maximize and steer the driving force. For example, the supporting "down" arm is driven backward to allow maximal force to be developed in the free arm as it rotates forward rapidly. The size of the first step is variable between athletes, For some, as much ground is gained in the first step as possible and foot placement follows a straight line. Full stride length is only possible when in an upright posture. The upright posture is an objective that is optimized with maximal horizontal power production critical to the first two or three strides. For others, a smaller first step works better to get the explosive rhythm. Perfect "steerage" of the driving force when running occurs with the eyes locked straight ahead to the finish. The head has no tilt. Hip torque efficiency and steerage of the driving force occur with the spine locked in the slightest of extension posture. The arms move about the shoulder with the elbow driving by the torso very tightly to eliminate any unproductive lateral forces. These upper extremity forces are driven through the locked torso (stiffened with the held breath and stabilizing muscle forces) to minimize any energy losses in the transmission. The swing leg is driven forward and upwards with an image of "punching" towards the finish. The driving leg is moved through to full extension, developing and steering maximal force to the ground. Teaching these mechanics to a developing sprinter is conducted following the Russian approach of grooving perfect motion and motor patterns only when the athlete is as fresh as possible. Ultimate sprint mechanics are impossible in the fatigued athlete.

The previous paragraph should heighten the importance of the torso, back and hips for all aspects of sprinting performance. To the surprise of some, the limiting variable of most sprinters is hip flexion power, not a deficit in extension power. Explosive hip mechanics with optimal forward projection requires a stabilized torso. Stabilization training with the breath held is very important. Many sprinters hold their breath to stiffen the torso/core for a substantial distance of the race. General training of the torso to the highest level of stability is also necessary to prepare the athlete to withstand the rigors of hip flexion torque training. Anyone familiar with sprint training knows the great number of back injuries associated with hip flexion training. Explosive force development in psoas loads up the lumbar spine in very high compression. The spine must be in a neutral posture to survive. Many techniques are useful and may begin with "dead bug" progressions (see Chapter 10). Other approaches include cable resistance loads around the swing leg and bounding. Both of these are progressed to high levels of dynamic correspondence where hip flexion is always accompanied with hip extension of the driving leg. The quick feet exercise is very helpful in some athletes (see chapter 11). Neuromuscular challenges are extended with downhill sprinting to condition top end swing leg recovery power. Focus is, as always, on impeccable technique.

Back troubles in the long distance runner

Efficiency in the long distance runner depends on a stiff torso. Suggesting that they "image" not having a joint between their shoulders and hips is a start. Training the weak link of torso stiffness and stability in their overall program is easily addressed. Another common practice among this group is an overemphasis on flexion stretches. They tend to overstretch the hamstrings at the hip, the spine and shoulders in flexion. Many have developed accentuated kyphosis. Interestingly, I would not suggest stretching beyond the range of motion needed for running. The great runners, to a large extent, run on their passive tissues. Some would do better with less stretching! I generally only suggest stretching to correct asymmetries. Here is why I take this approach. When I am asked to see the cross-country or long distance track athlete with back pain, I look for movement asymmetry in the torso. For example, upon right foot heel strike there may be torsional motion in the lumbar region. There could be several causes for this. Further screening is conducted to sort out the cause, which is then addressed. However, more core stiffness mostly always helps. Challenged breathing while performing torso stability work ensures the ventilation system and diaphragm function are not compromised with abdominal muscle contraction. The full side bridge during heavy breathing is an excellent start on this approach. Generally, the trick is to remove the cause of the back trouble in these special types of athletes, rather than create a new set of general training exercises.

The Rock Climber

Never having rock climbed myself, an analysis of the specific demands were in order. The athlete drew the body positioning and demonstrated good understanding of the need to direct the forces to cling to the wall. He drew and developed internal lines of drive that were properly controlled and directed to enable the body center of mass to develop clinging forces. Interestingly, the athlete had never considered the fundamental motion pattern, the most basic and innate of all gait patterns – the crawl. Grip strength was highlighted as another necessary attribute, together with general range of motion requirements for both hand and foot reach.

The best training in this case was facilitated with an artificial climbing wall which was made in his car garage. Several different rip shapes were purchased at an outdoor shop and mounted on the wall and ceiling to simulate the reaches and control of body postures required, combined with some basic training.

The "Big Three" were implemented to develop torso stability and control. The curl-up posture was progressed to include "crawling" motions – flexion of one leg through the hip with dynamic correspondence of the opposite side arm through the shoulder (see figure 16.3). Chin-ups with a variety of hand (and finger) grips were developed. The athlete was able to train some of the more compromised grips by performing these holds with squatting motions. Sumo style squats were performed to simulate the leg drives developed with the body close onto the rock face. These were progressed into single-leg variations with dynamic correspondence to better capture the crawling motion.

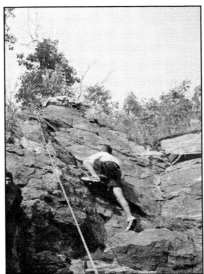 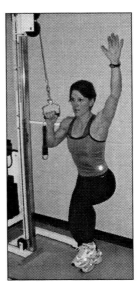

Figure 16.3 Rock climbing is a crawl pattern. A one-legged squat while pulling
down with one arm and reaching with the other facilitates
dynamic correspondence.

The champion squash player

A former champion squash player developed significant back troubles, to the point that training became impossible. This individual had been a former professional football player, playing tight end, and was a natural athlete. He was a tall fellow, with a lanky sort of build and tremendous reach which he used to his advantage on the squash court. But the reaching skill also caused back symptoms neutralizing this natural advantage. When I first saw him, his objective was simply to reduce pain during daily activity. However, we also set the long-term goal of regaining a national championship which was a very lofty goal given his morbid condition.

Starting with the back symptoms, the program was designed to first re-groove motion patterns where the back was locked and braced in a neutral posture. Back stabilization exercises were commenced, using the "Big Three". As symptoms resolved, lunging progressions were developed. These began with sagittal plane lunges and developed into "star" patterns with lateral and rearward motions. Arm swing was integrated with a racquet in the hand. One-legged squat progressions also assisted in developing the necessary leg strength and power throughout the range to enable spine conserving motion on the squash court.

Cable work completed his preparation before full fledged squash training.

The dancer building to the arabesque

A dancer, following injury, had difficulty achieving the arabesque to either side. She was unable to build the foundation of both motion and motor patterns and continued to struggle with the arabesque. We began with basic one-legged squats with forward, side and posterior projection of the leg. Performing the entire progression on the "star" on the floor was helpful in guiding symmetry and the ability to perform in either direction. Balance was developed in the squat program as was controlled range of motion, "dynamic flexibility", endurance and strength. The one-legged squats were modified into the "bowlers squat" (see figure 16.4) to begin developing the graceful twisting motion pattern, again to both sides. Finally, the full arabesque was achieved to either side.

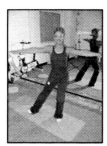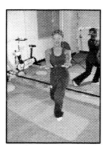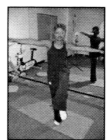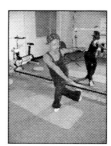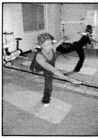

Figure 16.4 Progression of one-legged squats, to the bowlers squat, culminating in the arabesque.

Two former gymnasts and the spine instability legacy

I have been involved with a number of gymnasts in spine-related ways. Here is a typical case sent for referral. A 17 year old female reported pain over her lumbar area, mostly over the PSIS's and sacrum. She had participated in gymnastics from the age of 3 until she was 12 and had suffered ever since. No other clinical approach had helped her. Generally, the several physical therapists she had seen insisted on stretching her back together with recommending some extension based motions. She reported that these made her worse and was admonished for being non-compliant. Watching her sit, stand, open a door, walk and move to the floor and up again, it was clear that she overused her back. She underwent large spine motions with little control and allowed very large torques to develop about her spine. This was caused by her failure to direct forces through her back, reducing the moment arm. She also exhibited the classic pattern of using her back muscles for extension rather than the hip extensors. During provocation tests, she reported more pain on shear provocation when the legs were raised from the floor, which is unusual. Coupling this with intolerance of compression and extension motion to both right and left sides, together with her gymnastics history, I began to suspect a spondylolisthesis. As a matter of procedure, I never look at the radiology report or the actual pictures until after I have formed an opinion from assessing the individual. I use the images to only confirm or refute my impression. This is in contrast to many clinicians who put the films on the viewer immediately and begin diagnosis. Interestingly, a grade 1 spondylolisthsis was clear on the CT sagittal scout view – previously unnoticed by the radiologist.

Given that she was provoked by many motions and loads (compression, shear, mild extension, moderate flexion), we began the exercise program with motion/motor patterning. The first chore was to reduce spine motion in daily activity. Locking the "ribcage to the pelvis" with wall exercises began this process together with spine position awareness training in a standing posture. Gluteal re-patterning was also incorporated. Despite her robust overall appearance, her hip extensors were so poorly conditioned that after 4 reps of the glut medius exercise, with no resistance, the muscle cramped with exhaustion. This was a further demonstration of the severe gluteal dysfunction. Glut max patterning was prescribed and she was able to develop the gluteal dominant pattern quite quickly. The "Big Three" spine stabilizer exercises were prescribed (curl-up, side bridge, birddog) at an appropriate starting level. A one-legged squat matrix was also prescribed at this point, with forward, lateral and rearward foot projections. Special effort was required to groove the motion/motor pattern where a neutral spine curvature was maintained and the motion was entirely about the hip. No component of this program caused any pain. This was the first time that exercise had not hurt her for over 10 years.

I will mention another case at this point, because of the striking similarities. I was asked to provide expertise in a legal case involving a former gymnast (international competitor). She had retired some 15 years prior and had since married, had children and lost her fitness. Sitting at a stoplight while driving her car, she was rear-ended by another vehicle moving at a slow rate of speed. The collision caused her to become symptomatic in her low back. She was diagnosed with spondylolisthesis and underwent surgery where stabilizing hardware was implanted. In surgery, it was clearly visible that this was not a new injury, given the significant osteogenic activity. She was asked if she had back troubles when she competed. Her response? "Of course". It appears that many of these gymnasts have spondylolisthesis and pars fractures while they compete (as do cricket bowlers, for example). Yet they are so fit and so stable and have such wonderful buttressing motor patterns that they can control the pain and compete. In this case, she lost the motor patterns and fitness and a very minor physical insult caused her to become highly symptomatic. Her rehabilitation program was very similar to the one described in the previous paragraph.

Sciatic case: Flossing

A water-skier wanted a consult for sciatica. Analysing the demands of skiing, in particular the start and the slalom ski task, revealed the need for significant isometric bracing in the torso. Reviewing some videotape of the skier demonstrated a starting style where the lumbar spine was allowed to bend into what appeared to be quite close to full flexion. This spine posture technique was modified and grooved in the skier by building a ski simulator and practising the neutral spine posture within the skiing posture. After learning to avoid full lumbar flexion, the skier reported less discomfort.

The second part was to employ nerve flossing (see *Low Back Disorders*). The potential for nerve flossing was determined in the following way: First a lying leg raise and nerve tensioning test was performed coupled with cervical flexion to determine movement potential in the cord and nerve roots. While supine with the leg raised to the point of symptom onset, the leg was lowered slightly, the cervical spine was flexed to add tension and the leg was lowered further to change the tensioning from the caudal end. Alternating tensioning between the caudal end and the cranial end helps to determine if the cord and nerve roots are moving. In this case, the indication was that nerve flossing had potential. Nerve flossing began in the seated posture and progressed to full flossing with hip integration while side-lying on the floor. The sciatica was eliminated within a month.

The "Strongman" competitor unable to conquer the sticking points

Working with the strongmen is fun – I have never come across one who is not a gentlemanly giant! Of course, the key is to generate functional strength where the emphasis is on moving awkward objects. The best competitors are extremely cerebral in their analysis of each unique task. For example, when Bill Kazmeier dominated the competitions, he would go all out to win the first round, ensuring that he could choose his position in the order for the subsequent event. This allowed him the opportunity to study the techniques of the others. From his analysis, he found ways to enhance his own abilities to win. He has some terrific stories! These days, all of the principles for effective movement are needed for optimal performance as the events have become longer (think of the farmer's walk and the bus pulls, which are longer than ever). In addition to training for the actual events, strength training in body regions often ignored by others is commonplace among these special people. Grip strength, for example, with wrist pronation/supination is enhanced, which is important to ensure the optimal steerage of force. Finger strength for gripping odd-shaped objects could never be developed using conventional bars or handles. The feet are emphasized to optimize ground grip and steerage of force. But the point to be made here is about technique to conquer the sticking points.

Sticking points occur during every strongman event. The solution is to employ the techniques of superstiffness described in the previous chapter.

Consider the tire flip where a huge earth mover tire must be flipped end over end down the course. Hands are placed under the front edge of the tire and the lift is initiated. Joint mobility is needed to adopt a low squat. Several sticking points will be experienced. This is often the phase where injuries occur. For example, avulsion of the biceps tendon is not uncommon. This shows that overload occurred at a relatively weak joint. This could have been prevented by stiffening the elbow, cocontracting through the linkage, and driving with the hips. The major proportion of the force to the tire is accomplished through "chest drive" (see figure 16.5). In fact, there are all sorts of opportunities during these tasks to stiffen the body and position the hips to allow for hip drive. If you have the opportunity to analyze injuries from video tape, it is time very well spent. Then practice rapid stiffening in the postures where the sticking points may occur.

Finally, many strongmen come from a powerlifting background. They will probably continue with their training habits and spend an inordinate amount of time on the squat, deadlift and bench press. Of course these are, or should be, whole body exercises. The bench press requires tremendous back extensor and abdominal muscle activation. Nonetheless, the strongmen will probably need to direct more attention to "out of sagittal plane" challenges. It's hard to beat pushing a car with many positional techniques such as using one arm, pushing laterally, employing sidestepping, pushing facing backwards and running to the other end of the car to stop it (see figure in chapter 14).

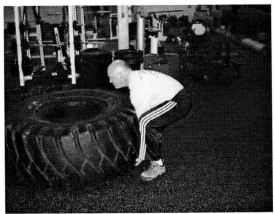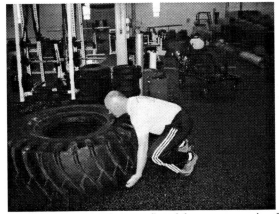

Figure 16.5 Art McDermott demonstrates poor technique (left panel) with compromised performance outcome, and excellent technique (right panel) where "chest drive" is used to flip the tire. The risk for biceps avulsion, which is so common, is eliminated. The risk of back injury is reduced. Hip drive is facilitated for optimal performance.

Blending speed, stiffness, strength and compliance for the martial artist

While speed, strength and impact stiffness are needed for many different sorts of athletes, the example of training martial artists will be used here. A devastating punch or kick must be fast. Of course, a burst of muscle activity is needed for initiation of movement at the hip and shoulder. Note that torso stiffening was a precursor to minimize energy losses and to buttress the reaction torques resulting from the extremity motion. Once the limb motion has begun, a relaxation phase is needed as the hand or foot speed is increased. Continued muscle activation and stiffness only hinders speed during this phase. Just prior to impact, a total body stiffness occurs to impact maximal energy to the opponent.

Too many martial artists (and other similar athletes) train in the sagittal plane. These individuals spend an inordinate amount of time using barbells and other resistive approaches and become "sagittally strong", but have weakness when taken outside of the plane. For example, jerk on the sleeve of a martial artist, gauge their reaction and assess lateral and torsional tasks. These may reveal weaknesses to be addressed in training.

Foundational exercises include the program for torso stability so that a stiff core facilitates efficient energy transfer and enables the spine to withstand the rigors of speed training. Exercises to train relaxed hand and foot "speed" are the focus with the rapid stiffening on impact. Begin with a lunge walk for warm-up with intermittent rapid body stiffening. Find the "soft spots" by vigorous tapping with a stick – better to deal with them in training than to have them discovered by an opponent's foot! Try to take steps landing on the heel for speed but also in some strides land on the toes for whole body stability – both of these foot postures will be needed. Then employ more rapid lunge position steps with a rapid return. Again, focus on technique with optimal stiffening prior to each rapid motion. Then graduate to resistance exercises. One effective exercise is a two-handed cable pull and push initiated in a lunge position. (see figure 16.6). While the rear foot heel may be off the ground, it must be driven flat to enable maximal force development in the stiffened linkage. Then the shoulders/arm/hand complex is "snapped". Training speed, stiffness and accuracy depends on attention to detail and optimizing the foundational biomechanical principles.

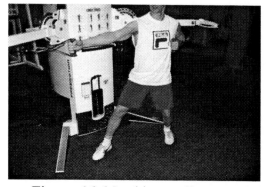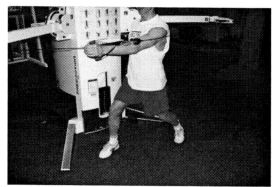

Figure 16.6 In this excellent martial artist, the torso is stiffened and the heel of the rear foot driven to the ground. The focus for the pulling arm is latissimus dorsi activation to torsionally buttress the torso to facilitate maximal power and speed development in the pushing arm. Total stiffness is practiced at full arm extension (and contact with the opponent).

Martial artists who kick with specific styles are some of the few who need extreme mobility and speed, together with the ability for extreme stiffness. An innate ability for this combination of demands is necessary, which may then be enhanced with training. The "axe kick" is an unusual demand in that the hip is flexed to its maximum, where an elastic rebound is created through the hip and spine (see figure 16.7). Carefully conceived progressions to train the elastic tissue synergy are necessary and depend on the injury/pain history of the individual's back.

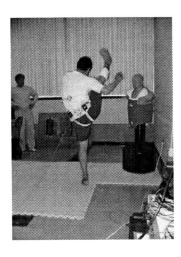

Figure 16.7 The impressive "axe kick" utilizes hip and back elastic recoil abilities.

A squat "clinic"

When I am asked to put on a course or seminar for athletes and coaches, I try and workshop a clinic with some specific patients or athletes. This is very helpful in demonstrating the level of detail and expertise needed to achieve the best results. One of my favorites is a squat clinic because squatting is a fundamental movement pattern. Everyone thinks they can perform one, yet there are so many technique components to correct in nearly everyone for immediate demonstrable gains. Here is the process.

I start with observation of the squat with various loads and from many vantage points, looking for fundamental motion patterns. Beginning with initial postures such as foot placement, I shift to examining motions such as the knee trajectory as it relates to the foot and hip. The knee, ankle and hip must move in a planar motion. Simple corrections may include modifying the direction of the foot (in line with the knee hinge), or perhaps hip orientation - usually external rotation is needed. Look for any knee buckling potential indicated by out of plane motion as the squat deepens. People usually comment on my rigour at this stage. Here, I move quickly around the athlete to assess this with my eye. I observe one leg from about 3 meters away in line with their knee hinge, then I walk quickly to observe the other leg in the plane of that knee hinge. This is followed with another quick walk to the side and then to behind the squatter to observe hip and spine motion patterns. In other words, I really work at it. Mediocre coaches are lazy.

Corrections for motion can include testing a small heel lift if a problem is isolated to immobility in one ankle. Interestingly, this sort of problem is seen more in the mid-range of the descent. The depth of the squat is largely determined by the hips. Here a hip assessment is performed (shown in my clinical textbook: *Low Back Disorders*) which involves acetabulum scouring to find the angles where restriction manifests. This is followed by the process of finding the optimal width of leg spread to enable a deeper squat. Here the athlete adopts a hands and knees, all fours posture, and the spine is set in a neutral position. The buttocks are rocked back to the heels. This indicates the depth of hip flexion possible before the back "breaks" or lumbar flexion is observed. Then the knees are spread further and the process repeated. Usually the hips are able to reach closer to the feet. Leg width is adjusted until the optimal depth is found. This hip-leg posture should then be tried in the actual squat. Another technique that helps at full descent is to have the athlete attempt conscious flexion at the hips. Several images help here but active flexion with psoas and iliacus is desired. This sometimes helps to 'get into the hole' at the full parallel squat.

Of course, a major motion pattern that must be addressed is that in the hip-spine. The back break angle is probably the single most important factor in injury risk. There are some athletes who appear to be immune to back injury with a flexed spine under load. But they are rare and occasionally are able to rise through the ranks with poor technique. For the majority of people, the squat should never go deeper than the point where lumbar flexion occurs. The basic motion is to squat "back" and not "down". This means that the trajectory of the hips is along a line that is about 45 degrees from vertical. It helps to place a target behind the athlete to which the buttocks are directed and eventually touched.

Motor patterns are the next item for consideration. Time and again there seems to be an overemphasis on knee extensors in many athletes. The usual weak link in those wanting to improve their squat is in the hamstrings, hip extensors and low back. Interestingly, some have the foundational strength in these areas but fail to employ it. Their technique is poor. Here the trick is to image "spreading the floor" with the feet through conscious hip abduction. The feet are also gripping the ground with the toes and heels for two reasons: First, the base of support is lengthened this way; second, this anchors the feet, which are being twisted in external rotation through conscious hip external rotation. This facilitates more gluteal activation and much better hip drive. Then focus is directed towards latissimus dorsi. This is a major back extensor that is not in the motor scheme of many athletes. Squeeze the scapulae together and pull the elbows in to facilitate the contraction in this muscle. Image and execute "bending the bar" using latissimus dorsi as this forms a second lifting cam with hip external rotation being the first. Develop the upper trapezius for "hanging" the shoulders and the supporting extensor musculature and the lower trapezius to create a "shelf" to rest the bar on.

Bar placement is important for competitive performance. The bar should be low down the back to minimize the horizontal distance to the hips and lumbar spine. This low placement reduces the reaction torque, reducing the hip-back extensor muscle force required to lift. Some lifters greatly benefit from thoracic extension mobilization exercises to assist advantageous bar placement (see chapter 10).

A final note is needed on preparing to lift. The warm-up should not involve any passive stretching. Active flexibility exercises are needed more for certain individuals. An excellent routine includes active wall squats to mobilize the hips and facilitate the squatting musculature (see figures in chapter 10). It is usually the hips that are the weak link for the squat. Others find "stomping the ground" is facilitating for the rooting mechanism prior to lifting. This is a generic start to a squat clinic. To go further into the process of technique correction and then technique optimization, I would need a specific individual.

A comment on forensic cases

Some of my activities as a consultant are directed toward legal cases. My expertise is used in several ways. Sometimes I am asked to provide expertise on injury mechanisms, perhaps on how a person could injure their back picking up a pencil (spine instability and buckling), or perhaps a case of injury allegedly linked to a machine. Perhaps it may be a contest on whether a person is malingering, or to comment on the extent of the pathology or loss in performance capacity from a back perspective. I will list my criteria and principles that determine whether I would become involved in a case. The case must be just – I have to believe that a true injustice will occur without my involvement. I must have confidence in the skill and expertise of the lawyers; I must not be "used". As has happened before, sometimes I am hired as a threat, so once the opposing lawyers see me appear they settle the case. For example, I have been asked to testify and as I stepped out of the cab from the airport, the lawyers settled on the courtroom steps. I was "used" only to call a bluff, and this is a waste of my time.

On occasion, I am asked to view a video tape, obtained usually by a private investigator, of a back patient performing a questionable activity. In one case, a woman was walking in town with a cane barely able to hobble, but a clandestine videotape of her on the weekend revealed her lifting an 80lb boulder from the ground and pushing it in a wheelbarrow up a hill with no limp. Case closed! In a similar vein, a pro athlete was unable to practice with the team but was caught on tape dog sledding. Dog sledding requires more hip flexor forces and higher spine loading than playing his sport. Case closed! It's not always so simple. In many instances, the expert on the opposing side will state there is no problem and that the athlete is malingering. When I watch athletes play (on submitted evidence tapes), I can see movement pathology apparently not seen by the opposing experts. I can see an athlete struggling with spine motion control to minimize the pain, and the back and hip loading patterns adopted to minimize pain, which compromise performance. I recall examining the tape of a soccer player where the hip flexion power loss when kicking was clear, as was the shortened stride when running, the spine posture, and the odd arm assistance and pathological motion when rising from the ground after falling. Hopefully, after reading this book, your "eye" will be tuned to seeing this as well.

Another "category" for my involvement is directed towards the issue of whether an athlete can play. Many of today's pro athletes' salaries contain clauses for payment even when injured and are "sold" to an insurance company. If the athlete claims they cannot play or perform then the insurance company has a great interest in reversing this. On occasion, I am asked to assess an athlete's back to determine if he/she is capable of withstanding the demand of the sport. This is difficult and interesting work and rarely results in a conclusive opinion. At this stage of my career, I am happy with this. Perhaps my role is seen more in offering a perspective to temper some of the absolute views offered by some other experts. While I get calls from lawyers every week, I rarely take the case. I hope this short expression of thoughts may be helpful to some of you who are asked to do this type of work.

Epilogue: Becoming the elite builder of ultimate backs

You now have a scientific approach to add to your skills for training backs. This approach evolved from my scientific, and clinical work and working with athletes and their conditioning coaches. It guides me in my daily interactions. Here is some final wisdom that will help you: In my dealings with patients and athletes alike, from the basket case bad back through to the celebrity athlete and business star, two guiding principles have been of great assistance. It is both humbling and intimidating to meet and work with some of these people – how does one handle the stress and potentially awkward situations? The first guideline that has been invaluable came from my father – "*Whoever you are speaking with at that moment – you are their equal*". Whether I am speaking with a highly recognizable sports figure, who is mobbed wherever they go, or consulting with a government minister or corporation CEO or sharing ideas with an undergraduate student, for that moment I am their equal. It works!

Anyone who performs scientific investigations is familiar with the peer review process. Scientific camps develop and turf is staked out. Challenging the status quo, holding your ground and standing by your data requires a certain constitution. The second guideline that has served me well is to *never be offended*. Criticism can be personal and not always constructive. No matter, take the criticism and consider it, for the possibility exists that it contains an element of truth (it usually does). You will become a better authority, and leader.

I listened to Bill Pearl speak a couple of years ago on the "integrity of training", which reinforced the notion that ultimate training produces ultimate results when conducted with integrity and discipline to maintain form, to listen to your body, to think and consider all information that you hear within an education that never ceases to expand and to help others when they will benefit from your expertise. *Integrity honors both your teachers and your students.*

As I mentioned many times throughout the book, body building principles and muscle development for aesthetics rather than for performance so pervades "Western" training. Always consider the objective of the approach and technique. *There is no such thing as a safe or dangerous exercise – only an ill-prescribed exercise for an individual.* If you are unsure of an approach but want to try it, monitor the athlete and if things do not progress as planned, don't be afraid to admit that perhaps a mistake was made.

There is no single fitness God - all approaches have a place at some point in time. Back troubles are sometimes easily corrected, and sometimes not. Complex presentations require multidimensional approaches. This book has provided you with another tool for your toolbox of approaches. You are well on the way to being a superstar consultant.

These guidelines have helped me and perhaps they will help you. As I am writing these final lines I am looking forward to the next few experiments and tests scheduled in the lab, and my travels where, no doubt, I will meet many of you lecturing on the latest discoveries to assist in building the ultimate back. I plan on writing three more books: One dedicated to the prevention of back troubles, one compiling provocative tests and functional screens, and one for the lay reader. We are also producing a DVD to accompany this text to demonstrate the techniques "live". Visit our website www.backfitpro.com for more info. Our journey continues.

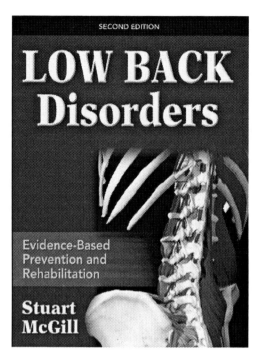

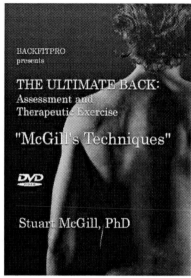

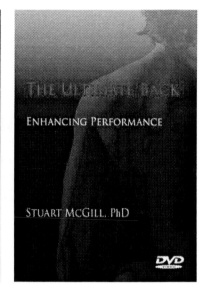

Dr McGill's other textbook is entitled *Low Back Disorders: Evidence Based Prevention and Rehabilitation* published by Human Kinetics. Companion DVD's are also available: that show the techniques live, "The Ultimate Back: Assessment and therapeutic exercise" and "The Ultimate Back: Enhancing performance". All are available from www.backfitpro.com

About the Author

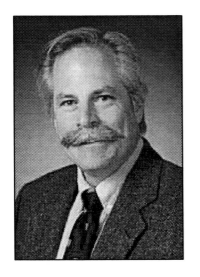

Stuart McGill is a Professor of Spine Biomechanics in the Department of Kinesiology at the University of Waterloo. He heads a team of scientists and graduate students who have authored hundreds of scientific publications that address the issues of low back function, injury prevention and rehabilitation and performance training. Collectively this work has received numerous scientific awards. He sits on the editorial boards of the journals SPINE, Clinical Biomechanics and Journal of Applied Biomechanics. As a consultant, he has provided expertise on low back issues to various government agencies, many corporations and legal firms and elite athletes and teams from many countries.

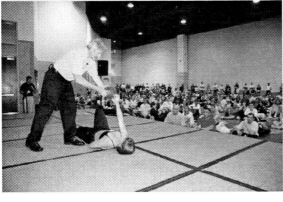

In addition to seeing patients sent for consult, he teaches clinical courses regularly around the world. They are listed on www.backfitpro.com.

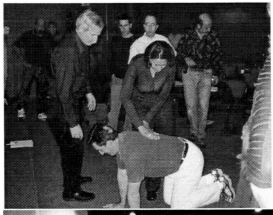

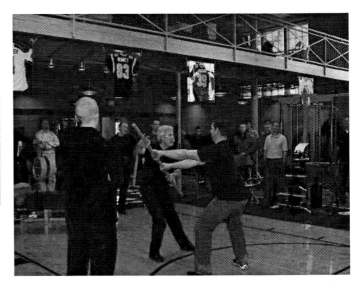